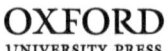
OXFORD
UNIVERSITY PRESS

Great Clarendon Street, Oxford, OX2 6DP,
United Kingdom

Oxford University Press is a department of the University of Oxford.
It furthers the University's objective of excellence in research, scholarship,
and education by publishing worldwide. Oxford is a registered trade mark of
Oxford University Press in the UK and in certain other countries

© Paul Fyfe 2015

The moral rights of the author have been asserted

First Edition published in 2015

Impression: 1

All rights reserved. No part of this publication may be reproduced, stored in
a retrieval system, or transmitted, in any form or by any means, without the
prior permission in writing of Oxford University Press, or as expressly permitted
by law, by licence or under terms agreed with the appropriate reprographics
rights organization. Enquiries concerning reproduction outside the scope of the
above should be sent to the Rights Department, Oxford University Press, at the
address above

You must not circulate this work in any other form
and you must impose this same condition on any acquirer

Published in the United States of America by Oxford University Press
198 Madison Avenue, New York, NY 10016, United States of America

British Library Cataloguing in Publication Data
Data available

Library of Congress Control Number: 2014947943

ISBN 978–0–19–873233–4

Printed and bound by
CPI Group (UK) Ltd, Croydon, CR0 4YY

Links to third party websites are provided by Oxford in good faith and
for information only. Oxford disclaims any responsibility for the materials
contained in any third party website referenced in this work.

By Accident or Design

Writing the Victorian Metropolis

PAUL FYFE

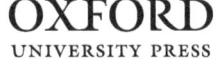

BY ACCIDENT OR DESIGN

Acknowledgements

As my friend David Kirby says, "Art is the deliberate transformed by the accidental." While I began this project deliberately, many such unexpected encounters with mentors, friends, and supportive environments along the way have transformed it into this book. The process has happily replayed the book's own arguments, set not in the Victorian metropolis but the institutions in which I have had the great pleasure to study and serve. They deserve more than the acknowledgements to follow. The project first took shape amid the remarkable community of nineteenth-century studies at the University of Virginia and the four faculty members who taught me most about how to read. (And then how to write about it.) To Chip Tucker, Karen Chase, Michael Levenson, and Jerry McGann, I owe the deepest thanks, by whose lights of acuity, imagination, and generosity I hope always to steer. Thanks also to the outstanding mentoring, teaching, and support of Stephen Arata, Jennifer Wicke, Andy Stauffer, Brad Pasanek, Cindy Wall, John O'Brien, Greg Colomb, Paul Cantor, Alison Booth, Jahan Ramazani, Clare Kinney, Vicky Olwell, Guinn Baker, Cheryl Lewis, and Randy Swift. My friends in UVa's graduate community pushed this book always to more ambitious and engaged terrain; thank you particularly Jim Cocola, Justin Neuman, Jill Rappoport, Heather Morton, John Murphy, Neil Hultgren, Michael Lewis, Pete Capuano, Lindsay Wright, Bethany Nowviskie, Brad Tuggle, Ashley Faulker, and Chris Ruotolo. This book would not have been possible without the unfailing support of the UVa English Department as well as a NINES Graduate Fellowship.

My colleagues in English and the History of Text Technologies program at Florida State University likewise significantly supported my research. As department chairs, Ralph Berry and Eric Walker provided clear-eyed professional guidance for the book's completion. I am grateful to the insights and encouragement of Meegan Kennedy, Anne Coldiron, Andrew Epstein, Paul Outka, Elaine Treharne, Cristobal Silva, Leigh Edwards, Barry Faulk, Gary Taylor, and Micah Vandegrift. I did not deserve the brilliance of Sarah Unruh, Cheryl Price, and John Handel, whose research assistance grounded the book's argument and expanded its reach. I also thank the Council on Research and Creativity for a First-Year Assistant Professor grant. The FSU Libraries provided special materials grants and unflagging helpfulness in all my pursuits. Tony Harrison and colleagues in the English department at North Carolina State University have NCSU have provided financial and intellectual support for this project and those it has lead to.

The Victorian studies community has been welcoming since the first time my dissertation director insisted I go talk to strangers at a conference. We are no longer strangers. Thanks to the many people who have responded to the following materials at conferences, in reviews, and in print. For their help, thanks especially to Richard Menke, Dan Novak, Jill Galvan, Alexis Easley, Ellen Rosenman, Paul Dobraszczyk, and Jim Mussell. Significant research for the project was facilitated by the excellent staff at the UVa Library, FSU Libraries, the British Library, the London Metropolitan Archives, The National Archives at Kew, and the Library at the London Transport Museum. Thanks also to Patrick Leary, the VICTORIA listserv, and the evolving scholarly community on social media in which I find daily affirmation of this field.

I am grateful to Jacqueline Baker at OUP for taking an interest in this project and smartly guiding it through its reviews. Two anonymous reviewers offered extremely constructive feedback during the process. Rachel Platt and Lucy McClune ably shepherded the book's administration; its production was expertly handled by Gayathri Manoharan, Jack Howells, and Ann Broughton. Thanks to the journal editors and publishers who have allowed materials to be adapted from "Accidents of a Novel Trade: Industrial Catastrophe, Fire Insurance, and *Mary Barton*" which appeared in *Nineteenth-Century Literature*, vol. 65, no. 3 (December 2010): 315–46; and from "The Random Selection of Victorian New Media" in *Victorian Periodicals Review*, vol. 42, no. 1 (Spring 2009): 1–23.

I could not have pursued literary scholarship without my parents Derek and Inger who unreservedly urged me and my siblings into open fields, to borrow a phrase from Gillian Beer. My dear children Camm and Anders were always with me, as was their mother—my friend, colleague, and most serendipitous encounter—Maggie Simon. This book is dedicated to my family.

Contents

List of Illustrations	ix
Introduction: A Tremendous Chapter of Accidents	1
Arguments from Design to Accident	4
The Accidental City	12
The Accidental Hermeneutic	20
Writing the Metropolis	25
The Chapters of Accident	27
1. Accidents in the News	31
New Chapters of Accident	33
The Column of Accidents	43
Courts of Inquiry	51
The Margins of Causality	61
2. Dickens and the Traffic of Accidents	67
The Knowledge of London	67
Boz on the Bus	71
The Traffic of Accidents	83
The Omnibus Genre	93
3. Industrial Accidents and Novel Insurances	100
Risk Writing in Crisis	103
Risky Descriptions	109
Novel Fields of Probability	116
Novel Compensation of Accidents	124
4. Street Literature and the Remediation of Accident	132
Profusion and Classification	138
Random Selection and Diffusion	143
The Remediation of Accident	149
Victorian New Media; or, Print 2.0	162

5. Chaos and Connections on the Victorian Railway	170
'This Lateral Babylon'	174
Accidental Junctions	181
Colliding Interpretations	193
Terminal Connections	203
Afterword: An Accidental Excursion	211
Bibliography	221
Index	241

List of Illustrations

1. 'Accident' in two databases of nineteenth-century British newspapers — 36
2. Advertisement by the West of England Fire and Life Insurance Office, Exeter, April 1847 — 115
3. 'A Railway Map of England' — 178
4. J. C. Bourne, 'Building Retaining Wall near Park Street, Camden Town, Sept 17th 1838' — 192
5. 'Scene of the Fatal Accident at Staplehurst' — 204
6. Front and back cover of *Mugby Junction*, the Christmas issue of *All the Year Round* for 1866 — 209
7. 'The Railway Juggernaut of 1845' — 212

Introduction: A Tremendous Chapter of Accidents

> God made the country, and man made the town.
> William Cowper, *The Task*, 1785
> On the banks of the Thames it is a tremendous chapter of accidents.
> Henry James, 'London', 1888

In the years between Cowper and James, London explodes. As do prevailing notions of how a metropolis even forms and develops. Sprawl, population, demographic diversity, economic muscle, skeletal poverty, global connectedness: the foundational metrics of urban studies are themselves a product of the nineteenth-century cities they attempted to measure. This book attends to other ways of understanding what seemed to many (then and now) like a unique phenomenon in the history of human settlement: the emergence of the modern metropolis.[1] In particular, it tracks a significant change in attitudes about metropolitan development or what might metaphorically be called the death of the urban planner.[2] When James describes London as 'a tremendous chapter of accidents', he is

---

[1] These terms have been the subject of extensive debate in urban and cultural studies. Rather than defining metropolitan modernity from the outset or claiming Victorian London as its exemplar, I am persuaded by Simon Parker's argument in *Urban Theory and the Urban Experience: Encountering the City* (Abingdon, Oxon; New York: Routledge, 2004) that Victorian London helped facilitate a broad self-consciousness about the urban condition. From a similar angle, Alexander Welsh argues that 'the discovery of the city as a problem ... coincided with the rise of modern historicism'; see *The City of Dickens* (London: Clarendon, 1971), 31. If scholars have been debating metropolitan modernity ever since, they extend the inquiries, theorizing, and self-scrutiny of nineteenth-century urban observers, inhabitants, and artists. As such, this book begins with their keywords about the metropolis and its distinguishing problems.

[2] Urban experience ranks high in J. Hillis Miller's argument about the nineteenth-century disappearance of God: 'Life in the city is the way in which many men have experienced most directly what it means to live without God in the world'; see *The Disappearance of God: Five Nineteenth-Century Writers* (Cambridge, MA: Belknap Press, 1963), 5. This book changes the terms of Miller's argument from disappearing God to a missing designer and attempts to offer more specific contexts for such a transformation.

commenting on its architecture, ruminating on the design of buildings and the aggregation of strangely mingled styles. But in effect, James also sums up a century's worth of questions about the increasingly uncertain origins of urban species. Cowper could echo Virgil to quip, 'God made the country, and man made the town'—though by the end of the eighteenth century this cultural geography is already old-fashioned with its moral, even Manichean contrasts. The famous quote also attempts to answer an implied question about design: who made what? Certainly by the early nineteenth century, no one was quite so sure, particularly concerning the unprecedented form of what Friedrich Engels called 'the great towns'. Divinely ordained? Definitely not. But man made? Was such a sprawling, labyrinthine Babylon really something man had wrought?

Babylon and the labyrinth were favourite metaphors for nineteenth-century London. So too were metaphors of city as organism, whether bodily system or rancorous tumour. In the 1820s, William Cobbett famously diagnosed the metropolis's unnatural growth with its nickname 'the Great Wen'.[3] Also circulating was the characterization of the city as a ceaseless living stream of traffic and strangers, each an atom unto themselves, swirling in a social maelstrom. In 1865, John Ruskin would say of the city that 'existence becomes mere transition, and every creature is only atom in a drift of human dust, and current of interchanging particles... for a city, or cities, such as this no architecture is possible—nay, no desire of it is possible to their inhabitants.'[4] For Ruskin, the built environment of the city is entirely lacking in design; the urban has no planner. London was the signature but not the exclusive example of this phenomenon. Visiting the greatest of the industrialized great towns in the 1840s, Engels argues, 'it is precisely Manchester that has been built less according to a plan and less within the limitations of official regulations—and indeed more through accident—than any other town.'[5] Writers on England's rapid urbanization were often stunned by its apparent randomness:

> The discontinuities and obscurities, the apparent absence of large, visibly related structures, the disorganizations and disarticulations, seem to compose

---

[3] William Cobbett, 'Sussex Journal', *Cobbett's Weekly Register*, 12 January 1822, 92.
[4] John Ruskin, 'The Study of Architecture in Our Schools', in *On the Old Road. Volume 1—Art* (Sunnyside, Kent: George Allen, 1885), 378.
[5] Friedrich Engels, *The Condition of the Working Class in England*, ed. Victor Kiernan (Harmondsworth, Middlesex; New York: Penguin, 1987), 86. Henderson and Chaloner translate the sentence differently: 'Yet Manchester is the very town in which building has taken place in a haphazard manner with little or no planning or interference from the authorities.' See *The Condition of the Working Class in England*, trans. W. O. Henderson and W. H. Chaloner (New York: Macmillan, 1958), 56.

the structure of a chaos, a landscape whose human, social, and natural parts may be related simply by accidents, a random agglomeration of mere appearances.[6]

Accidentally composed, such an urban landscape becomes illegible, argues Steven Marcus. What all of these characterizations share—and what their diversity also suggests—is a deep uncertainty about how the metropolis comes into being, about its il/logical, un/motivated, or chaotic processes which certainly seem beyond human making or control.

The persistent accidentalness within Victorian writing about the metropolis tells another story: not about incoherence or illegibility but about change. This book challenges the geographical and disciplinary scope of the nineteenth-century's transforming ideas about change—and especially the role of chance within it. The conventional genealogies of such transformations cluster into three domains: the development of statistics and mathematical theories of probability, the arrival of an aesthetic modernity of contingency and shock, and evolutionary biology's emphasis on random mutations and the chances of survival. Each of these critical narratives makes claims about the new enfranchisement of chance over the course of the nineteenth century. But, as this book argues, the metropolis ought to rank among the primary arenas for this intellectual history. It was ground zero for some of the most important interdisciplinary thinking about causation in the nineteenth century. *By Accident or Design* offers a different vocabulary for the century's shifts towards probabilistic or relativistic paradigms by grounding them in the material contexts of the Victorian metropolis and, in particular, the increasingly conspicuous accidents that marked its characteristic dynamics of order and dispersion.

By Accident or Design looks to moments after the town was no longer evidently man-made but before it was reconceived as systemically independent, emergent, or globally interconnected. Examining representations of metropolitan life in text and image from 1830–70, this book locates in the Victorians' eroding certainty about the built environment a productive play between concepts of design and chance. Those decades mark several major changes in metropolitan infrastructure—including the arrival of the omnibus, the railway, massive urban improvement projects, and significant industrial development—which not only shaped a generic category of the modern city, but underscored its troubling instabilities in often spectacular ways. The accidents they generated became a focus of writing about the metropolis as well as a backdrop for thinking about the

---

[6] Steven Marcus, 'Reading the Illegible', in *The Victorian City: Images and Realities*, ed. H. J. Dyos and Michael Wolff (London: Routledge & Kegan Paul, 1973), I, 257.

contingencies of human design, whether expressed in cities or in forms of printed representation.

Attending to omnibus collisions, pedestrian mishaps, fires, industrial catastrophe, and railway crashes, this book investigates a representative set of urban accidents not merely to characterize the changing experience of metropolitan life but to explain why these phenomena captured Victorian attentions, to show their prevalence and particular uses in discourse, and to propose their close relations to some of the signature genres and circulatory patterns of metropolitan writing. Through its series of case studies, this book pursues two interdependent goals: to establish the mid-century metropolis as an important domain of probability thinking and to demonstrate alternate, even accidental literary histories for the most conspicuous forms of its representation, from the newspaper to the realist novel. This study of accidents offers an alternative critical vocabulary for the cultural contingencies, generic development, and complex circulation of some of the major forms of Victorian print culture. Those textual forms describe and index how Victorians came to perceive not just the emergent metropolis but perhaps modernity itself.

ARGUMENTS FROM DESIGN TO ACCIDENT

From his later perspective, Henry James can suggest that 'the most general appeal of the great city remains exactly what it is, the largest chapter of human accidents. I have no idea of what the future evolution of the strangely mingled monster may be.'[7] To Cobbett's metaphor of a monstrous organism, to Ruskin's apprehension of random atomic collisions, James contributes the ascendant language of Darwinism, wherein chance mutations generate the enormity and strange mingling of the city whose future course is neither teleological nor predictable. Darwin's development theory presents one of several important contexts for the paradigmatic transitions this book hopes to complicate. Then as now, Darwin earns a lot of attention for his role in turning Victorian attitudes towards an understanding of systemic contingency. *The Origin of Species* inspired reactions in precisely these terms, as anxious contemporaries seized upon how 'Darwin seemed to risk turning the world into an accident'.[8] For example, as William Denton sniped in *Is Darwin Right?* (1881), 'this is no hap-hazard world, nor is man a mere come-by-chance. We are not the

---

[7] James, 'London', 232.
[8] George Levine, *Darwin and the Novelists: Patterns of Science in Victorian Fiction* (Cambridge, MA: Harvard University Press, 1988), 93.

accidental result of a million accidents, each fortunately, yet accidentally, contributing to the grand result'.[9] Though Darwin said no such thing, he has been entangled ever since in arguments about causation and design, in which Darwinism seems to invoke 'the law of higgledy-piggledy' governing an accidental world.[10]

By contrast, in *The Origin of Species*, Darwin addresses the role of chance within the laws of variation quite directly:

> I have hitherto sometimes spoken as if the variations—so common and multiform with organic beings under domestication, and in a lesser degree with those under nature—were due to chance. This, of course is a wholly incorrect expression, but it serves to acknowledge plainly our ignorance of the cause of each particular variation.[11]

From this perspective, 'chance is the name we give to as yet unknown laws', as Gillian Beer has explained.[12] Darwin gently suggests that natural selection is less as a matter of chance than human ignorance about causation. As in the *Origin*'s famous final sentence, Darwin went further to press the compatibility of natural selection with divine creation, translating our ignorance of causes into a sense of faith and wonder.[13] Of course, this in no way attributes those causes to a divine agent, and Darwinian biology was instantly perceived as challenging traditions of natural theology which credit a divine creator for the world's design.[14] Natural selection not only removed agency and knowable causation, it seemed to invite operations beyond human prediction or discernment, in keeping as much with randomness as with faith. Thus, George Levine argues that 'Darwin abjured chance but required it for his argument' which ultimately presents 'a very strange combination of the random and the orderly'.[15] So too does chance spur the 'Darwinian imagination'

---

[9] William Denton, *Is Darwin Right? or, The Origin of Man* (Wellesley, MA: Mrs E. M. F. Denton, 1881), 109, <http://books.google.com/books?id=_d04AAAAMAAJ>.
[10] Charles Darwin, 'Darwin, C. R. to Lyell, Charles', 10 December 1859, Letter 2575, Darwin Correspondence Project, <http://www.darwinproject.ac.uk/letter/entry-2575>.
[11] Charles Darwin, *The Origin of Species*, ed. Gillian Beer (Oxford: Oxford University Press, 1996), 108. For a good survey of the issue of chance in Darwin and in evolutionary theory more broadly, see Roberta Lynn Millstein, 'The Chances of Evolution: An Analysis of the Roles of Chance in Microevolution and Macroevolution' (Ph.D. Dissertation, University of Minnesota, 1997), <https://webspace.utexas.edu/deverj/personal/test/chance.pdf>.
[12] *Darwin's Plots: Evolutionary Narrative in Darwin, George Eliot, and Nineteenth-Century Fiction*, 3rd edn (Cambridge: Cambridge University Press, 2009), 79.
[13] Darwin, *The Origin of Species*, 396. Gillian Beer notes how this sentence was revised in different editions; see *Darwin's Plots*, 48.
[14] Levine, *Darwin and the Novelists*, viii.
[15] Levine, *Darwin and the Novelists*, 19, 93.

that Levine finds operating in a variety of cultural, generic, and narratological spheres, structured by a 'contest between design and chance'.[16]

Darwin's complex wrangling with questions of design, chance, and change has at times overshadowed other domains and earlier contexts in which similar cultural work was being done. As Levine reminds us, '[t]here were many evolutionisms before Darwin and there have been many since.'[17] In analogous ways that predate Darwin, observers of the Victorian metropolis were fascinated by the accidents that seemed to characterize its haphazard speciation and which gradually suggested other kinds of organizing principles at work: the aleatory, meaning dependent on uncertain contingencies, like throwing dice; and the stochastic, meaning patterned or structured by these aleatory processes. Even Darwin's route to the Galapagos went through the metropolis, in part because it linked the English to global or imperial expansion, and in part because 'metropolis' had a working definition in nineteenth-century biology as the most concentrated location for a given species which could be anywhere: country, city, wilderness, archipelago. The metropolitan concept travelled, radiating its questions about 'the difficult relations between design and causation, futurity and chance'.[18]

In this sense, the metropolis does not just shadow the century's better-known debates about design between evolutionism and deistic religion: it shares a lexicon and conceptual framework with which to confront such questions. Throughout the nineteenth century, theologians and religious defenders deployed 'the argument from design' as a fundamental principle of interpreting the complexity and contingency of the natural world. Inspired by Bishop (Joseph) Butler's 1736 work *Analogy of Religion, Natural and Revealed to the Constitution and Course of Nature*, natural theology claimed—as would its contemporary offspring, intelligent design theory—that the improbably perfect structures of the natural world could only prove the existence of God as divine craftsman. William Paley in *Natural Theology* (1802) points to natural structures like the eye and biological systems like the circulation of the blood to underscore their thoughtful mechanisms, an intentionality of design which natural theology converts into religious faith. At certain points, Paley relies on mechanical and industrial analogies to underscore the purposeful design of human invention and infrastructure. As we would never expect the random appearance of watches, factory equipment, or city water systems

---

[16] Levine, *Darwin and the Novelists*, 13, 62.
[17] Levine, *Darwin and the Novelists*, 3.
[18] Gillian Beer, *Open Fields: Science in Cultural Encounter* (Oxford, NY: Oxford University Press, 1996), 276.

nor attribute them to any 'principle of order, acting blindly and without choice', so we should trust the prior design of the natural world, however seemingly unmotivated or imperfect.[19] As Paley explains, chance is merely a factor of our ignorance. Chance exists, but only as a necessary aspect of greater and usually providential design:

> There must be *chance* in the midst of design: by which we mean, that events which are not designed, necessarily arise from the pursuit of events which are designed. One man travelling to York, meets another man travelling to London. Their meeting is by chance, is accidental, and so would be called and reckoned, though the journeys which produced the meeting were, both of them, undertaken with design and from deliberation. The meeting, though accidental, was nevertheless hypothetically necessary.[20]

We need not be troubled. When accident simply means 'by chance', the argument works fine. But it comes under greater stress when accident suggests injurious mishaps or design failures, as increasingly textured urban and industrial life in the years following the publication of *Natural Theology*.

The *Bridgewater Treatises* of the 1830s carried on Paley's efforts to justify the works of God to man, enlisting prominent authors to directly engage the challenges of materialistic science. But similar tensions arise within these arguments from design. For instance, Sir Charles Bell, in the fourth treatise titled *The Hand: Its Mechanism and Vital Endowments as Evincing Design* (1833), marvels at the intricate perfections of the human hand as evidence for God's creation and stewardship. Ironically, Bell's physiological intimacy with the human hand stemmed from his surgical work treating the injuries of factory workers who suffered accidents on the job. As a deeply religious man with sincere commitment to the argument from design (he later edited and illustrated an edition of Paley's *Natural Theology*), Bell focused his treatise on the hand precisely to engage concerns about the supersession of human manufacture by machines.[21] Bell's argument put him in the middle of the 'machinery question', as he, like Paley, used analogies to transpose the purposeful intentions of industrial mechanisms onto natural ones. But accidents could unsettle the argument

---

[19] William Paley, *Natural Theology: Or, Evidences of the Existence and Attributes of the Deity, Collected from the Appearances of Nature* (Houston, TX: St. Thomas Press, 1972), 52.
[20] Paley, *Natural Theology*, 378.
[21] My thanks to Peter Capuano for sharing work-in-progress about the significance of the hand and representations of manufacture in 'Maneuvering between Early Nineteenth-Century Science, Religiosity, and Industrialization', 2013. See also Peter Capuano, 'On Sir Charles Bell's The Hand, 1833', *BRANCH: Britain, Representation and Nineteenth-Century History* (Romanticism and Victorianism on the Net, 2012), <http://www.branchcollective.org/?ps_articles=peter-capuano-on-sir-charles-bells-the-hand-1833>.

in each domain. If unintentional injuries offered the surgeon a closer look at God's handiwork, they also underscored the problem of how to interpret seemingly chance events like industrial accidents as part of a divine telos.

The trouble with accidents is whether or not they happen by chance. Or, instead, whether they indicate a larger purpose or plan which we do not initially recognize. Many religious thinkers dealt with the problem of chance by simply denying it, as did Paley. Bishop Butler underscored the human ignorance of causation, particularly in cases of natural disaster: 'we call the events which come to pass by them, accidental: though all reasonable men know certainly, that there cannot, in reality, be any such thing as chance'.[22] In *Grammar of Assent* (1870)—a complex defence of faith as more than a matter of logical inference—John Henry Newman claims that marvels and coincidences must be 'beyond the operations of chance' and 'cannot be properly resolved into the mere accident of concurrent causes, but must in reason be considered the warning voice of God'.[23] In the fragment of his *Bridgewater Treatise* (1837), Charles Babbage seeks to demonstrate 'Nature's God' by arguing that anything aberrant, arbitrary, or impossibly complex only seems that way because of our limited cognitive horizon.[24] Given enough iterations, all such phenomena will resolve into 'some few and general principles, by which the whole of the material universe is sustained, and from which its infinitely varied phenomena emerge as the necessary consequences'.[25] In other words, anything seemingly random, whether an individual event or a series, would actually resolve into patterns given a large enough view, revealing general laws established by God.

Such arguments paralleled a line of deterministic thinking in continental mathematics developed by figures including Pierre-Simon Laplace, Carl Friedrich Gauss, and Adolphe Quetelet. From the positivist perspective of Laplace, chance merely indicates the lack of obtainable knowledge about the world. As Theodore Porter explains, chance for Laplace means 'not the irreducibly random, but the fortuitous production of patterns

---

[22] Joseph Butler, *The Analogy of Religion Natural and Revealed to the Constitution and Course of Nature* (Dublin: George Ewing, 1736), 188–9, <http://find.galegroup.com/ecco/infomark.do?&source=gale&prodId=ECCO&userGroupName=tall85761&tabID=T001&docId=CW121666346&type=multipage&contentSet=ECCOArticles&version=1.0&docLevel=FASCIMILE>.

[23] John Henry Newman, *An Essay in Aid of a Grammar of Assent* (Oxford: Clarendon Press, 1985), 276.

[24] Charles Babbage, *The Ninth Bridgewater Treatise: A Fragment*, 2nd edn (London: John Murray, 1838), 33, <http://books.google.com/books?id=y_ERAAAAYAAJ>.

[25] Babbage, *The Ninth Bridgewater Treatise*, 32.

through the interaction of a multitude of independent causes'.[26] We misrecognize chance as such only because we simply do not know about the multiplicity of causes which are nonetheless determinable. Given sufficient knowledge (or even omniscience), chance instead resolves into patterns of regular distribution, which Laplace and Gauss made famous as the 'central limit theorem' (the bell curve), and which Quetelet regularized as the error law or the law of averages. In physics, James Clerk Maxwell was arriving at similar conclusions with the kinetic theory of gases, which accepted the unpredictability of molecular motion in its statistical models.[27] Accidents—as events which may manifest the principle of chance—are thus epiphenomenal to the operations of probabilistic laws which could be described statistically. Scholars including Porter, Thomas Kavanagh, Mary Poovey, and Ian Hacking have extensively written about the development of statistics and its transformation into probability theory.[28] This so-called 'probabilistic revolution' culminates by the end of the nineteenth-century, according to Hacking, in the 'taming of chance', subordinated to deterministic and predictive models.

The interpretation of accidents follows a similar trajectory, subject to changing forms of deterministic explanation over the nineteenth century, beginning with the paradigmatic legacy of fate, fortune, and Providence. The chapters to come will engage with such concepts in more detail, specifically in how they reckon (or fail to reckon) with man-made rather than natural events, including the seemingly random elements of urban and industrial experience. The poet and Evangelical Hannah More furnishes a brief example with her poem 'Turn the Carpet; or, the Two Weavers', published in the extremely popular series of *Cheap Repository Tracts* in the 1790s. In it, More promotes a faith in design that keeps with natural theology, using an elaborate figure of a carpet on the loom. One of the poem's weavers is troubled by the apparent randomness of the textile, which seems to have '[n]o plan, no pattern'. But his companion suggests

---

[26] Theodore Porter, *The Rise of Statistical Thinking, 1820–1900* (Princeton, NJ: Princeton University Press, 1986), 72.
[27] Porter, *The Rise of Statistical Thinking*, 114.
[28] Porter, *The Rise of Statistical Thinking*; Thomas M. Kavanagh, *Enlightenment and the Shadows of Chance: The Novel and the Culture of Gambling in Eighteenth-Century France* (Baltimore, MD: The Johns Hopkins University Press, 1993); Mary Poovey, *A History of the Modern Fact: Problems of Knowledge in the Sciences of Wealth and Society* (Chicago, IL: University of Chicago Press, 1998); Ian Hacking, *The Taming of Chance* (Cambridge; New York: Cambridge University Press, 1990); Ian Hacking, *The Emergence of Probability: A Philosophical Study of Early Ideas About Probability, Induction and Statistical Inference*, 2nd edn (Cambridge; New York: Cambridge University Press, 2006).

that turning over the carpet reveals the patterns on its finished side. Metaphorically, that means moving from this world to the next:

> But when we reach that world of light,
> And view these works of God aright;
> Then shall we see the whole design,
> And own the workman is divine.
> What now seem random strokes, will there
> All order and design appear.[29]

Unlike Bell's *Bridgewater Treatise*, More's poem does not attempt to resolve the manufactured irregularities of this world for the living. Rather, it promotes faith in a governing Providence whose designs we cannot know until after death. Randomness remains in this world, though stabilized by a compensatory model of God's providence. That faith would be severely tested when the 'random strokes' of machines resulted in grievous injury, which few wanted to attribute to God's plan or to the fates of undeserving individuals or workers as a class. Rather, providential understandings of accidents became part of a larger discourse involving the insurance industry, in which random events are not fated but displaced into an emerging notion of risk.

What became known as 'risk management' is a crucial context for the nineteenth century's changing definitions of accidents and how to interpret them. According to some scholars, the development of risk signals something much bigger. Risk is the signature concept of cultural modernity according to Anthony Giddens, replacing notions of fortune, fate, and providence with a diffused awareness of contingency, and compelling people to subscribe to the institutions which define and manage it.[30] Ian Baucom offers a powerful account of that transformation starting from the 1781 massacre aboard the slave ship *Zong*, in which white slave owners, by throwing more than a hundred slaves into the sea, converted living humans into lost property and recovered its value by an insurance contract. For Baucom, the *Zong* incident marks the onset of our own capitalist

---

[29] Hannah More, *Turn the Carpet; or, the Two Weavers: a New Song in a Dialogue Between Dick and John* (London: J. Marshall, 1796), 6, <http://find.galegroup.com/ecco/infomark.do?&source=gale&prodId=ECCO&userGroupName=tall85761&tabID=T001&docId=CW3316021656&type=multipage&contentSet=ECCOArticles&version=1.0>.

[30] Anthony Giddens, *The Consequences of Modernity* (Palo Alto, CA: Stanford University Press, 1990), 30, 48. While Giddens is less precise than others about where or when this occurs, he does suggest that risk responds to the pace, scale, and dynamism of the late nineteenth-century city, as well as the collapse of categories of external and manufactured risks. Giddens, *The Consequences of Modernity*, 6; Anthony Giddens, *Runaway World: How Globalisation Is Reshaping Our Lives* (New York: Routledge, 2000), 44–5.

modernity, shaped by new actuarial, evidentiary, and typicalizing treatments of risk and loss from late eighteenth-century marine insurance to twentieth-century speculative finance. This story is not about commodities but about property whose value only exists by imagining its potential destruction.[31] Writing about risk helped both to define and manage that proleptic loss; as Elaine Freedgood has shown, it was occurring in a diverse set of nineteenth-century contexts including popular narratives of adventure tourism, balloon flight, and global travel. As they stabilized notions of danger, they helped constitute 'modern cosmologies' of risk in which modernity was unevenly articulated.[32]

As an important site for the production and management of risk in the nineteenth century, the financial system provoked broad discussions about speculation and safety, especially concerning the moral appropriateness of investments and the interpretation of financial disasters. From the establishment of the London Stock Exchange (1808) to joint stock companies (1844) to legislation of 'limited liability' (1856), developments in the British financial system made it progressively easier for the general public to participate. Alongside, attitudes were changing about the social acceptability of financial speculation, to where even the parochial ladies of Elizabeth Gaskell's *Cranford* (1851), though vehemently opposed to the vulgarity of money, could still be upright women of business with investments in the funds or in joint stock banks.[33] As happens to Miss Mattie, they could also lose those investments in moments of financial panic. Market crashes, bank failures, and financial panics all provoked contested interpretations about how the financial system actually worked. As a system, it was complex, obscure, and occasionally punctuated by catastrophe. Poovey suggests that 'every piece of writing about finance in this period was an attempt to understand and interpret something that was only partially visible and constantly in a state of change'.[34] In times of disruptive change, financial professionals tried to reassure the public that crashes or downturns were just aspects of a larger and coherent system, working against more sensational accounts which emphasized those events as singular catastrophes.[35] In other words, financial catastrophes became

---

[31] Ian Baucom, *Specters of the Atlantic: Finance Capital, Slavery, and the Philosophy of History* (Durham, NC: Duke University Press, 2005), 138–9.
[32] Elaine Freedgood, *Victorian Writing About Risk: Imagining a Safe England in a Dangerous World* (Cambridge; New York: Cambridge University Press, 2000), 2.
[33] Elizabeth Gaskell, *Cranford*, ed. Elizabeth Porges Watson (New York: Oxford University Press, 2011), 119.
[34] Mary Poovey, ed., *The Financial System in Nineteenth-century Britain* (New York: Oxford University Press, 2003), 4.
[35] Timothy Alborn, 'The Moral of the Failed Bank: Professional Plots in the Victorian Money Market', *Victorian Studies* 38, no. 2 (1995): 199–226.

public occasions to interpret the very dynamics of causation and design that interest this book: whether things happen or entities form by design, chance, or some systemic admixture. Even the language of financial downturn suggests its consonance with this study of accidents, relying on metaphors of crashes, disasters, failures, and sudden ruin. For instance, after an 1825 disaster provoked 'agitation and alarm in the city', anxious crowds filled the streets to wonder about just what had caused it.[36] Though 'city' refers specifically to London's consolidating financial district, its panics and crashes had broader urban effects, generating a kind of heuristic speculation that relates to the puzzles of metropolitan causality at large.[37]

This small but representative set of contexts were all simultaneously active in perceptions of the nineteenth-century metropolis, itself emerging as a category defined by and redefining concepts of design and accident. But the metropolis deserves its own special place in these cultural, literary, and intellectual histories. Amid the disorientation of new urban centres, the Victorians conceived a non-deterministic organizing principle with which to imagine novel forms of probability. The major experiments in this field were conducted by a diverse cohort of metropolitan citizens, observers, and writers, specifically as they confronted the development of their cities by accident or design. The dominant questions facing early Victorian social statisticians and political economists and imaginative writers concerned how to measure, organize, and represent urban randomness, or, by contrast, how to resist the fatalism of a deterministic system. What were the logics of urban phenomena and populations? Did chance play a part, or could it be eradicated? In what conceptual frameworks or textual representations might either be possible? These were also the questions facing insurance agents, urban antiquarians, industrial workers, literary critics, novelists, journalists, philosophers, railway directors, and biologists. The accidents of the metropolis offer an overlooked historical context in which a variety of cultural actors reconsidered the civic, epistemological, and ethical significance of causation.

THE ACCIDENTAL CITY

The modern city preoccupied its contemporaries as 'a special problem', according to James Winter: 'Out of this perception of crisis arose a

---

[36] 'The Money Market', *The Times*, 14 December 1825, 2.
[37] On the term 'city' as a specific reference for London's transforming financial centre, see Garrett Ziegler, 'The City of London, Real and Unreal', *Victorian Studies* 49, no. 3 (Spring 2007): 431–55.

consciousness that a new kind of human arrangement, the metropolis, was coming into being, the defining feature of which would be sustained growth and an ever-increasing complexity in the interaction of its separate functions'.[38] As Steven Johnson has argued, the nineteenth century saw the development of a modern form of urban existence before anyone was sure it was actually going to work.[39] Its construction could seem like degeneration, its growth like haphazard sprawl, its expanding populace like a bewildering mix of privilege and abjection. Charles Dickens complained in *Bleak House* (1852–3) that London is 'a shameful testimony to future ages, how civilisation and barbarism walked this boastful island together'.[40] The Victorians reached for representations of the city that could accommodate its paradoxical extremes, deploying a dizzying array of discursive and representational modes to grapple with the uncertainties of who or what was making the town. As Caroline Arscott and Griselda Pollock explain, '[t]he debate was not about a place, but about a process'.[41] That disputed process is not merely urbanization, but an inchoate notion of unplanned change. 'Change in London was happening so quickly that it seemed by enchantment rather than man-made', Lynda Nead suggests.[42] Metropolitan change seemed driven by something else, whether the aggregate effects of its fragmented municipal authorities, the enchantment of urban-industrial capitalism, or the ignorant armies of benighted chance. Seeming to grow spontaneously, it was also 'spontaneously combusting, its houses and streets continuously on the verge of falling down or blowing up'.[43]

Whatever it was, '[t]hat huge fermenting mass of human-kind', as Wordsworth called London in *The Prelude*, seemed to roil with processes for which adequate causal explanations did not yet exist.[44] In 1840, William Cooke Taylor speculated that England's changing cities were revealing 'a system of social life constructed on a wholly new principle, a principle as yet vague and indefinite but developing itself by its own

---

[38] James Winter, *London's Teeming Streets, 1830–1914* (London: Routledge, 1993), 4.
[39] Steven Johnson, *The Ghost Map: The Story of London's Most Terrifying Epidemic—and How It Changed Science, Cities, and the Modern World* (New York: Riverhead, 2006).
[40] Charles Dickens, *Bleak House* (Oxford: Oxford University Press, 1987), 151.
[41] Caroline Arscott and Griselda Pollock, 'The Partial View: The Visual Representation of the Early Nineteenth-Century Industrial City', in *The Culture of Capital: Art, Power, and the Nineteenth-Century Middle Class*, ed. Janet Wolff and John Seed (Manchester; New York: Manchester University Press, 1988), 197.
[42] Lynda Nead, *Victorian Babylon: People, Streets, and Images in Nineteenth-Century London* (New Haven, CT: Yale University Press, 2000), 29.
[43] Nead, *Victorian Babylon*, 94.
[44] William Wordsworth, *The Prelude, or, Growth of a Poet's Mind: An Autobiographical Poem* (London: Edward Moxon, 1850), 197.

spontaneous force and daily producing effects which no human foresight had anticipated'.[45] This vague principle was elaborated by the *Illustrated London News* in an 1866 article using slightly different terms:

> The metropolis may really be said to exist, rather than to live.... London is an inorganic mass of humanity, from which the one thing that humanity most needs—to wit, government by an intelligent will—is utterly absent.... It resembles a crowd, the very size of which deprives it of all self-guidance and control. Large human interests, merely for want of some methodising energy, lie weltering in perpetual chaos. Light, air, water, health, locomotion, order—to say nothing of convenience, beauty, grandeur, moral influence—all are mere matters of chance in what may be called the metropolitan districts.[46]

The *ILN* has to scramble for a conceptual vocabulary to accommodate whatever 'methodising energy' lurks between metropolitan chaos and governance. It tries comparisons to an unruly crowd and unsanitary spaces, explaining the lack of metropolitan governance through a familiar set of Victorian social evils. Fermenting, transitional, spontaneous, indefinite, accidental: this vocabulary was invoked throughout the century to explain the making of metropolitan form and the functioning of metropolitan life. Those concepts were often politically freighted with presumptions about sanitation and ordered governance, as the *ILN*'s diction suggests, but these biases were not the rule. What composed the broader pattern—and what this book argues is crucial to the texts and conceptual legacies of the nineteenth-century city—were the uncertain relations of chaos and method, chance and design, which have interested urban observers ever since.

In his foundational study *The Country and the City*, Raymond Williams observes that the nineteenth-century metropolis reveals 'a contradiction, a paradox: the coexistence of variation and apparent randomness with what had in the end to be seen as a determining system'. For Williams, this interplay of randomness and determinism shows up conspicuously in literary representations of London which evince 'this double condition: the random and the systematic, the visible and the obscured, which is the true significance of the city, and especially at this period of the capital city, as a dominant social form'.[47] This 'double condition' is not the dynamic

---

[45] William Cooke Taylor, 'The Moral Economy of Large Towns', *Bentley's Miscellany*, 1840, 597.

[46] 'Metropolitan Municipalities', *Illustrated London News*, 5 May 1866, 430. For a brilliant reading of the politics of the crowd in the nineteenth century, see John Plotz, *The Crowd: British Literature and Public Politics* (Berkeley, CA: University of California Press, 2000).

[47] Raymond Williams, *The Country and the City* (New York: Oxford University Press, 1973), 154.

of country and city, but the perplexing coexistence of urban randomness and design. This book pursues the conspicuous embodiments of this 'double condition' in accidents, in events which fascinated the Victorians for keeping seemingly exclusive kinds of causation in suspense. *By Accident or Design* argues that accidents provide an explanatory framework for the paradoxes of urban modernity, elaborated in an interdisciplinary context of Victorian metropolitan writing with lasting consequences for understandings of causation and design.

Victorianist scholars have explored the dimensions of the city's 'double condition' in fascinating ways, mapping them onto the dynamics of urban representation.[48] Among the most robust of these studies is Nead's *Victorian Babylon*. In it, Nead demonstrates what dialectics drove metropolitan development, showing how the Victorians knew and represented the city between extremes of civilization and barbarity, metropolitan improvement and demolition, light and darkness, order and anarchy. According to Nead, these are the paradoxical conditions of London's urban modernity.[49] This book proposes a set of related concepts which the metropolis would continually collapse: design and chance. Doing so builds upon the rich critical history of urban dialectics while also looking to exceed the binary of a 'double condition'. This crucial meeting point is the accident itself. As a phenomenon to interpret, accident holds questions about design and chance in suspense. To adapt a phrase from Walter Benjamin, accident is 'the figurative appearance of the dialectic, the law of the dialectic at a standstill'.[50] As I will show, the Victorians used repre-

---

[48] A few notable examples: Alexander Welsh renovates the Augustinian antinomy between contrasting visions of the earthly city and the city of God to describe the Victorian metropolis in *The City of Dickens*. David Pike demonstrates two primary ways of representing the nineteenth-century city, from above and from below, deriving from a metaphorics of the devil and the vertiginous metropolis in *Metropolis on the Styx: The Underworlds of Modern Urban Culture, 1800–2001* (Ithaca, NY: Cornell University Press, 2007). James Buzard argues that metropolitan knowledge oscillates between insider and outsider perspectives, producing a modern notion of culture through reciprocal 'autoethnography'; see *Disorienting Fiction: The Autoethnographic Work of Nineteenth-Century British Novels* (Princeton, NJ: Princeton University Press, 2005). Tanya Agathocleous explains how Victorians depended on a dynamic between particularity and totality, the street-level detail and the panoramic, in working through the apparent impossibility of resolving metropolitan vastness and effectively substituting cosmopolitan London for the world at large. See *Urban Realism and the Cosmopolitan Imagination in the Nineteenth Century: Visible City, Invisible World* (Cambridge; New York: Cambridge University Press, 2011).

[49] Nead, *Victorian Babylon*, 8.

[50] Walter Benjamin, *Charles Baudelaire: A Lyric Poet in the Era of High Capitalism*, trans. Harry Zohn (New York: Verso, 1997), 171. Benjamin proposes this ambiguous, dream-like middle-state as the realm of the commodity, the arcades, and the whore—some of the signature features of the urban modernity he theorizes and which have been justly critiqued.

sentations of accidents to model an emerging urban modernity and to study its dialectics at such moments of arrest.

The Victorians were drawn to accidents for their substantial explanatory power in confronting the increasingly complicated de/generation of the modern city. But accident offered more than a metaphor to describe the disorderly complexity of Victorian London. It was also a very material reality during the nineteenth-century's industrial transformation of metropolitan life, manifesting, for example, as collisions of vehicles, pedestrian misfortunes, workplace accidents, factory fires, railway disasters, the unnerving problem of collapsing buildings, gasworks explosions, and all the unexpected encounters and coincidences that the city foregrounds in novel ways. That said, 'accident' did not exclusively signify a calamity or a technological or industrial event. It retained a range of philosophical and theological connotations including happy coincidence, providential arrangement, unintended happening, error, and meaningless attribute. By the mid-nineteenth century, these very significations were shifting, largely because of the conspicuousness of hazardous or technological accidents as such, which are the primary concerns of this book. The unstable definition of accident between 1830–1870 is precisely what helped Victorians to interrogate metropolitan upheaval from multiple viewpoints— philosophical, legal, actuarial, and theological—resulting in complex notions of probability that have yet to be adequately recognized.

Through accidents, we can see Victorian writers coming to grips not only with the chance happenings and hazards that increasingly marked metropolitan life, but with a set of concepts and discursive practices developing alongside them, including the rise of accident news in the modern newspaper, the statistical and sociological cataloguing of urban types, the definition of new forms of risk by the insurance industry, and the management of industrial and technological accidents made conspicuous by the railway. If these seem like disparate domains, they all share a vocabulary of accident which testifies to the widespread reckoning with design and chance in metropolitan contexts. If they seem loosely connected to the metropolis as such, they likewise testify to its dispersed ubiquity in the nineteenth century—as well as, perhaps, in our own. The nineteenth-century city has never lacked critical attention; indeed, the idea of the city 'has been ubiquitous in cultural analysis of the Victorian period'.[51] As a result, scholars in the wake of Paul Gilroy have turned away from

---

But his interest in the 'standstill' recommends a different way of thinking about how the Victorians encountered their urban Babylon.

[51] Katharina Boehm and Josephine McDonagh, 'New Agenda. Urban Mobility: New Maps of Victorian London', *Journal of Victorian Culture* 15, no. 2 (August 2010): 196.

the exclusive notions of metropolitan intellectual and cultural history, and towards the peripheries, global margins, contact zones, and cosmopolitanisms that have been wrongly eclipsed by a metropolitan legacy.[52] My project is neither to enshrine the metropole nor the empire it helped constitute, but rather to illuminate the contradictions and uncertainties by which Victorian writers experienced and represented them.

In acknowledging the problems of metropolitan totality and exploring its internal contradictions, this book promotes what has been called a 'new agenda' of scholarship on the city, shifting away from 'the construction of power, meaning and identity through representation' and toward the material histories and phenomenologies by which the metropolis and its discursive contours were experienced.[53] The oft-reported chaos of nineteenth-century cities demands reconsideration in terms other than the influential notion of modernity bequeathed by Georg Simmel and Benjamin: the metropolis as the domain of shock, chance encounter, random associations, alienation, and wandering. In the last two decades, scholars from Victorian studies have brought strong critiques to this legacy, particularly through feminist deconstruction of the *flâneur* and the recognition of other social actors and modes of urban interaction.[54] Victorianists have proven adept at exploring the social construction of space and the routines and imaginative trajectories of different constituents within them.[55] Their efforts parallel the turn to social geography in urban theory as in the work of Henri Lefebvre, Edward Soja, David Harvey,

---

[52] Paul Gilroy, *The Black Atlantic: Modernity and Double Consciousness* (Cambridge, MA: Harvard University Press, 1993); Mary Louise Pratt, 'Arts of the Contact Zone', *Profession* (1991): 33–40.

[53] Boehm and McDonagh, 'New Agenda'; Alastair Owens et al., 'Fragments of the Modern City: Material Culture and the Rhythms of Everyday Life in Victorian London', *Journal of Victorian Culture* 15, no. 2 (August 2010): 212.

[54] See Elizabeth Wilson, *The Sphinx in the City: Urban Life, the Control of Disorder, and Women* (Berkeley, CA: University of California Press, 1992); Judith R. Walkowitz, *City of Dreadful Delight: Narratives of Sexual Danger in Late-Victorian London* (Chicago, IL: University of Chicago Press, 1992); Deborah Epstein Nord, *Walking the Victorian Streets: Women, Representation, and the City* (Ithaca, NY: Cornell University Press, 1995); Deborah L. Parsons, *Streetwalking the Metropolis: Women, the City, and Modernity* (Oxford; New York: Oxford University Press, 2000).

[55] See Sharon Marcus, *Apartment Stories: City and Home in Nineteenth-Century Paris and London* (Berkeley, CA: University of California Press, 1999); Pamela K. Gilbert, *Mapping the Victorian Social Body* (Albany, NY: State University of New York Press, 2004); Pike, *Metropolis on the Styx*; Seth Koven, *Slumming: Sexual and Social Politics in Victorian London* (Princeton, NJ: Princeton University Press, 2004). This is not to exclude the generative work on urban spaces in other fields or cultural eras, such as Miles Ogborn, *Spaces of Modernity: London's Geographies, 1680–1780* (New York: Guilford Press, 1998); James Chandler and Kevin Gilmartin, eds, *Romantic Metropolis: The Urban Scene of British Culture, 1780–1840* (Cambridge; New York: Cambridge University Press, 2005).

and Neil Smith.⁵⁶ Particularly useful to literary scholars has been Michel de Certeau's more encompassing notion of walking as a social practice, a strategy of everyday life that encodes its own urban theories contingent on specific agents and their social pathways and imaginative horizons.⁵⁷ *By Accident or Design* is indebted to de Certeau and the work he inspires on the textures of the metropolitan everyday, the particular routines and ruptures that do not amount to cultural totalities. I argue that the Victorians used such tropes, manifesting in accidents and their interpretation, to intervene in exclusionary discourses of urban knowledge. Countering empiricist and managerial attitudes on the rise, the Victorian writers I consider accentuated the randomness or accidentalness of the metropolis to other ends, specifically to challenge positivistic and politicized notions about causation, dis/order, and change.

This book does propose a constitutive role for accident in shaping the modern city and its signature forms of representation, and recommends these contexts in explaining large-scale epistemological and cultural change in the nineteenth century. But such a change is neither hegemonic nor historically even. Rather, it is subject to the very array of contradictions and instabilities described herein. Whether it constitutes 'modernity', it does so in the sense promoted by scholars like Nead, Freedgood, and Miles Ogborn who attend to the particularities and contradictions of urban modernity without underestimating the degree of its changes.⁵⁸ Nead describes the need for scholars

> to pay particular attention to the local elements that constitute modernity and to the tensions and irregularities that create modernity's conditions of existence... These are the varied strands that make up London's modernity in this period, which advance and stall, and are predictable only in their unpredictability.⁵⁹

Accidents are strung with the tension of regular irregularities, the predictable unpredictability of metropolitan modernity as Nead suggests. Ogborn recommends an investigation of 'the peculiar combination of routinisation and dynamic change' which marks modernity's spatial, institutional, and

---

⁵⁶ Henri Lefebvre, *The Production of Space* (Oxford; Cambridge, MA: Blackwell, 1991); Edward W. Soja, *Postmodern Geographies: The Reassertion of Space in Critical Social Theory* (London; New York: Verso, 1989); David Harvey, *Consciousness and the Urban Experience: Studies in the History and Theory of Capitalist Urbanization* (Baltimore, MD: Johns Hopkins University Press, 1985); Neil Smith, *Uneven Development: Nature, Capital, and the Production of Space* (New York: Blackwell, 1984).

⁵⁷ Michel de Certeau, *The Practice of Everyday Life*, trans. Steven Rendall (Berkeley, CA: University of California Press, 1984).

⁵⁸ Ogborn, *Spaces of Modernity*, 14.   ⁵⁹ Nead, *Victorian Babylon*, 5.

textual forms.⁶⁰ That 'peculiar combination' characterizes a great deal of how the Victorians perceived and debated their changing metropolis, from its quirky neighbourhoods to the iron-and-glass fantasies of improved urban life. *By Accident or Design* illustrates that dynamic across a range of metropolitan contexts and discourses but not to substitute one transcendental interpretive pattern for another. Instead, its examples constitute what Ogborn calls 'a haphazardly layered topography; not a hierarchy of levels, but a complicated and shifting space of connections and simultaneity'.⁶¹ Ogborn's topography recalls the urban theorist Manuel Castells for whom the metropolis is not a place but a 'space of flows', constituted neither entirely by geographic nor political determinants, but manifesting in complex networks of information and cultural representation.⁶²

This is a notion of urban modernity informed by what succeeds it, including ideas about spontaneous metropolitan development as so energetically articulated by Jane Jacobs and then Richard Sennett, by postmodern architects like Bernard Tschumi, and by contemporary theorists of complex systems who use the city to explain chaos theory and emergence.⁶³ But this book is not a normative prescription for spontaneous metropolitan growth, rather a historical reminder of the dialectical co-development of the city as accidental as well as designed. As Elizabeth Wilson has cautioned, postmodern perspectives can implicitly rely on 'market-led initiatives', capable of reinforcing the asymmetrical urban development and global hierarchy spawned by the modern networked

---

⁶⁰ Ogborn, *Spaces of Modernity*, 6.   ⁶¹ Ogborn, *Spaces of Modernity*, 235.
⁶² Manuel Castells, *The Informational City: Information Technology, Economic Restructuring, and the Urban-Regional Process* (Oxford; Cambridge, MA: Blackwell, 1989). Though Castells links this metamorphosis to the late twentieth-century information economy, the Victorian metropolis was itself expanding its networks of communication and global influence enough to warrant consideration in the same terms.
⁶³ See Jane Jacobs, *The Death and Life of Great American Cities*. (New York: Random House, 1961); Richard Sennett, *The Uses of Disorder: Personal Identity & City Life* (New York: Knopf, 1970); Bernard Tschumi, *Architecture and Disjunction* (Cambridge, MA: MIT Press, 1994). In *Emergence*, Steven Johnson finds within the nineteenth-century city '[t]hat mix of order and anarchy [that] what we now call emergent behavior'. As Johnson knows, a varied nineteenth-century cohort or urban observers and writers make these ways of thinking possible. See *Emergence: The Connected Lives of Ants, Brains, Cities, and Software* (New York: Scribner, 2001), 38. Peter Ackroyd offers a contemporary and rhapsodic version: '[s]ometimes it even seems to me that the city itself creates the conditions of its own growth, that it somehow plays an active part in its own development like some complex organism slowly discovering its form'; see 'London Luminaries and Cockney Visionaries', in *The Collection* (London: Chatto & Windus, 2001), 342. Taking on the challenge of describing this 'somehow', one recent book in complex-systems theory uses chaos theory to model cities as self-organizing phenomena; see Peter M. Allen, *Cities and Regions as Self-Organizing Systems: Models of Complexity* (Amsterdam: Gordon and Breach, 1997).

metropolis. As a result, 'we are in danger of forgetting that the unplanned city still *is* planned'.[64] If the legacy of the Victorian metropolis includes hegemonic notions of modernity or emergent theories of postmodernity, then Victorian metropolitan writing can refocus the historical contours and contradictions in which their formative ideas were rooted.

THE ACCIDENTAL HERMENEUTIC

Just as accidents helped the Victorians interrogate a strange new metropolitan condition, they also exposed difficult questions about causality, about how and why things happen. A coincidental meeting, an omnibus or railway crash, a factory fire: the accident presents a 'hermeneutical challenge', requiring an interpretive effort to reason through or deduce its causation and significance.[65] It has not always done so. As argued in numerous studies of chance and histories of probability, accident and chance are subject to shifting frameworks of interpretation. Ross Hamilton's extensive *Accident: A Philosophical and Literary History* begins with Aristotle who defines the accidental as the mutable or inessential qualities in contrast with definite essence or substance.[66] As Michael Witmore argues, an early modern 'culture of accidents' brought new attention to their interpretation and to the potential uses of accidents in narrative and performance to encode significance. As late sixteenth-century theology came to theorize God's providential actions and empiricism elevated the value of the particular over the universal, the accident was increasingly perceived as disclosing hidden forms of meaning.[67] Theologies of divine providence remained among the dominant ways of interpreting accidents and framing them in narrative throughout the eighteenth century and into the nineteenth.[68] As more mathematical notions of probability developed in step, the interpretive possibilities of accidents expanded to include new understandings of agency and narrative which came to accept chance as a structuring condition.[69]

---

[64] Wilson, *The Sphinx in the City*, 151, 152.
[65] Brian Richardson, *Unlikely Stories: Causality and the Nature of Modern Narrative* (Newark, DE: University of Delaware Press, 1997), 13.
[66] Ross Hamilton, *Accident: A Philosophical and Literary History* (Chicago, IL: University of Chicago Press, 2007), 1.
[67] Michael Witmore, *Culture of Accidents: Unexpected Knowledges in Early Modern England* (Palo Alto, CA: Stanford University Press, 2001).
[68] See Thomas Vargish, *The Providential Aesthetic in Victorian Fiction* (Charlottesville, VA: University of Virginia Press, 1985); Levine, *Darwin and the Novelists*.
[69] Useful studies of the relations between probability and literature include: Sandra MacPherson, *Harm's Way: Tragic Responsibility and the Novel Form* (Baltimore, MD: Johns

The meaning of accident was likewise transitioning in the century and texts with which this book is preoccupied. For Levine, mid to late Victorian literature discards providence for a more relativistic worldview wherein 'the providential function of chance in narrative is transformed into meaningless accident'.[70] Levine does not mean to imply that accident is meaningless, but rather that it becomes unhinged from interpretive frameworks which had previously warranted its meaning. Or, from a different perspective, accident becomes available for as-yet unarticulated paradigms, such as the 'relativity imagination' which Christopher Herbert tracks to diverse Victorian contexts well before, as historians of science would have it, early twentieth-century physics unleashes chance from deterministic paradigms.[71] Anticipating and helping to produce the relativity imagination, nineteenth-century writers 'began to configure chance as a radical indeterminacy principle, and so, as far more than simply a name for human ignorance of divine intentions or operative laws'.[72] Victorian cultural production anticipates and complicates the paradigmatic changes in probability thinking by the century's end. *By Accident or Design* suggests that the Victorian city plays a crucial role in these changes.

Hopkins University Press, 2010); Douglas Lane Patey, *Probability and Literary Form: Philosophic Theory and Literary Practice in the Augustan Age* (Cambridge; New York: Cambridge University Press, 1984); Robert Newsom, *A Likely Story: Probability and Play in Fiction* (New Brunswick, NJ: Rutgers University Press, 1988); Kavanagh, *Enlightenment and the Shadows of Chance*; David F. Bell, *Circumstances: Chance in the Literary Text* (Lincoln, NE: University of Nebraska Press, 1993); J. Jeffrey Franklin, *Serious Play: The Cultural Form of the Nineteenth-Century Realist Novel* (Philadelphia, PA: University of Pennsylvania Press, 1999).

[70] Levine, *Darwin and the Novelists*, 207. For a related look at nineteenth-century American literature and its deep reckoning with chance, see Maurice S. Lee, *Uncertain Chances: Science, Skepticism, and Belief in Nineteenth-Century American Literature* (New York: Oxford University Press, 2012).

[71] Christopher Herbert, *Victorian Relativity: Radical Thought and Scientific Discovery* (Chicago, IL: University of Chicago Press, 2001). Herbert's perspective is a valuable corrective to a dated but persistent simplification that only with twentieth-century modernism can writers register the cultural impact of what science has revealed. For example, that is the unfortunate presumption of Stephen Kern: 'In the nineteenth-century novel, chance or coincidence was invariably a sign of some transcendent controlling destiny if not divine plan. In the modern novel, chance is more often evidence of life's fundamentally stochastic nature and the absence of any ultimate designing mind.' See *A Cultural History of Causality: Science, Murder Novels, and Systems of Thought* (Princeton, NJ: Princeton University Press, 2004), 11.

[72] Jason Puskar, *Accident Society: Fiction, Collectivity, and the Production of Chance* (Palo Alto, CA: Stanford University Press, 2012), 7. Puskar argues that American writers used that principle to produce a sense of causeless accidents, to exceed notions of contractual liberal individualism, and to enable new forms of collectivity. Leland Monk also considers the effects of chance as radical indeterminacy in literary contexts; see *Standard Deviations: Chance and the Modern British Novel* (Palo Alto, CA: Stanford University Press, 1993).

Hamilton rightly argues that 'to envision the changing interpretation of accident as a series of historical ruptures' is an oversimplification.[73] By sketching out such a series, I do not endorse a neat history of accident's changing interpretation, but emphasize that accident's interpretation is historical. According to Roger Cooter and Bill Luckin, accidents 'have not been seriously or substantially historicized'—and they ought to be, with due recognition of the complexities and limitations of doing so.[74] Hamilton is also sceptical of Foucauldian 'ruptures' and wants instead to appreciate the continuities of accident's metaphysics since Aristotle. But accident practically demands thinking about rupture: not necessarily ruptures of history, but the history of rupture and its interpretation. From this perspective, we might reconsider how Foucault uses accident in his influential notion of genealogy:

> to follow the complex course of descent is to maintain passing events in their proper dispersion; it is to identify the accidents, the minute deviations... that gave birth to those things that continue to exist and have value for us; it is to discover that truth or being do not lie at the root of what we know and what we are, but the exteriority of accidents.[75]

Foucault's notion of 'the exteriority of accidents' as opposed to 'truth or being' invokes Aristotle and inverts his philosophy, elevating the accidental above the essential and discarding teleological, evolutionary, or linear histories for the radical breaks and exceptions which constellate narratives of power. Interestingly, Foucault does so through a language of accidents, deviations, and dispersion. This book takes Foucault quite literally, seeking to 'identify the accidents' not merely as metaphorical breaks within historical or evolutionary narratives, but as phenomena that focus teleological narrative and radical divergence at a dialectical standstill—a 'double condition' at the level of theories of history.

This theoretical condition is what draws this study to the nineteenth century. Victorianism is the conflicting story of progress and deviation writ large, an age that alternately judges itself exceptional and historically contingent. Judith Green suggests that 'the accident is made possible at

---

[73] Hamilton, *Accident*, 2.

[74] Roger Cooter and Bill Luckin, eds, *Accidents in History: Injuries, Fatalities, and Social Relations* (Amsterdam; Atlanta, GA: Rodopi, 1997), 1. Cooter and Luckin note 'the paradox that compounds the difficulty of historicizing the accident—the fact that accidents may seem to be random and arbitrary, yet at the same time be expected or preordained'; *Accidents in History*, 3. This 'paradox' is precisely the 'double condition' that links the metropolis to the study of accidents.

[75] Michel Foucault, 'Nietzsche, Genealogy, History', in *Language, Counter-Memory, Practice*, ed. Bouchard, Donald F., trans. Donald F. Bouchard and Sherry Simon (Ithaca, NY: Cornell University Press, 1977), 146.

the interplay of beliefs in probability and determinism'.[76] If so, then the very epistemological instabilities characteristic of the nineteenth century— 'strapped across two systems, the teleological and the stochastic'—suggest the usefulness of accident as an interpretive and historical framework.[77] In *Cooking with Mud*, David Trotter takes a similar approach to his argument about 'mess' in the hands of artists and painters between 1860–1900: mess makes thinking about chance possible.[78] I hold that accidents likewise make thinking about design and chance possible, which ranks among the reasons why accidents were sources of such fascination (and messes) around the same time. According to Baucom, the actuarial thinking characteristic of both risk management and the historicist mind 'do not simply happen to emerge at the same historical moment but to some degree license, depend upon, and ensure one another'.[79] That linkage was hardened in the nineteenth century as accidents in contemporary understanding were transformed from private, fairly insignificant happenings to public, systemic concerns.[80] In Cooter's phrase, this was 'the moment of accident'.

So what *is* an accident? Hamilton holds to a trans-historical metaphysical definition deriving from Aristotle, whose notion of the accident is two-fold: as the non-essential, mutable quality of a given thing or idea, and as an accidental event.[81] It is the latter definition, according to Hamilton, which has predominated in theory and cultural studies, especially in the last hundred years. Hamilton wants to revive the word's double senses and reanimate accident as an ontological term, as something potentially constitutive of the being of things. Witmore also takes issue with accident as 'event'; he wants to 'cease to think of accidents in epistemological terms, as spontaneously contrived events that disclose hidden forms of order, and instead begin to understand them as occasions for storytelling and the expression of immanent forms of value'.[82] Taking a completely different approach, Green rejects metaphysical conceits to identify accidents, as we have come to know them, as the 'remnants of a modern classificatory system' of Enlightenment determinism. According to Green, 'An accident

---

[76] Judith Green, 'Accidents: The Remnants of a Modern Classificatory System', in *Accidents in History: Injuries, Fatalities, and Social Relations*, ed. Roger Cooter and Bill Luckin (Amsterdam; Atlanta, GA: Rodopi, 1997), 40.
[77] *Open Fields*, 276.
[78] David Trotter, *Cooking with Mud: The Idea of Mess in Nineteenth-Century Art and Fiction* (Oxford; New York: Oxford University Press, 2000), 10.
[79] Baucom, *Specters of the Atlantic*, 41.
[80] Roger Cooter, 'The Moment of the Accident: Culture, Militarism and Modernity in Late-Victorian Britain', in *Accidents in History: Injuries, Fatalities, and Social Relations*, ed. Roger Cooter and Bill Luckin (Amsterdam; Atlanta, GA: Rodopi, 1997), 109.
[81] Hamilton, *Accident*, 1–2.   [82] Witmore, *Culture of Accidents*, 10.

was an event for which there was no motivation, but which lay on a boundary between the need for a cause, as all [measurable events] must now be accounted for, and the lack of a "real" cause as defined by the new scientific principles of statistics'.[83] In other words, accidents became 'random' only to fill the gaps of a logical framework devised to account for causality. In Green's view, accidents are themselves historical accidents, by-products of rationalization whose apparent contingency has been exploited by a variety of rhetorical and theoretical frameworks.

Accident's problematic and contested definition is precisely the point: whether in the form of inessential qualities, chance coincidences, performances, material calamities, or epistemological bandages, accidents consistently cross a variety of cultural domains. As Witmore explains, 'what makes the accident a powerful focal point for cultural interest in this or any other historical period is the way in which it puts this plural sense of cultural value into play, allowing such value to be shifted, contested, or openly debated in either narrative or dialectical form'.[84] The moment of accident, to adapt Cooter's phrase, is the moment of interpretation. Put differently, accident is the interpretive moment of chance, contested in methodological collisions then as well as now. The interpretation of accident also concerns the credibility and authority to do so, and in the nineteenth century, varied cultural and professional domains were emerging to stake their claims. In this sense, accident opens a window onto several important discourse formations as well as the active interdisciplinary (or predisciplinary) efforts which so often characterize how Victorians creatively engaged the significant questions of their era.

By Accident or Design does not set out with strict definitions of its keywords, nor does it aim to settle their definitions by its conclusion. It neither attempts to be a history of urban-industrial accidents in the nineteenth century nor a philosophical history of accident. Instead, it historicizes specific forms and patterns of their usage to establish conceptual fields in which the Victorians grappled with the complexities of metropolitan space, mass phenomena, and probability. It selects a set of contexts where accidents focused people's attention on the metropolis, particularly for its dynamics of randomness and determinism, its curious evolution by accident and/or design. Accidents facilitate the imaginative breakthrough in reconceptualizing the metropolis as an

---

[83] Green, 'Accidents: The Remnants of a Modern Classificatory System', 49.

[84] *Culture of Accidents*, 14. Lee makes a similar argument about nineteenth-century American writers and their deep reckoning with chance, 'marked by contingency, approximation, fallibilism, pluralism, open-endedness, and the suspension of judgment' which proved 'the reach of probabilistic explanation [by] the looseness of its grasp'. See *Uncertain Chances*, 6.

emergent phenomenon. Thus, the metropolis provides underappreciated ground for some of the most innovative and interesting thinking about uncertainty in the Victorian age, manifesting not only in literary domains, but across a spectrum of disciplines, commercial pursuits, and material practices so concerned.

WRITING THE METROPOLIS

As Simon Parker suggests, the Victorians pioneered the notions that would become modern urban theory, but their methods were hardly methodologies, their disciplinary commitments rarely discrete.[85] As such, this book investigates 'metropolitan writing' as an intentionally broad category, open to the borrowings, coincidences, and conversations that occurred across many different discursive domains. In its apparent tumultuousness, the metropolis invited writers to join an interdisciplinary fray where probability and chance were being negotiated, including in such yet-to-consolidate fields as urban demography, actuarial statistics, industrial safety, civic improvements, and even natural history. The metropolis has always been successful at mixing intellectual pursuits as well as challenging its observers to articulate new forms of inquiry and representation. Victorian writers on the metropolis are practically interdisciplinary by default, though many of them realized specific opportunities to engage with the often-competing discourses by which the Victorians were coming to know the city. Victorian metropolitan writing—by which I take a generous measure of different generic forms from the literary sketch to the novel, from broadsheet ballads to journalism in illustrated periodicals—is thus integral in defining the cultural legacy of the Victorian metropolis as well as many of the intellectual revolutions it provoked.

This book qualifies metropolitan writing as both source material and evidence of metropolitan accidentalness at the levels of form and circulation. In other words, writing—particularly in so-called literary manifestations or genres predicated on notions of design—offers a uniquely reflexive context for thinking about intention and deviation, design and accident. Just as this book argues that accidents provided the Victorians a lexicon for complex and inchoate notions of probability, it also offers accidents as a vocabulary for talking about form and genre—how patterns of textual and literary communication arise, change, and function. The

---

[85] Parker, *Urban Theory and the Urban Experience*, 27–9.

'hermeneutical challenge' of accidents lends itself not only to philosophical questions but also to formal ones, particularly those arising in the 'new formalism' which Victorianist scholars have done much to promote. In an important article in *Victorian Studies*, Caroline Levine suggests that 'we need a vocabulary that conceptualizes contests and encounters among different forms of order', and recommends an encompassing 'strategic formalism' for the purpose.[86] While Levine joins a number of prominent Victorian neoformalists in this enterprise, she underscores why formal attentions might especially qualify for a study of accidents: literary forms, she argues, reveal the 'surprising, aleatory, and often confusingly disorderly ways' that social dialectics work.[87] *By Accident or Design* takes Levine's insight one step further: forms which are explicitly concerned with the accidental and the aleatory exhibit a fascinating self-awareness about their own making and cultural implications.

Accident invokes the narrative and dialectical structures by which cultural value is defined, giving rise to a hermeneutic well suited for considering literary, textual, and discursive forms. Does form result from premeditated design? Does it disclose a hidden order? Are forms incidental, even coincidental, occurring as an immanent instance of meaning or even by chance? Trotter claims that 'the hardest thing of all to think about is chance, which denies the very form and purpose of thought itself'.[88] But accidents are events which are simultaneously interpretive, providing the heuristic forms which make such difficult thinking possible. Thus, form is an interpretive strategy for Victorian writers to reckon with similar dynamics in the metropolis. Form is the creative perception of planning and aleatoric change that metropolitan accidents seem to express.

'It would be a highly interesting application of the mind to trace the discoveries made in science and the arts through ages and through accidents'. So quips the editor on a front-page article of the *Belfast News-Letter* in 1839 entitled 'Accident the Father of Improvement'.[89] This rumination is itself prompted by an accident: in this case, a train ran off its rails but continued travelling on an adjacent roadway without its passengers noticing—until it stopped. Though the article begins as a conventional accident report (the renewable fodder for so much newspaper journalism), it evolves into speculation about a grander theme: the 'improving' powers of accident. The article both cheers the ideology of Progress and ironically

---

[86] Caroline Levine, 'Strategic Formalism: Toward a New Method in Cultural Studies', *Victorian Studies* 48, no. 4 (Summer 2006): 630.
[87] Levine, 'Strategic Formalism', 626.   [88] Trotter, *Cooking with Mud*, 10.
[89] 'Accident the Father of Improvement', *Belfast News-Letter*, 19 February 1839. For a similar perspective in an American context, see Charles Collins, 'The Value of Accident', *The Atlantic Monthly*, February 1870.

undermines its sources, not necessarily attributable to ingenious inventors or to Providence. Instead, '[t]he most stupendous discoveries in science, in arts, in navigation, and commerce, have been made by accidents'. In capsule form, the *Belfast News-Letter* article suggests the ubiquity of accidents, their circulation in Victorian print media, and the questions they prompted about how things develop and change, particularly those things—like the discovery of steam, manufacturing, and transport—which profoundly changed the dimensions of urban-industrial experience.

By Accident or Design looks to the fascination, ambivalence, and even opportunism that metropolitan accidents provoked. Unlike the *Belfast News-Letter*, its goal is not a revisionist history of industry, but an alternative genealogy of the modern metropolis and some of the major forms of Victorian writing about it. The readings to follow of Dickens, Gaskell, Oliphant, Collins, Trollope, and Eliot, as well as various journalists, commercial agents, anonymous street balladeers, artists, and engravers, suggest that, through metropolitan accident, the Victorians reimagined the formative possibilities of chance. This book explores several contexts for where and why this happened, paying close attention to the particular historical and discursive contexts in which ideas about chance, accident, and risk were taking (and sometimes losing) shape. The chapters each concentrate on a conspicuous domain of metropolitan accidents, including: traffic, industrial catastrophes, the railway, building construction, and the chance vagaries of urban experience. In each, I suggest how Victorian metropolitan writing engages and often competes with other discourses emerging to compensate for accidents, manage chance and risk, and organize metropolitan knowledge to accommodate its singularities. These contexts inform the development of some of the signature forms, genres, and patterns of transmission in metropolitan writing, which assimilate the accidental into their own imaginative horizons and textuality.

THE CHAPTERS OF ACCIDENT

I begin, in Chapter 1, with a survey of the rising tide of accidents which, thanks to the increasing popularity and distribution of the newspaper, were so frequently in the public eye. Nineteenth-century newspapers offer useful documentation about accidents and the changing ways they were perceived. More interestingly, they show how accident reporting significantly reshapes the formats, distribution patterns, and cultural functions of newsprint. Thus, this chapter sets the interpretive agenda this book pursues throughout: a recursive argument for accident and the writing it fascinates and transforms. If the nineteenth century was the age of newspapers, as John Stuart Mill once said, then accidents can go a long way toward defining the newspaper's epochal success and distinctiveness as a form of communication. I argue that a kindred set of underappreciated newspaper contents—accident columns, coroners' inquests, and miscellaneous or extraordinary news—reveals how the newspaper cultivates and circulates sometimes aberrant notions of causality. As the newspaper insinuates itself into the daily lives of Victorian readers of all kinds, so too does its generic accidentalness become integrated into a sense of the metropolitan everyday. Ultimately, the newspaper fashions itself into a periodical encounter with uncertainty, part of a broader cultural inquiry into causality manifesting in the contents, formatting, and reading experience of metropolitan news.

Chapter 2 zooms in on an early example of such reporting to consider the chaotic influx of horse-drawn omnibuses and cabs to London in the 1830s. Having newly unseated the hackney coach monopoly, these vehicles caused all manner of accidents in their competitive scramble, drawing the attention of journalists including the aspiring Charles Dickens in his guise of 'Boz'. I argue that such accidents are crucial to understanding the sketch genre Boz pioneers, as well as the imaginative legacy of London that Dickens would bequeath. These early sketches (later edited and collected as *Sketches by Boz*) inaugurate Dickens's reputation as an imaginative pedestrian, but they also establish what Ana Parejo Vadillo has called a 'Victorian aesthetics of transport in the development of a new urban epistemology'.[90] Hardly just a *flâneur*, Boz is better understood in the context of commercial transportation, competing for the primary vehicle (generic, metaphorical, or wheeled) in which to pursue 'the knowledge of London', as the taxi licensing examination was soon to become known. At a time when discursive practices of 'knowing' London were largely in flux, Boz harnesses the sketch for its generic sympathies with an almost chaotic system of transport. Against the statistical and proto-sociological epistemologies emerging in his day, Boz pioneers an urban knowledge that is insistently accidental, linked to the instabilities which urban transport materially embodies and thematically reveals.

Expanding the book's metropolitan horizon to England's northern industrial cities, Chapter 3 explores a crisis in accidents on the rise in the 1840s: urban-industrial disasters and fires in particular. They preoccupied a range of observers who comprise a nascent field of risk management,

---

[90] Ana Parejo Vadillo, *Women Poets and Urban Aestheticism: Passengers of Modernity* (Basingstoke, Hampshire; New York: Palgrave Macmillan, 2005), 25.

including the struggling fire insurance industry and novelists like Elizabeth Gaskell, whose 1848 novel *Mary Barton: A Tale of Manchester Life* tries to define accidents, liability, and compensation on its own terms. Industrial accidents sparked a contest on this unsettled field, as insurers and novelists each adapted the other's strategies for their own under/writing of risk. I demonstrate how changing concepts of accident characterize the unstable political landscape of the industrial north, measure the increasingly material pressures on property and life, and inform practices of writing, especially those that novelists shared with the insurance industry. The salient contingencies of the Victorian novel may derive from such historical circumstances in which writers like Gaskell absorb accidents as a practice of the genre.

Accidents were favourite subjects for the enterprising publishers of broadsides and ballads—ephemeral publications that were often sung and sold on the streets themselves. Such street literature, as discussed in Chapter 4, was part of a surge of cheap, popular literature or 'reading for the million' as it was variously called by middle-class writers who sneered at the seeming randomness of its production, contents, and circulation. Wilkie Collins, Margaret Oliphant, E. S. Dallas, and Bennett Johns all imagine cheap literature as so many species of strangely fecund and chaotic forms—a perception which ironically authorizes their 'random selection' of the same materials to read. Their reviews also reveal an anxiety about the ungovernable change of Victorian print culture into a mass media, particularly as the literary economy seems transformed by chance. But randomness expresses an important feature of Victorian print media at mid-century: how it becomes a chaotic system organized by the contingencies of modern urban life. The remediation of accident—from an event to an ephemeral print form marked as 'random'—reveals how Victorian popular print became the 'new media' of its moment, an accidental media with surprising relevance to new media today.

In the decades between 1840 and 1870, nothing symbolized accidents as strongly as the railway. Just as significantly, the railway seemed an engine of metropolitan transformation, turning the country into one immense city. These reputations are linked. Chapter 5 suggests that railway accidents became an important site of representation for the Victorians to explore the signature conceptual distortions of the metropolis. Indeed, journalistic reports and Victorian fiction overrepresent railway accidents in relation to their historical occurrence. But railway accidents were overreported because of their conceptual utility in trying to understand—and paradoxically recover—what had been erased by the 'machine ensemble', in Wolfgang Schivelbusch's phrase. If many writers, including William Aytoun and George Eliot, blame the railway for erasing the local or destroying perception and the possibilities for narrative, then railway accidents tell a different story. Their representations instead creatively recover what the railway seemed to annihilate, including notions of space, time, place, and the contingent network of interconnection that patterns the mundane. Dickens and Trollope, in their evolving relationship to the railway over its most tumultuous decades, reveal how accidents facilitate an awareness of stochastic complexity to complement the realist project of mid-Victorian fiction.

Much of early to mid-Victorian print culture traffics in accidents: as a characteristic of its production and distribution; as subject matter responding explicitly to phenomenal events; and as aspects of the chaos which people imagined to be a vital aspect of urban change. *By Accident or Design* points to writers who were fascinated with change in modernizing cities, particularly as they simultaneously invited and defied new attempts to design urban spaces and exchanges. Early to mid-Victorian metropolitan writing does more than catalogue the city's 'tremendous chapter of accidents'. It comes, in a variety of senses, to embody those chapters, to accept the uncertainties of it subjects into textual structures which disclose their lack of predictive or managerial control. These works are stitched with the interpretive possibilities of chance, a pattern simultaneously perceived within and imposed upon the metropolis. If C. S. Peirce declared a 'universe of chance' at the end of the century,[91] the modernizing Victorian city was its micro-cosmos, stretched by the gravities of chance's contested interpretations and constellated with texts in swerving orbits. But all was not random. By tracing representations of accidents, we can see how Victorians figured the phenomenal, epistemological, and ethical significance of chance alongside concepts of design, agency, and responsibility. Accidents offered the Victorians access to the dialectics of chance and purpose, chaos and order, through which to reconfigure literary forms and grasp their urgent work of knowing.

He could not think of anything further that could be done; so ... he went out into the street; and there he stood still, to ponder over probabilities and chances.

(Gaskell, *Mary Barton*)

---

[91] Porter, *The Rise of Statistical Thinking*, 150.

1
Accidents in the News

> A newspaper without an account of one or more accidents... is scarcely ever taken up.
>
> *Chambers's Edinburgh Journal*, 1854[1]

As England's great towns swelled in size and complexity, so grew a general sense of their capacities for the unpredictable. The metropolis seemed a tremendous chapter of coincidences, crimes, collisions, and catastrophes, but that did not simply reflect the everyday experiences of its inhabitants. Rather, it indexed the Victorians' expanding print culture which took the metropolitan everyday as its subject and materially circulated in the everyday transactions of its readers. The history of the Victorian metropolis is inextricable from the confederation of diverse textual practices by which it was represented and consumed. Its reputation as a tremendous chapter of accidents is consolidated by metropolitan writing—like the literary sketch, the novel, the broadside ballad—which exposes and embodies the phenomenal status of an urban entity between accident and design. Most people would only have encountered major accidents through such textual manifestations. In the nineteenth century, the chapter of accidents par excellence was the newspaper.

'Cab Accident'. A reader of *The Times* of 25 May 1843 would find this simple title atop a short column of news of fascinating and fearful accidents. The first paragraph reports on a coroner's inquest on the body of a woman killed when her cab flipped sideways after a wheel flew off. The driver was apparently sober and driving moderately, but fled the scene. In the next paragraph about a 'Fatal Accident', a cistern explodes in a Woolwich dockyard. In 'Wonderful Escape', four drunken men ride along in a cattle wagon when one falls overboard, getting perilously caught in ropes above the wagon's rail. His companions fail to notice; a passer-by stops the cart. 'How to Prevent Accidents on Railways' offers sarcastic advice about

---

[1] 'Insurance Against Accidents of All Kinds', *Chambers's Edinburgh Journal*, 19 April 1854, 254.

running a bad business: with fewer customers, fewer accidents. Such assorted news items came in packs. 'Destructive Fires in the Metropolis' heads a series of reports in the *Bristol Mercury* on 26 August 1843. Many of them report on coroners' inquests. Another details fire damage to St Olave's church, while another paragraph highlights the wedding which took place, to the delight of an onlooking crowd, during the fire in St Olave's church. The singularity of these events is belied only by the continual appearance of such news in these papers and others throughout the century.

Accidents were increasingly in the news and in newspapers. I make that distinction to plot two concurrent and converging trajectories: the increasing conspicuousness of accidents and the rise of the modern newspaper. While news of wonder and miscellaneous events were acknowledged aspects of newspapers over the long eighteenth century, historians have marginalized accident news in favour of other narratives about the newspaper's development, more concerned with its changing business operations, its emergent generic features, or its historical continuity or distinctiveness. But part of what distinguishes the Victorian 'age of newspapers' is its reliance upon the content sketched above.[2] The newspaper rose to its epochal prominence in large part by accident—which is to say by its increasing dependence upon such news in a great variety of forms, including accident reports, coroners' inquests, 'accidents and occurrences' columns, and the *faits divers* of miscellaneous news items. Those contents surged during the nineteenth century. Moreover, they conveyed to the newspaper a similar causal flexibility that characterized its representations of the accidental metropolis. In general, accidents provided for the up-to-the-minute novelty, spectacle, and dramatic interest that earned newspapers the attention of so many readers. In formal terms, they also supplied content which newspapers could readily manipulate into paragraphs, recurring columns, and illustrated formats, providing the necessary recurring structures of a genre which also insisted on its periodical newness. The nineteenth-century newspaper press contributed to the impression of increased accidents of all kinds. In turn, such accidents reshaped the newspaper as well as the heuristic reflexes of those readers into whose daily lives the newspaper would so thoroughly diffuse.

Matthew Rubery has claimed that 'the transformation of news during the nineteenth century profoundly influenced literary narrative in ways that have yet to be recognized'.[3] This chapter will also propose such narrative influences, but the transformation of news tells more stories

---

[2] John Stuart Mill, *On Liberty and Other Essays*, ed. John Gray (Oxford; New York: Oxford University Press, 1991), 101.

[3] Matthew Rubery, *The Novelty of Newspapers: Victorian Fiction After the Invention of the News* (Oxford; New York: Oxford University Press, 2009), 4.

than about the novel, particularly about changing attitudes to the metropolis and causality. In the sections to follow, I spotlight three genres of news writing—accidents/offences news, inquest reports, and the miscellany of *faits divers*—which have been largely overlooked by cultural histories of newspapers and journalism. By grouping these categories into 'accident news', I am not suggesting they entirely report accidents (though they largely do), but that they express the unsettled causalities which the term accident was coming to embody. Dallas Liddle has called for scholars to expand 'our knowledge of the historical discourse genres published *in* periodicals—the forms taken by articles themselves'.[4] This chapter recovers subgenres of accident news and their conspicuous patterns of circulation to reveal how newspapers participate in and potentially steer a broader cultural inquiry into causation.

While the Victorian newspaper offers an extensive textual archive for the accidents of its technologizing age, it also represents their material expression within periodical print culture. Hilary Jewett has argued that 'the accident scene becomes a particularly self-referential site of knowledge production'.[5] In a similar sense, the newspaper becomes a self-referential scene of accident for metropolitan writing. The patterns and styles of accident coverage within the newspaper press show transformations in what 'accident' even signifies. They reveal some of the primary cultural domains in which that definition was negotiated. And they suggest the prominence of the newspaper as a source and competitive genre for other forms of writing so concerned. Accident news brings into focus how the Victorian newspaper—even considering its various metropolitan, local, and periodical kinds—fashioned itself into a periodical encounter with uncertainty. Accident news, whether comic or sad, invited newspaper readers into 'serious considerations' about agency, causality, and institutional responses to calamities. Those considerations were significantly shaped by the emerging generic and circulatory patterns of newspapers with lasting effects upon notions of the accidental metropolis they engendered.

NEW CHAPTERS OF ACCIDENT

One important qualification to begin with: 'newspaper' compresses some notably different enterprises, such as the metropolitan daily, the evening

---

[4] Dallas Liddle, *The Dynamics of Genre: Journalism and the Practice of Literature in Mid-Victorian Britain* (Charlottesville, VA: University of Virginia Press, 2009), 155.
[5] Hilary Jewett, 'The Scene of the Accident in the Nineteenth Century' (Ph.D. Dissertation, Yale University, 1996), 56.

news sheet, the Sunday paper, the illustrated weekly, the advertiser, and so forth—all of which evolved over time or even between editorships. The term also collapses geographic distinctions, political affiliations, and the particular differences and concerns of the metropolitan, regional, and local press. Margaret Beetham suggests that any periodical is an 'open form' with fluid boundaries, a generic and temporal amoeba which is difficult to delimit.[6] And yet, as Aled Jones claims, for the Victorians 'the newspaper was a separate and distinct form of printed text... explained primarily in terms of its economy, the regularity of its production and the fragmentary nature of its content'.[7] Accident news offers another way of understanding the Victorian newspaper's 'distinctive identity as a form of communication',[8] because, as I will show, accident as a concept, news classification, and information commodity tends to float across the distinctions that are otherwise important to observe. Furthermore, accident news has particular patterns of usage and circulation only revealed by examining newspapers in the aggregate. Of course, the very notion of an aggregate is problematic, as the archive is incomplete and overlooks how even its elementary units may not be stable entities.[9] Notwithstanding these limitations, the mass of available media still suggest meaningful patterns about accidents and the generic entity of the newspaper they helped to construct.

In the most basic sense, accidents were news because they were new. While accidents appeared in the miscellanies of eighteenth-century papers, they became an ever more conspicuous feature of nineteenth-century newspapers in part because there were simply more accidents to report, particularly in the terms by which accidents were increasingly defined. The density of urban living, the rapid pace of construction, the influx of new forms of horse-drawn urban transport into the streets, railways, expanding shipping commerce, steam-powered factories and gasworks, industrialized labour, and the lagging oversight in almost every case all contributed to the prominence of Victorian accidents. Sociologist Roger Lane suggests that very little has been written about the history or sociology of such accidents even though they are potentially measurable

---

[6] Margaret Beetham, 'Towards a Theory of the Periodical as a Publishing Genre', in *Investigating Victorian Journalism*, ed. Laurel Brake and Aled Jones (New York: St. Martin's Press, 1990), 29.

[7] Aled Jones, *Powers of the Press: Newspapers, Power and the Public in Nineteenth-Century England* (Aldershot, Hampshire: Ashgate, 1996), 3.

[8] Jones, *Powers of the Press*, 3.

[9] For example, as Laurel Brake has shown, individual issues of newspapers can vary widely depending on time and place of publication, and chronology may not even be the best index of a newspaper's use. Laurel Brake, 'The Longevity of "Ephemera": Library Editions of Victorian Periodicals and Newspapers' (presented at the North American Victorian Studies Association, Yale University, 2008).

and useful as indices to social and especially industrial change.[10] How to measure them is a problem, as accidents hardly exist outside the discourses which define and account for them. Roger Cooter complains of accident reports that 'even if the categories could be segregated and standardized, and the statistics regarded as "accurate" there would be little point, since the meaning of an "accident" itself has no stability... accident statistics must be treated as subjective attempts at the construction of evidence'.[11] With this as a proviso, Cooter still gives counting a try. He observes in the London *Times*, 'the number of reports of accidents of all kinds rose from an average of 300 per annum (from the 1830s) to well over 500 (after 1870)'.[12] Cooter's numbers draw his attention to the latter part of the century as 'the moment of accident', a conclusion seemingly supported by a keyword search for 'accident' across two major databases of nineteenth-century British newspapers. Over 90 per cent of results in *19th Century British Library Newspapers* and *British Newspapers 1800–1900* occur after 1850. But by looking to net results instead of gross, the numbers tell a different story. The percentage of accident results relative to all other content rises substantially through the 1860s and then drops off. The charts in Figure 1 track date-limited searches for 'accident*' (the asterisk functioning as a search wildcard) as a relative measurement of all other indexed newspaper items in each database.[13]

If newspapers were merely historical data, it would seem that accidents were more prevalent during the mid-nineteenth century than ever before. Swelling between the 1830s and 1890s, the curve of 'accident' appears compellingly proportional with the Victorian era itself—which is one of the major arguments of this book. But such quantitative exercises risk some serious tautologies: industrialization increased in real numbers accidents, machines to cause them, and newspaper pages on which to print reports of them. It overlooks all the particular conditions of the query and the source database, including what newspapers (and what issues of those papers) are included, the fidelity of its optical character recognition, the

---

[10] Roger Lane, *Violent Death in the City: Suicide, Accident, and Murder in Nineteenth-Century Philadelphia* (Cambridge, MA: Harvard University Press, 1979), 35.
[11] Roger Cooter, 'The Moment of the Accident: Culture, Militarism and Modernity in Late-Victorian Britain', in *Accidents in History: Injuries, Fatalities, and Social Relations*, ed. Roger Cooter and Bill Luckin (Amsterdam; Atlanta, GA: Rodopi, 1997), 111.
[12] Cooter, 'The Moment of the Accident', 108.
[13] These queries were run a year apart through different entry points to the database. The first tests used the 'keyword' search function on '19th Century British Library Newspapers', *Gale Cengage Learning*, 2007, <http://infotrac.galegroup.com/itweb/viva_uva?db=BNCN>. That search option was not available for the subsequent queries, which used 'document title' to search 'British Newspapers 1800–1900', *British Library*, 2009, <http://newspapers11.bl.uk/blcs/>.

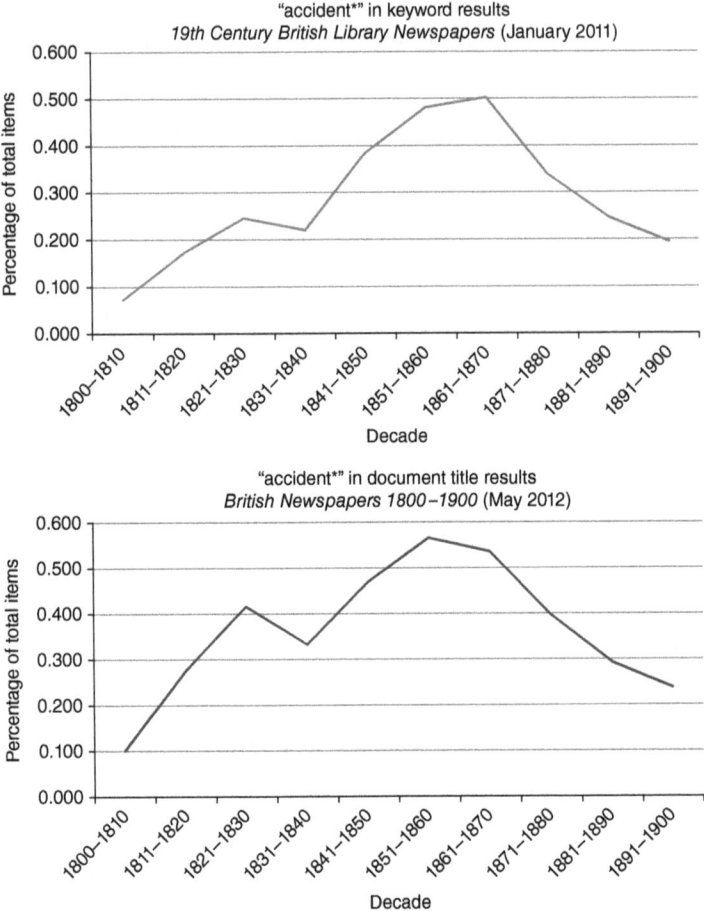

Fig. 1. 'Accident' in two databases of nineteenth-century British newspapers

integrity of its metadata, the output of its search results, and so on. This 'data' also overlooks how periodical sources can vary even at the level of the single issue, and more generally how newspapers are evolving cultural forms.[14] Finally, quantitative methods for studying accidents already presume they are entities which can be counted, which is the legacy, not

---

[14] For a rich discussion of the problems and possibilities of accessing digitized newspapers, see James Mussell, *The Nineteenth-Century Press in the Digital Age* (New York: Palgrave Macmillan, 2012). Joel Wiener goes so far as to say, 'I am *almost* prepared to conclude that newspapers are too speculative, too problematic, to be used as sources at all'; see 'Sources for the Study of Newspapers', in *Investigating Victorian Journalism*, ed. Laurel Brake and Aled Jones (New York: St. Martin's Press, 1990), 155.

accidentally, of the rise of statistics in the nineteenth century. A countable accident has already been modernized.

The curve makes more sense as an interpretive visualization, suggestively tracing an attention to accidents that parallels their unstable evidentiary status across the century. It registers a historical pulse and sends us to investigate. What did an accident even signify? In its own construction of accidents, the newspaper was responding to sea changes in attitudes about accidents and the 'the field of discourses' which conceptually produced them, including probability and risk.[15] During these shifts, accidents were unhinged from the cosmological frameworks that had either dismissed them as inessential or warranted their significance in terms of fate or providence. Instead of 'expressing hidden meanings of nature or ineffable intentions of the Deity', accidents were increasingly perceived as constitutive aspects of human design.[16] George Landow finds this in representations of shipwrecks: by the late-eighteenth century such accidents became dissociated with their religious significance: 'a transition from a Christian to a post-Christian framework of interpretation marked by the attribution of responsibility to external forces rather than to the fallen individual'.[17] Wolfgang Schivelbusch locates this transition in the nineteenth century with the emergence of the 'technological accident'. In contrast to the 'preindustrial' accident caused by external forces (such as natural disasters), 'after the industrial revolution, destruction by technological accident comes from the inside. The technical apparatuses destroy themselves by means of their own power'.[18] For Schivelbusch, industrial accidents come to embody modernity's dialectics of progress and destruction, taking the measure of the growing gap between those poles. Furthermore, the technological accident raises questions about its own production: is it too a human invention? Is it built into its systems? The history of Schivelbusch's primary example, the railway accident, shows a consistent relation between accidents and resulting safety measures to prevent, expunge, or minimize them. In other contexts too, accidents impelled 'a clear and legitimate relation between sensation, exposure, and

---

[15] Judith Green, *Risk and Misfortune: A Social Construction of Accidents* (London; Bristol, PA: University College of London Press, 1997), 203.
[16] Anthony Giddens, *The Consequences of Modernity* (Palo Alto, CA: Stanford University Press, 1990), 30–1.
[17] See Rubery, *The Novelty of Newspapers*, 29; George P. Landow, *Images of Crisis: Literary Iconology, 1750 to the Present* (Boston, MA: Routledge & Kegan Paul, 1982), 17.
[18] Wolfgang Schivelbusch, *The Railway Journey: The Industrialization of Time and Space in the 19th Century* (Berkeley, CA: University of California Press, 1986), 133.

reform'.[19] But just as accidents spur the search for a specific cause, they also highlight the ineradicable instabilities within human design.

From this perspective, the curve spikes not because 'technological accidents' proliferate, but because of the proliferating discursive approaches to understanding them. A 'technological' interpretation is merely one among many overlapping views at the time. The seeming uncertainty of accident allowed for some curiously hybrid attempts to rationalize it. For example, in 1848, the Reverend Fountain Elwin published a sermon, 'Personal Danger, and Providential Deliverance', following his escape from a serious accident on the Great Western Railway. Though the sermon draws from providential theology, it also tellingly accepts accidents as a constitutive feature of industrial materiality. Elwin reads the accident as a sign of the perpetual instability of earthly bodies, a systemic condition not unlike the technological accident itself. Elwin also describes the afterlife in terms of 'assurance' and the 'property' of which 'we are not yet in possession'.[20] His lesson about providence shades into the language of insurance, part of a regime including statistics, risk management, and liability law which moved the interpretation of accidents into more secular realms.

These fields encouraged actuarial notions of what was typical and expected, offering a way of understanding seemingly extraordinary or aberrant events within a framework of their periodic recurrence. Chapter 3 considers the functions of insurance in more detail, though they also suggest why newspapers seized on the reporting of such accidents to consolidate their own generic identity. Although accident reports do feature in newspapers before the nineteenth century, they flourish with the abstraction, secularization, and critical distance that new notions of risk or the technologized accident make possible. Accident can only become a spectacle with the abatement of traditional forms of moral judgment, 'a prerequisite for the public's fascination with catastrophe'.[21] Like the emerging business of risk management, newspapers seized the opportunity to represent and interpret such accidents. Scholars have argued that newspapers came to express a secularized religion, a mythology, and an imagined community—all of which displace providential

---

[19] Ian A. Burney, *Bodies of Evidence: Medicine and the Politics of the English Inquest, 1830–1926* (Baltimore, MD: Johns Hopkins University Press, 2000), 47.

[20] Rev. Fountain Elwin, *Personal Danger, and Providential Deliverance. A Sermon Preached at the Octagon Chapel, Bath, on the Occasion of a Fatal Accident Which Happened to the Express Train, on the Great Western Railway, May 10, 1848* (London: J. Hatchard and Son, 1848), 4, 5.

[21] Rubery, *The Novelty of Newspapers*, 29; John Fowles, *Shipwreck* (London: Cape, 1974), 9.

outlooks while still maintaining a collective interpretive structure which could accommodate events like accidents.²² As the technological accident draws attention to the system which produced it, so the Victorian newspaper can be similarly characterized by its increasing reliance upon and production of accident news.

We can see all this in the evolving attention to accidents in nineteenth-century British newspapers. For example, scanning the thousands of articles with 'accident' in the title in the *19th Century British Library Newspapers* database, a conspicuous pattern emerges that seems to support (and expand) Schivelbusch's claims. A philosophical and providential understanding of accident gets replaced by industrial, technological, commercial, and also professional contexts for interpreting them. During the first half of the century, the majority of headlines use a simple, regular construction:

- Shocking Accident
- Dreadful Accident at Liverpool
- Afflicting Accident
- Melancholy Accident
- Distressing Accident
- Fatal Accident at Lochend

The '[Adjective] Accident' headline might suggest the early fascination with accidents as such, registering the shock of their mere occurrence. These headlines seem impressionistic, closer to the eighteenth-century cosmologies which had underwritten the affective or moral meaning of such events, as if the accident was something not only to report but to wonder at, to interpret.²³ Especially when compared with accident

---

²² C. John Sommerville, *The News Revolution in England: Cultural Dynamics of Daily Information* (New York: Oxford University Press, 1996), 10; James W. Carey, *Communication as Culture: Essays on Media and Society* (Boston, MA: Unwin Hyman, 1989); Benedict R. Anderson, *Imagined Communities: Reflections on the Origin and Spread of Nationalism* (London: Verso, 1983).
²³ Bob Clarke claims that such headlines are 'melodramatic' and 'mirrored the new taste for melodrama in the popular theatre'; see *From Grub Street to Fleet Street: An Illustrated History of English Newspapers to 1899* (Aldershot, Hampshire; Burlington: Ashgate, 2004), 244. But he consigns such headlines to the new Sunday papers, implying a class preference for lower forms of news and popular entertainment. The consistency of such headlines in *The Times* (and elsewhere) suggests otherwise. Furthermore, 'melodrama' may not be the most useful interpretive category. Consider Clarke's own examples, 'taken at random' from a 2 December 1838 issue of *Bell's Life*: The Late Brutal Murder at Preston, Drunkenness and Determined Suicide, Dreadful Accident on the Liverpool and Manchester Railway, Shocking Coach Accident. They suggest a pattern that, while potentially present in melodrama, makes more sense in terms of the dynamics of motive/chance, design/accident, that so conspicuously textured Victorian newspapers of all kinds.

headlines from the 1860s and 70s—the decades when, by the numbers, accidents were most prominently in the news—which consistently emphasize their circumstances and frequently specify a vehicular or industrial context:

- Fatal Omnibus Accident
- Railway Accident
- The Fatal Boat Accident at...
- Disastrous Steamboat Accident
- Railway Accidents [stand-alone newspaper section]

The affecting adjective gets retrained on these vehicles to the point where omnibuses, railways, steamboats all seem like accidents waiting to happen.[24] From its earlier condition of free-floating wonderment, accident becomes systematized, accepted as a structuring feature of mechanisms. The affective distress of accidents moves into the material of industrial and transport technologies.

By the mid-nineteenth century, accident opens a new chapter of signification. In parallel with the technologizing of the accident, we can also track its loosening associations with cosmological meanings including Christian providence and a general sense of fate or destiny. Consider the phrase 'chapter of accidents' itself. Brewer's *Dictionary of Phrase and Fable* defines it as 'metaphorically, the sequence of unforeseen events'.[25] The *Oxford English Dictionary* suggests 'the unforeseen course of events' and 'the chapter of possibilities'.[26] Those meanings are entirely consistent with usages in the eighteenth century, such as:

- 'But, O Providence, how unscrutable are thy ways! how fertile in surprizes is thy chapter of accidents here!' (John Cleland, *The Romance of Day*. London, 1760.)
- 'he received him with more signs of affection than civility, bidding him not to be cast down, but trust to the chapter of accidents, as he

---

[24] In Patrick Studer's terminology, the headlines shift from thematic to performative, from general announcements to speech acts more concerned with details. See 'Textual Structures in Eighteenth-Century Newspapers: A Corpus-Based Study of Headlines', *Journal of Historical Pragmatics* 4, no. 1 (2003): 32–5.

[25] Ebenezer Cobham Brewer, 'Chapter of Accidents (A)', *Dictionary of Phrase and Fable* (Philadelphia, PA: Henry Altemus Company, 1898), <http://www.bartleby.com/81/3380.html>.

[26] 'The Chapter of Accidents', *Oxford English Dictionary* (Oxford University Press, 1989), <http://www.oed.com/view/Entry/30613?rskey=s3HOXw&result=2&isAdvanced=false#eid216078486>.

had always done.' (*Cleanthes and Samantha. A Dramatic History.* London, 1764.)
- 'let us trust to time and the chapter of accidents; or rather to that Providence which will not fail' (Tobias Smollett, *The Expedition of Humphry Clinker.* London, 1771.)
- *The Chapter of Accidents: A Comedy in Five Acts* (Sophia Lee. London, 1780.)
- 'Never of any importance, the chapter of accidents alone could have elevated it to the rank of being represented in the House of Commons.' (John Robert Scott, *Parliamentary Representation.* Dublin, 1790.)
- 'Nonconformists has [sic] always been dispersed all over the empire, and had trusted for liberty to the chapter of accidents.' (Robert Robinson, *Ecclesiastical Researches.* Cambridge, 1792.)

As a definition, the 'unforeseen course of events' already deracinates the phrase of its cosmological associations. But 'chapter of accidents' means more, having abundant and sometimes contradictory relations with providence, fate, and meaningless chance. Tracking the phrase through the nineteenth century, those meanings do not disappear; the 'chapter of accidents' continues to be used in similar ways. What changes is the consistency of its relations to providence and fate. For instance, by the late nineteenth-century it becomes nearly a journalistic cliché in reports of horse races.[27] Some race horses were even named 'Chapter of Accidents'—a seemingly unfortunate moniker, but certainly truth in advertising about games of chance. More typically, the phrase described strange race outcomes or the collisions or falls of horses and riders (especially in steeplechases). While this is a small and specific example, it captures two larger semantic turns underway: the distancing of 'chapter of accidents' from providence or fate, and its usage for material collisions or calamities.

While never shedding its metaphorical usages, 'chapter of accidents' in the nineteenth century takes on conspicuous reference to catastrophes and series of calamitous events.[28] This lexical shift parallels how accidents

---

[27] As Lucy Brown points out, the 'general scale of sports reporting grew substantially in the last thirty years of the nineteenth century.' See *Victorian News and Newspapers* (Oxford; New York: Oxford University Press, 1985), 244.

[28] In 1911, *The Century Dictionary and Cyclopedia* adds to the definition, 'A series of mishaps; a succession of mischances', but its examples do not depart from the metaphorical. See William Dwight Whitney and Benjamin Eli Smith, 'Chapter, N.', *The Century Dictionary and Cyclopedia* (New York: The Century Co., 1911), 925, <http://books.google.com/books?id=ownpAAAAMAAJ>.

themselves were newly defined as material and technological actualities, as Schivelbusch suggests. Examples run the gamut of nineteenth-century print culture, such as in juvenile and didactic fiction (*The First (Second and Third) Chapter of Accidents and Remarkable Events, Containing Caution and Instruction for Children* (1801)), farcical plays, comic songs ('The Chapter of Accidents' (1819–44?), to be discussed in Chapter 4), and books of domestic utility (*A Chapter of Accidents; or, the Mother's Assistant in Cases of Burns, Scalds, Cuts, etc.* (1860)). But the most significant engine of this lexical transformation was the periodical press, particularly the newspaper. There, the 'chapter of accidents' became legible as part of its very form.

In 1851, *Chambers's Edinburgh Journal* uses the phrase to describe both the vagaries of fate and the Victorian newspaper: 'The chapter of accidents is a chequered page—sometimes comic passages—more often scenes of sadness, inviting the most serious considerations. A newspaper without an account of one or more accidents of the latter kind is scarcely ever taken up.'[29] Not only does the article suggest the ubiquity of accident news in the press, it hints at how pages of newsprint are 'chequered' or marked by 'chapters of accident'. That marking could be quite literal, such as by headlines:

- 'A Chapter of Accidents'—a passenger's account of a railway accident (*The Times*, 5 November 1845, 8).
- 'A Chapter of Accidents'—'There have been several remarkable accidents of late; not only from the rail whence we get such an unfailing supply, but from fire' (*The Leader*, 7 January 1854, 9).
- 'A Catalogue of Accidents'—the strange history of an accident-prone family, inaugurated by a fatal railway accident (*Illustrated London News*, 29 August 1857, 226).
- 'A Chapter of Accidents. Narrow Escape'—another account of a railway accident (*The Times*, 1 October 1868, 9).
- 'A Chapter of Accidents'—involving a horse and cab (*Ipswich Journal*, 29 September 1883).

As newspapers increasingly became attuned to accident news, they seized upon the prevailing 'chapter' or 'catalogue' metaphor to organize the abundance of their reports. Such usages do not eclipse how the phrase continued to signify 'unforeseen events', even within these articles themselves. However, they do suggest how the cosmological in/significance of

---

[29] 'Insurance Against Accidents of All Kinds', 254.

'chapter of accidents' is blurred by more technological or material significations. The titles also suggest how the proliferation of accidents required cataloguing them within a chapter or enfolding them in news sheets—which is entirely consistent with the etymology of the phrase. Brewer's *Dictionary* explains that '[t]he Roman laws were divided into books, and each book into chapters. The chapter of accidents is that under the head of accidents, and metaphorically, the sequence of unforeseen events'.[30] The book or chapter links the thematic categorization of accident to its bibliographic status. Newspapers elaborate that correspondence in the nineteenth century, using accidents as featured subjects as well as a category of news defined by bibliographic divisions or 'heads' of printed text.

THE COLUMN OF ACCIDENTS

The Victorian newspaper transforms accidents into the particular features of its chequered pages. Not chapters but columns of accidents were legion in the nineteenth-century press. If accidents had always been a source of fascination, a topic for reporting, and even a generic feature of the periodical press, they did not become 'news' until their conceptual split with eighteenth-century cosmologies provided the critical distance to make them into public and printed spectacles. Accompanying this split is the broadening focus of the nineteenth-century newspaper in general, a 'shift from the eighteenth-century newspaper's emphasis on foreign intelligence, parliamentary reporting, and political commentary to the broadly accessible *omnium gatherum*'.[31] As the newspaper steadily diffused into the everyday practices of its readers, so was the newspaper infused with various quotidian topics from 'every' kind of angle. With more as well as miscellaneous content, newspapers needed topical structures to impose categorical familiarity and formal structures to offer visual cues to its increasingly complex usage. These dynamics of miscellaneity and seriality (unfamiliar topics presented in consistent forms) are at heart of the development of the press.[32] If, as Lucy Brown argues, successful 'news' works the continuity of a story, then newspapers made the discontinuous stories of accident into continual features of the paper.[33] A newspaper's own bibliographic division of a chapter of accidents, as it were, occurred not only in article titles,

---

[30] Brewer, 'Chapter of Accidents (A).'
[31] Rubery, *The Novelty of Newspapers*, 9.
[32] Mussell, *The Nineteenth-Century Press in the Digital Age*, 24.
[33] Brown, *Victorian News and Newspapers*, 96.

but in recurring sections or columns or peripheral spots that aggregated various stories. By tracing these parts, we can see how accident was variously construed and how it materially affected the forms of writing about it.

Many nineteenth-century newspapers had versions of an 'accident' column. But the category could get blurry, as seen in the inconsistency of column titles and the placement of accident news therein. *The Morning Chronicle* sets a pattern with 'Accidents, Offences, &c.' alternating with 'Offences, Accidents, &c.' (1812–18). That pairing of accident and criminality was common for grouping violent or injurious events. It also conjoins different notions of causation about hazardous or disorderly things, happening by accident and/or by criminal design. The 'Accidents and Offences' column was used widely in the Victorian press, including in *The Charter, Illustrated London News, The Era, Lloyd's Illustrated Newspaper, Reynolds's Newspaper*, and *The Examiner*. The column headings in some of these newspapers were curiously variable, in the case of *The Examiner* oscillating through:

- 'Accidents, Offences, &c.' (1808–34)
- 'Offences, Accidents, &c.' (1834–5)
- 'Accidents and Offences' (1835–6)
- 'Accidents' and 'Offences' and 'Occurrences' in separate columns (1844 and following)
- 'Accidents Occurrences and Offences' (1845–52)
- 'Accidents and Occurrences' (1859–61)
- 'Chapter of Accidents' (1861–5)

The evolving columns in *The Examiner* present a fascinating trajectory of accident in newspapers, from its close relation to police reporting, to its more general status as a notable occurrence, to the self-referential 'Chapter of Accidents' column that enfolds all kinds of news within its own category of 'unforeseen events'. That column housed reports on railway accidents, pedestrian or strange incidents, lost hot air balloons, coroners' inquests, omnibus accidents, and so on. The very mark '&c.' testifies to the category's unpredictable seriation. The *Penny Illustrated Paper* offers a similarly interesting trajectory, in which accident news variously appears in columns including 'Law and Police', 'Accidents, Inquests, &c.', 'Accidents', and 'A Chapter of Accidents'. In so doing, these newspapers reinvigorate the textual origins of the 'chapter of accidents' metaphor as it comes to shape their thematic interests and publication formats.

Journalism about accidents almost inevitably becomes such a miscellaneous chapter, as Jewett suggests of accident reports themselves: 'While there is an imperative behind the reports to produce sequential and causal knowledge of what actually happened, the collecting of details in newspapers and pamphlets constantly undermines that effort'.[34] Even more generally, Brown argues that the Victorian newspaper had 'weakness in generalizing and sifting capacities' and often failed to assemble disparate news into a coherent story across issues. Brown suggests this reflects 'the haphazard and casual way in which news, outside certain standard topics, tended to be put together'.[35] As we shall see, accident news for Brown falls 'outside certain standard topics' which newspapers treated more coherently. But, as Jewett implies, the haphazardness of accident reporting is related to its very topic—the problematic inquiry into lost causes, the logical challenge of 'generalizing' from the resolutely singular, and the 'sifting' of much borrowed content into coherent narratives. All that is possible is collage: 'The newspaper itself becomes a new scene [of accident] where narratives accumulate and clash'.[36] A history of British newspapers in 1901 suggests that the new abundance and technologizing of information had made 'accidents of transmission' more prevalent than ever.[37] That phrase can mean more than just typos and story errors. It characterizes how accidents and inconsistency became consistent features of newspaper media.

If an 'Accidents' column encompassed a miscellaneous category of reported events, then so could accident news appear within a surprising number of different news categories. As Jones suggests, 'for much of the nineteenth century, formats of news presentation remained fluid, and the frontiers between them porous'.[38] For example, before the short-lived weekly *The Charter* established an 'Accidents and Offences' column, its relevant news frequently appeared within columns like 'Varieties' and 'Waifs of the Week'—waifs in the sense of ephemeral things blown by the wind. The penny *Reynolds's Newspaper* also had an 'Accidents, Offences &c.' column whose news frequently strayed into other columns including 'Police', 'Miscellaneous', and 'Railway Accidents'. *Cobbett's Weekly Political Register* sometimes included such news in 'Domestic Affairs'. *The Era* scattered it through 'The Railway Chronicle' and 'Chit Chat'. These column titles all suggest particular logics for understanding accident: as a domain for the police or governance, as representing the aberrant events of the everyday, and as associated with technologies like

---

[34] Jewett, 'Scene of the Accident', 57.
[35] Brown, *Victorian News and Newspapers*, 253, 254.
[36] Jewett, 'Scene of the Accident', 58.
[37] *Progress of British Newspapers* (London: Swan Electric Engraving Company, 1901), 198.
[38] Jones, *Powers of the Press*, 115.

the railway or with urban-industrial hazards. Before exploring those contexts in fuller detail, two things are worth noticing: the ubiquity of accident news in so many categories by which these texts defined the 'news', and, relatedly, the inconsistent diffusion of accident into various domains for understanding them. The conceptual career of the term was itself quite a chapter.

From another perspective, accident news also made a lot of economic and production sense. In other words, accident news flourished in nineteenth-century newspapers because it was cheap, easy to come by, readily reproducible, and flexible to place. As Brown argues, the 'news' does not necessarily reflect the characteristics of its readers, nor does it always follow a particular editorial vision; mostly, 'news was assembled from what was easily available in the office'.[39] Brown usefully complicates the imaginary 'model situation in which a newspaper collects information, prints it, and sells it to its own customers'.[40] While 'interpretation and control' were vital concerns for editors and newspaper owners, Brown recommends other influence models for what makes the news, especially its abundant supply and frequent republishing across different papers.[41] Accident news was available from a variety of sources. It came, for example, from police courts, which had been newly opened to the press in the wake of the Peterloo trials. As Brown explains, 'the major Sunday papers—*Reynolds's*, *Lloyd's* and *News of the World*—subsisted, essentially, on police court reporting, an attractive recipe for success, being cheap, simple to organize, and popular'.[42] It frequently came from coroners' inquests, which the Peterloo trials also underscored as a domain requiring political transparency and press coverage.[43] It came from insurance companies, who frequently sent their own accident reports to the papers—complete with totals of damages which might frighten new clients to market. It came from 'penny-a-liners' who, as *Chambers's* derisively explained, 'are the stragglers of the London press—the foragers for stray news—the narrators of fires, street accidents, suicides, murders, police cases, and all the odds and ends that fill up the columns of newspapers'. These writers, *Chambers's* continues, 'are perpetually going about in watch for what the chapter of accidents may throw in their way'.[44] It came from freelance writers like '"Fire" Fowler' who actually bunked with the Metropolitan Fire Brigade

---

[39] Brown, *Victorian News and Newspapers*, 100.
[40] Brown, *Victorian News and Newspapers*, 112.
[41] Brown, *Victorian News and Newspapers*, 244.
[42] Brown, *Victorian News and Newspapers*, 96.
[43] Burney, *Bodies of Evidence*, 28.
[44] 'Penny-a-Liners', *Chambers's Edinburgh Journal* NS 57 (1 February 1845), 65.

in order to always be first on the scene and with a report.[45] After mid-century, it could come from international press agencies like Havas, Wolff, and Reuters, or British outlets like the Central News and the Press Association, which harvested and distributed news of all sorts centrally and at a discount.

Perhaps the most abundant supply of accident news was other newspapers. In an era of widespread republishing and shameless copying, accident and offences news stands out. It offered convenient packages of texts in paragraph form to republish and circulate. Often these were copied word for word. Stereotyping made possible the lifting of entire columns of texts between in-house papers or different newspapers with cooperative agreements. Many papers tried to mask this wholesale repurposing by not copying lead articles and features which could be easily recognized in comparing separate texts.[46] By default, marginal or miscellaneous news was more likely to be recirculated. It is also widely accepted that provincial newspapers heavily copied the London press.[47] Brown argues that such copying was not reciprocal and that provincial news rarely made it back into metropolitan papers. However, her own examples suggest a pattern she overlooks: half of the 'provincial' stories she finds in *The Times* in October 1864 and October 1894 could have appeared in any 'chapter of accidents' column: inquests, explosions, railway accidents, shipwrecks, miscellaneous curiosities like a stranded whale.[48] Brown dismisses these as simply 'miscellaneous', but they suggest instead how miscellany was largely informed by the cluster of concerns that newspapers categorized as accidents and how that category had a privileged position in the recirculation of news.

Consider also the example of Anthony Hewitson, the chief reporter for the *Preston Times*, who noted some of his activities in his diary for 1865:

Wed Sept 27: [Railway crash] 'Just got to place in time to obtain particulars, which I sent off to 14 newspapers . . . Returned in evening & telegraphed half a column about accident to The Times'.

---

[45] Brown, *Victorian News and Newspapers*, 133; Clarke, *From Grub Street to Fleet Street*, 244.

[46] Brown, *Victorian News and Newspapers*, 116–18.

[47] A fairly representative summary: 'until 1870 the provincial press—urban, regional and local—remained heavily dependent on metropolitan papers and sources for news, still largely deploying scissors and paste journalism.' See 'Metropolitan Press', *Dictionary of Nineteenth-Century Journalism* (ProQuest LLC, 2011 2005), <http://gateway.proquest.com/openurl?url_ver=Z39.88-2004&res_dat=xri:c19index-us&rft_dat=xri:c19index:DNCJ:955>.

[48] Brown, *Victorian News and Newspapers*, 255–7, 258–9.

Thu Sept 28: 'Got particulars of 16 cows being seized in cattle plague. Wrote it out for 20 papers'.

Wed Dec 6: 'I reported an inquest on two children (ages between 5 & 7) suffocated in a house in Mellings Yard, Friargate during their mother's absence. Sent report to 15 newspapers'.[49]

In addition to writing for his own paper, Hewitson freelances content and sells it wholesale for ready printing elsewhere. Andrew Hobbs cites Hewitson in arguing for the prominence of the provincial news network, supplying its own print outlets as well as metropolitan papers. But like Brown, Hobbs overlooks the *kinds* of news Hewitson circulates in these networks, suggesting only that these three examples from his diary are 'typical'. Instead, this news is better understood as neither provincial nor miscellaneous, but as clustering in topics concerning *atypical* causality and comprising an information commodity for ready transmission. Perhaps for reasons of the cheapness, ubiquity, miscellaneity, and sometimes 'low-life' character of such contents, critics have not attributed them much significance.[50] Their significance lies elsewhere: as expressions of causal inquiry and reflections on metropolitan concerns. This is not news of the city per se, but news which characterizes metropolitan interests—particularly in the atypical. As both Brown and Hobbs implicitly suggest, metropolitan papers absorb such news more consistently than any other kind, suggestive of a conceptual as well as economic affinity.

For the newspaper business, the metropolis provided the economics of agglomeration: a networked concentration of news, reporting agents, production infrastructure, and consumers. In this sense, the 'metropolis' is a conceptual effect of newspapers themselves, partly shaped by the editorial emphases of their contents.[51] In their pioneering volume *The Victorian City*, H. J. Dyos and Michael Wolff argue that '[t]he true verbal and graphic equivalent of urbanism is journalism proper, the best lens we have for a close-up of the Victorian city, of its disconnections, intimacies, conflicts, aberrations, incidents'.[52] As some of the most conspicuous

---

[49] Quoted in Andrew Hobbs, 'When the Provincial Press Was the National Press (*c.*1826–*c.*1900)', *International Journal of Regional and Local Studies* 5, no. 1 (Spring 2009): 27.

[50] Clarke, *From Grub Street to Fleet Street*, 244.

[51] In their landmark collection of essays on the Victorian periodical press, Joanne Shattock and Michael Wolff take this relationship as a given: 'Journalism is the verbal equivalent of urbanism and Victorian Britain was also the first "journalizing" [as well as "urbanizing"] society'; see *The Victorian Periodical Press: Samplings and Soundings* (Leicester, Leicestershire: Leicester University Press, 1982), xiv.

[52] H. J. Dyos and Michael Wolff, 'The Way We Live Now', in *The Victorian City: Images and Realities*, ed. H. J. Dyos and Michael Wolff (London: Routledge & Kegan Paul, 1973), II, 899–900.

incidents in the Victorian city and its news, accidents became an important thematic and material dimension of newspapers while newspapers accentuated the accidental as a dimension of metropolitan life, resounding in the very terms Dyos and Wolff use to describe it. I would emphasize other aspects of the newspaper's metropolitan imagination, particularly the extraordinary everyday, the surprising risks of quotidian urban life, and the technological accidents of metropolitan industries and transport infrastructure. I would also offer several caveats. Newspapers flourished in population-dense environments and within the communication and transport networks which made the metropolis their hub. But of course the newspaper was an importantly provincial as well as metropolitan phenomenon, as Hobbs and others claim.[53] The imagined communities it may have engendered were local as well as national or imperial. From another angle, accidents were also the conspicuous province of non-urban news, such as the regular reports of shipwrecks.[54] But I would argue that accidents mapped out the conceptual geography of the metropolis just as influentially as they shaped the newspapers which developed in step.

The metropolis and its emerging capital and transport networks seemed to uniquely generate accidents. For example, within *The Examiner*'s column 'Chapter of Accidents' (20 May 1865), a report about a gentleman getting knocked down by an omnibus begins, 'One of those fatal accidents so common in overcrowded London occurred last week'. The article explains the singular and sadly fatal accident as 'one' in a pattern common to London. Another issue's 'Chapter of Accidents' column reports in a similar strain on fires: 'On Tuesday morning, one of nine fires in London was that which broke out about two o'clock, at the railway works of the Brighton Railway Company' (30 August 1862). Fire was such a significant problem that *Lloyd's Illustrated Newspaper* devoted a semi-regular column to 'Fires in the Metropolis'. Several newspapers created columns just for 'Railway Accidents', including the *Illustrated London News*. As I will show in the next chapter, even serial columns on London's scenes and characters, such as Dickens's pseudonymous *Sketches by Boz*, emphasized particular accidents and the accidental as the occasions for their own reports.

Lloyd's also produced a column simply named 'The Metropolis' which aggregated paragraphs on various London subjects. 'London' columns had

---

[53] For a critique of metropolitan bias in histories of the press, see Andrew Hobbs, 'The Deleterious Dominance of *The Times* in Nineteenth-Century Scholarship', *Journal of Victorian Culture* 18, no. 4 (2013): 472–97.

[54] Rubery argues for another context: 'shipwrecks were the most regularly reported disaster for most of the nineteenth century'; see *The Novelty of Newspapers*, 26.

featured in earlier newspapers, such as the *Daily Gazetteer* whose 1762 'LONDON' column included what Clarke calls 'the usual mixture of crimes, accidents, marriages, and deaths'.[55] Other newspaper historians are similarly uninterested in such columns, or what Michael Harris dismisses as the 'highly miscellaneous "London" section' frequently used by cut-price papers.[56] But accident news helps reveal the explanatory power of such sections for the metropolis they indexed. For example, included in *Lloyd's* 'Metropolis' column for the 15 January 1843 issue were: antiquities discovered during the excavation for the metropolitan sewer; planning the construction of the Fleet Prison; 'A Narrow Escape', concerning a collapsing building in Wapping; and a fire at the Fountain Tavern and Coal Hole in the strand, about which '[n]o idea could be formed as to how the fire originated'. That issue alone condenses how 'The Metropolis' seemed like the ever-changing aggregate of planned and unpredictable things. *The Era* also had a column for 'The Metropolis' (1838–42) whose contents seemed to overlap with related columns, especially 'Accidents and Offences'. The first appearance of 'The Metropolis' column in *The Era* on 30 December 1838 included paragraph reports about:

- the Harrowgate Affair
- Christmas Day observances (and crimes)
- 'Infamous Publications'
- 'Curious Question of Identity'
- 'Serious Accidents': including an intoxicated cab driver, an unfortunate lover who fell off a roof trying to reach his sweetheart, another vehicular crash, and a runaway chaise whose horse collided with a post
- 'Death from Locked Jaw', declared an 'Accidental Death' by the coroner's jury
- 'Singular Suicide', judged the result of 'Temporary mental Derangement' by the inquest
- 'Horrible Deaths by Fire', all declared 'Accidental Death' by the coroner's jury

Accidents of all kinds abound. In mid-May 1842, 'The Metropolis' column was re-named 'The Synopsis', though its contents retained the same character. Such a synoptic view presents a grim picture of the

---

[55] Clarke, *From Grub Street to Fleet Street*, 84.
[56] *London Newspapers in the Age of Walpole: A Study of the Origins of the Modern English Press* (Rutherford; Cranbury, NJ: Fairleigh Dickinson; Associated University Presses, 1987), 164. See also Clarke, *From Grub Street to Fleet Street*, 181.

metropolis, largely textured by uncertainty and injury, with accidents indiscriminately diffused through public, private, and commercial domains, and signifying a new urban cosmology of risk.

'The Metropolis' column also suggests the prominence of the coroner's inquest in newspaper reports on fatal accidents. In this context, the coroner's inquest is doubly significant: as the source of information and testimony about accidents themselves, and also as one of the most conspicuous public forums for adjudicating what is 'accidental' at all. A coroner's inquest occurred whenever a death seemed overly sudden or suspicious, including circumstances of uncertain natural death, crime, and death by accidents of all sorts.[57] Newspaper reports on coroners' inquests were just as conspicuous as accident news—and just as categorically slippery, appearing throughout the same closely related columns: 'Accidents', 'Offences', 'Law and Police', 'Inquests', and 'Metropolis' columns, generally speaking. *The Penny Illustrated Paper* even consolidated the topics into 'Accidents, Inquests, &c.' (roughly 1861–6), uniting two of the most sensational phenomena in the imagination of the Victorian news-reading public. Within the newspapers' chapters of metropolitan accidents, the coroner's inquest became the familiar scene of their interrogation.

COURTS OF INQUIRY

In *Bodies of Evidence*, Ian Burney argues that the coroner's office was the site of an important nineteenth-century contest over governmentality. Burney focuses on the competing authority of legal versus medical expertise, which manifests a broader struggle over the significance and control of the coroner's inquest. Having originally been instituted in the late twelfth century, by the 1830s the coroner's inquest had paradoxically come to represent both an ancient political institution, as gradually built and impregnable as the English constitution, and an open forum for public representation and participatory governance. Coroners were elected officials, their juries of 12–24 persons were (male) members of the public, and inquests were typically held in public houses. Dickens famously lampooned the practice of holding inquests in pubs, but Victorian writers mainly took shots at inquests for other reasons.[58] Inquests pop up throughout Victorian fiction not merely as scenes of

---

[57] Burney, *Bodies of Evidence*, 3.
[58] As Dickens's narrator quips, 'The Coroner frequents more public-houses than any man alive.' See *Bleak House* (Oxford: Oxford University Press, 1987), 197. But Dickens's

crimes or testimony, but as evidence of their insufficiency to establish causes, contexts, and relations, which novels (at least) implicitly claim as the domain of narrative.[59]

Novelists were not alone in suspecting the inquest of failing to tell the whole story. That sense of insufficiency also informed legal critiques of inquests which, as Burney shows, complained that inquests were rumour mills at best and never arrived at conclusive evidence. The inquest's goals were open-ended 'information gathering rather than a formally structured proceeding against a named suspect'. Not only was this 'a more amorphous standard for instigating inquiry', it undermined the legal standing of what the inquest turned up, as it was 'largely unfettered by the development of rules of evidence affecting other courts'. As such, coroners' inquests had an 'air of indeterminacy' and were seen 'as episodic, contingent affairs, dictated to by circumstance rather than legal form'.[60] Furthermore, the verdicts delivered by inquest juries seemed to many—legal conservatives and statisticians in particular—to fail the very goals of the inquest itself: to explain the cause of uncertain death. Sir John Jervis, in his standard work on the coroner, insisted that verdicts must be 'made with certainty', 'stated *positively*', and 'be *single*' to avoid any possible uncertainties.[61] But even such singular, certain, positive claims might not prove themselves as fact. William Ogle, the successor to William Farr in the statistical department of the General Records Office (GRO), complained that verdicts like 'natural causes' or 'visitation of God' or 'accidentally, casually, and by misfortune' were not causal statements at all: 'It is using a phrase instead of giving a fact'.[62]

---

characterizations aside, it wasn't until the last quarter of the nineteenth century that pub inquests came under sustained scrutiny. Burney, *Bodies of Evidence*, 83.

[59] Alicia Garnica, 'The Curious Life of the Corpse in Nineteenth-Century English Literature and Culture' (Ph.D. Dissertation, University of Southern California, 2009). A good example can be found in Elizabeth Gaskell's *North and South*, when Mr Thornton, in his capacity as magistrate, heads off a coroner's inquest on the body of Leonards. Mr Thornton knows that Leonards died after scuffling with Margaret Hale's fugitive brother and falling to the tracks at a railway station. The 'cause' of death remains uncertain—either by the accidental fall, by homicide, or by aggravating a pre-existing condition. But Thornton is out to protect Margaret, whose delicate relations with these men must be the novel's inquiry, rather than the coroner's or his jury. As Mr Thornton tells his own mother: 'I tell you, mother, that there was no inquest—no inquiry. No judicial inquiry, I mean'. See *North and South*, ed. Patricia Ingham (London: Penguin, 1995), 305.

[60] Burney, *Bodies of Evidence*, 6–7.

[61] John Jervis, *Sir John Jervis on the Office and Duties of Coroners: With Forms and Precedents*, ed. C. W. Lovsy, 3rd ed. (London: Sweet, Maxwell, and Stevens & Sons, 1866), 294.

[62] Quoted in Burney, *Bodies of Evidence*, 68.

What coroners' inquests did do, as even their critics allowed, was to focus people's attention on problems of causal interpretations and the authority to make them, whether vested in political officials, experts, juries, or emerging discourses of validation. What makes the inquest unique is how very unspecialized it could be, in several senses. First, it invited amateur and expert perspectives at the same time: 'the peculiar expert-popular hybrid' of coroner, lay jury, and witnesses.[63] Second, it offered verdicts which could not attain the legal, factual, or statistical integrity that certain professional camps would have wanted. Coroners' inquests by contrast had narrative objectives, producing testimonies and phrased verdicts which seemed like a 'chaos of individuation' to those who would standardize or catalogue the results.[64] Third, by the 1830s, the inquest had formalized a rhetoric and practice of openness: to jurors, to the community in public houses, and just as significantly to the press.

Arguments about the necessary publicity of inquests were rooted in early nineteenth-century reformist politics. I want to consider the newspapers' involvement in publicizing inquests from a different angle. Beyond issues of access, newspapers made inquests into a particular and widely distributed reading practice. As Aled Jones claims, 'journalism nurtured the analytical skills of the readers that enabled them to make their own sense of the fragmented world portrayed in the news-sheets'.[65] Reports of inquests interpellated the readers of newspapers into the same position as the non-specialist jury, tasked with the analysis of testimony and evidence. For newspaper readers, inquest reports did have sensational and voyeuristic appeal, but newspaper accounts were also structured procedurally, offering summaries or even transcripts of testimonies with the coroner's interjections.[66] Though it is almost tautological to say, the great majority of these reports ended with the jury's conclusions. What was the cause of death? As *The Examiner* reports near the end of a piece on 'Dreadful Fires' (20 November 1841, 748), 'The point which [the jury] wished particularly to get at was, whether the fire originated from accident

---

[63] Burney, *Bodies of Evidence*, 82.
[64] Burney, *Bodies of Evidence*, 65.   [65] Jones, *Powers of the Press*, 91–2.
[66] While separate editorials about verdicts could be quite pointed, newspapers had a legal interest in keeping their summaries or transcripts free from comment. As Jervis explains, it had been illegal to publish evidence from inquests in advance of any official court trial to follow, partly for the protection of those involved, as the inquest is an exploratory rather than final proceeding. However, Jervis also suggests that by the late nineteenth century, times had changed: 'different notions now prevail upon this subject... it appears at this day to be generally admitted that the publication even of ex parte proceedings, if done fairly and honestly, and without being accompanied by unfounded or unjust comments, would not wisely be made the subject of prosecution'. See *Jervis on Coroners*, 272.

or design'. The verdict discloses an interpretation that recasts all the preceding information in terms of causality. The reader has implicitly been weighing the evidence too, suspended between the prescribed verdicts with which anyone could become readily familiar. Did this death happen by accident or by design? Even while verdicts aimed at single, positive certainties tantamount to legal facts, inquest reports indulged a different genre as short, contingent narratives.

Reports of coroners' inquests proliferated because of their very resonance with news itself, including: their relative immediacy—occurring quickly and on the spot, mostly because of the necessity to view a body in rapid decay; the narrative or uncertain evidence that legal critics cited as problematic; the overlaps of inquests with news of accidents or metropolitan events; and the ready availability of inquest content. The coroner's inquest was the most significant legal forum for adjudicating fatal accidents and the newspaper promoted it into an ever-more public position. If it is unlikely someone could find a 'newspaper without an account of one or more accidents', rare too would be the newspaper without an inquest *accounting* for such accidents. Brown and Clarke claim with justification that the Sunday papers (*Lloyd's*, *Reynolds's*, and the *News of the World*) were especially indebted to coroners' inquests as a cheap source of news, but such reports abound across the spectrum of the Victorian newspaper press.[67] Some unscientific but suggestive examples: a full third of issues of *The Times* in 1835–6 had articles with coroners' inquests referenced in headlines. Moving into the body text, inquests appear in all but two issues of *The Times* in January 1845 and all but three in February. In *The Morning Chronicle*, coroners' inquests show up in two-thirds of issues in May 1834 and closer to five-sixths of issues that August. All but three issues (94 per cent) of the weekly *Examiner* for the entire year of 1840 mention inquests. All but two issues (98 per cent) of the then twice-weekly *Manchester Times* in 1846. All but three issues (98 per cent) of the then thrice-weekly *Leeds Mercury* in 1858. About 95 per cent of all issues of the *London Dispatch* (1836–9). The same for early issues of *Lloyd's Illustrated Newspaper*. In the *Illustrated Police News*, you can hardly find anything else.

While newspapers conspicuously covered accidents, offenses, and deaths, they also made conspicuous the interpretation of such events as a public inquiry, directed by coroners and by the reading experience of published transcripts and summaries. Clearly there are important distinctions that such a synopsis overlooks, such as the political slants of certain

[67] Clarke, *From Grub Street to Fleet Street*, 246.

papers at certain times, their circulation, and their readerships. On the other hand, the conspicuousness of inquest reporting across the board may suggest a broader logic at work: a generic experience, or the newspaper genre as shaped by a dynamic of reported factuality and suspended causality. From this perspective, even the news of non-fatal accidents outside the purview of coroners' inquests begins to draw upon the same logic. Reading the 'Accident' column becomes a forensic exercise in assigning causality. At the bottom of the accident-heavy 'Metropolis' column is an implied verdict waiting to be pronounced, not just about specific cases but about the city they seemed abundantly to populate.

Coroners' inquests and the newspaper shared a rhetoric of political openness as well as formal strategies. Each claimed privilege as a public investigator of causality. And each transformed what might be singular or aberrant events into systemic concerns. Consider this exchange in the 1 August 1846 issue of *The Times*: a letter to the editor, highly critical of the contingency and publicity of inquests, claims that legislation should not be based on 'the fallacious test of a solitary accident' or by 'that idle clamour miscalled public opinion' but by reasoned judges. In response, *The Times* argues that '[t]here is nothing unnatural or extraordinary in the circumstance that a particular incident should forcibly concentrate public attention on a system, and precipitate a decision on its merits' which otherwise would have remained unknown. The exchange suggests how coroners' inquests spark disputes about the relation of 'solitary accident' and system, as well as who has the authority to articulate that logic.

Through the inquest, newspapers found a unique opportunity to convert themselves into public courts of inquiry. So too would newspapers come to lend their sympathy and support for expanding the coroner's inquisitorial horizon. In 1833, the conservative *Morning Post* strongly objected to any new functions for inquests, complaining that jurors have 'taken it into their heads to imagine that no inquiry can be too large, or too delicate, or complex for their faculties', including critiquing the government itself. The editors go even further: 'we venture to say that in no single instance has it ever yet contributed to the wholesome ends of public justice, welfare, and security of the community'.[68] That sentiment is wholly opposed to what the *Illustrated London News* (*ILN*) opines in a leading editorial in 1845:

> Of all the various and useful institutions which the people of the British Empire enjoy, there is not one which is more in accordance with common

---

[68] Quoted in Burney, *Bodies of Evidence*, 39. The editorial was also reprinted in *True Sun*, 21 May 1833, 4.

sense, more conducive to the security of the person, and more consonant with the true interests of society generally, than that of the 'Coroner's Inquest'.[69]

Leading the article (as well as the issue's editorial content), such a statement serves to justify the *ILN*'s own extensive coverage of coroners' inquests (not sensational but useful and good for society) and makes claims for the *ILN* as a populist, useful institution allied to the goals of inquests in general. The article explains how inquests have traditionally been confined to fatal disasters and then turns to a recent expansion of the coroner's purview. The article's goal is

> to direct public attention to an application of the principle of the 'Crowner's Quest' which has lately been made in the City of London; and which, developing as it does the advantages of the system, ought, we would suggest, to be adopted universally throughout the empire.[70]

While the *ILN* is characteristically not shy about the importance of its own opinion, this statement underscores how newspapers enable an analogous public diffusion through the routes of metropolitan and imperial expansion. The *ILN*'s advocacy comes at a particular moment of uncertainty in the otherwise historically stable office of the coroner, facing the special problems of the nineteenth-century metropolis and its array of phenomena begging for adjudication as to whether they were accidental or designed. In this case, the problem is not suspect bodies, but 'the frequent occurrence of destructive and extensive fires in many of the principal towns of the United Kingdom'. The *ILN* claims that this is 'just as fit a subject for immediate investigation, for the purpose of ascertaining whether the calamity was caused by accident or design, as sudden loss of life'. Having advertised the integrity of coroners' inquests, the *ILN* now stumps for expanding their investigative horizon in full support of a controversial move by the Coroner of the City of London, William Payne.

No one died in the extensive house fire in Aldermanbury, August 1845, that caught Payne's attention. With no fatalities, no bodies to view, the event fell outside the conventional jurisdiction of the coroner's office. But Payne was dissatisfied by the increasing number of fires in London which were not only outside the purview of the coroner but outside practically *any* legal purview: 'No one had the power to inquire into the causes of a fire—not even a magistrate, unless a party was in custody charged with

---

[69] 'Of All the Various and Useful Institutions', *Illustrated London News*, 30 August 1845, 134.
[70] 'Of All the Various and Useful Institutions'.

causing it'.[71] Payne's next move was controversial but not without precedent. Citing ancient legal statutes, Payne argued that coroners were originally tasked with duties more extensive than resolving unnatural deaths, specifically the investigation of extensive loss of property by fire.[72] Payne admitted these powers had been long dormant, but present circumstances demanded restoring them to current practice. So, beginning with the Aldermanbury case, Payne began to convene juries to hear testimony about fires in London, 'so that they might come to a proper verdict, whether it was caused by accident or otherwise'.[73] At a stroke, Payne converted the coroner's inquest into a general court of inquiry. Like the *ILN*, *The Times* enthusiastically endorsed Payne's actions which 'plainly prove that the coroner's duty is to enquire, on behalf of the Crown, into a variety of matters affecting the public peace and safety; and in the event of fires, and colliery explosions, and railway crashes, we should be well pleased to see this officer instituting an investigation'.[74] No longer limited to viewing a corpse, the coroner would assume a responsibility which the *ILN* and *The Times* agreed was sorely lacking: the need to adjudicate questions about causality more broadly, especially concerning the accidents which urban-industrial modernity seemed to increase.

Payne's actions represent the disembodiment of accident, as it were. But enthusiasm for increasing his authority would not have solved the problem of causality. These cases—and the newspapers' reports about them—could simply end with 'accidentally caused'. That was the verdict settled on the Aldermanbury fire. It closes a case, but, like coroners' inquests more generally, the verdict of 'accident' settles almost nothing. It only answers the original uncertainty by displacing it into a category, filing it within the chapter of accidents. Instead, 'accident' materially settles another problem: not causation but liability. The recent prevalence of fires was not the problem; the problem was property. Payne later cited the new opportunities for arson within an emerging (and tenuous) regime of fire insurance. Time and again in his position he must have seen the paradox that insurance causes fires. In Chapter 3, I will elaborate further on the unique problems of fire insurance and its own definitions of

---

[71] 'Of All the Various and Useful Institutions'. It is worth noting that the *ILN* copied this directly from 'The Late Fire in Aldermanbury', *The Times* (London), 22 August 1845, 3.
[72] Indeed, though investigating unnatural death was the most frequent task for early coroners, their duties extended to 'inquiries into treasure trove, wreck of the sea, and the finding of royal fish...abjurations of the realm...appeals and outlawries; and rapes'. See Burney, *Bodies of Evidence*, 24.
[73] 'Of All the Various and Useful Institutions'.
[74] 'The Step Taken by Mr. Payne', *The Times* (London), 27 August 1845.

property and causation. Suffice it here to say that Payne also saw a need to define fires in terms of accidents or criminal design, a need that emerged from the conspicuousness of urban catastrophe as well as material imperatives for legal and commercial protections of property at risk. In this context, Payne's innovation was entirely consistent with the coroner's original function 'as a local agent securing the king's interest in the revenues deriving from the administration of justice'.[75] By the 1840s, revenues from the administration of justice in cases of fire had been significantly displaced into the insurance business.[76] So instead, in a letter to the Lord Mayor of London, Payne appealed to a policing function of coroners' inquiries 'into the origin and causes of fires' which would have 'the most important and beneficial effect in checking incendiarism, as well as detecting offenders'.[77]

Considering how police and property were consolidating in the modern capitalized state, it is curious that Payne's innovation met with such internal resistance. He conducted several courts of inquiry on fires from 1845–51, but ran into ungenerous scepticism about padding his paid-per-inquiry bill—the common attack on overreaching coroners—as well as passive resistance in the form of his bills not getting paid, as Payne reported in his letter to *The Times*.[78] Payne also faced more philosophical resistance to enlarging the juridical horizon of the coroner beyond the situation of a dead body. As Burney has argued of Thomas Wakely, Payne was 'swimming against a strong judicial current' which was resistant to any 'new form of inquisitorial excess'.[79] In 1851, legal officers of the City of London declared that the coroner had no power to hold other inquests, effectively quashing the practice. But the issue was revived in the 1880s, as still 'the origin of many fires [remained] undiscovered'.[80] Eventually the City of London Fire Inquests Act of 1888 mandated that fires be reported to the coroner, authorizing him to open inquests as necessary. Payne was ahead of his time.

---

[75] Burney, *Bodies of Evidence*, 23.

[76] Though not exclusively. As Elisabeth Cawthon demonstrates, the ancient monetary award of the 'deodand' was resurrected in the 1830s and 40s, as coroner's courts 'began to levy deodands in a more sophisticated manner—to indicate quite specifically the "sense of misconduct" of a negligent party of an accident'. See Elizabeth Cawthon, 'New Life for the Deodand: Coroners' Inquests and Occupational Deaths in England, 1830–46', *The American Journal of Legal History* 33, no. 2 (1989): 138.

[77] William Payne, 'Letter to the Right Hon. John Musgrove, Lord Mayor of London', 22 April 1851, Original Fire Inquests. CLA/041/F1/01/01/068 1845–1885, Corporation of London Records Office.

[78] William Payne, 'Inquests on Fires', *The Times* (London), 28 June 1851, 7.

[79] Burney, *Bodies of Evidence*, 53–4.

[80] Duty Keeper of Records, 'Original Fire Inquests', 7 December 1976, Original Fire Inquests. CLA/041/F1/01/01/068 1845–1885, Corporation of London Records Office.

In his own time, Payne brought into focus a particular and unsettled contest over the assessment of accidents. Why, at this moment, did the legal community remain so sceptical? Could it really have been about the relatively insignificant monies required to hold additional inquests on fires? Opposition was more likely the result of ingrained legal scepticism about opening coroners' courts at all. Widening the horizon of inquests would blur the coroner's requisite expertise and potentially weaken the office's connections with vital statistics and the governance of a polity of bodies. In effect, judgments about testimony and evidence would be newly asserted by lay jurors from all kinds of backgrounds. The clarity of an inquest's verdict would tend toward individuated chaos. And if a coroner's job required the assessment of every disturbing phenomena of uncertain or unnatural cause, the bill might get expensive indeed.

In Payne's case, the legal establishment was a powerful minority. But he elsewhere garnered broad support. Those constituencies reveal a widespread concern with investigating accidents and doing so in a public forum. Payne's own jurors became strong supporters of the cause. In a March 1846 fire case, the jurors delivered a verdict of suspected incendiarism as well as a unanimous resolution of thanks:

> That the best and sincerest thanks are due from, and are hereby given by, this jury to Mr. W. Payne, coroner for the city of London, for the lengthened, patient, and complete investigation as to the cause of the fire at No. 6, Gracechurch-street, on Sunday morning last, and we further desire to express our great satisfaction at the revival by that gentleman of the ancient practice of holding courts of inquiry on all such fearful occasions in the city of London, which, we doubt not, will be productive of most important results.[81]

In producing a formal statement of thanks, the jury also produced a detailed paragraph that was ready for journalistic uptake, anticipating its circulation through the media already consuming its verdicts. And so the resolution appeared in newsprint. Newspapers were also quick to offer their own editorial praise of Payne's innovation. The *ILN* was one of numerous papers which were favourably impressed by these new courts of inquiry, including:

- *The Times*, 27 August 1845
- *Illustrated London News*, 30 August 1845
- *Dorset County Chronicle*, 2 October 1845
- *Lincoln, Rutland, and Stamford Mercury*, 6 March 1846

[81] 'Alleged Incendiarism', *The Times* (London), 19 March 1846, 5.

- *Morning Post*, 18 March 1846
- *Western Luminary*, 26 May 1846
- *Maidstone Journal*, 8 June 1847
- *Lincolnshire Times*, 25 April 1848
- *Sheffield Times*, 2 December 1848
- *Jersey Times*, 20 February 1849
- *The Times*, 10 October 1849
- Report of the Government Board of Health (247–57), 28 May 1850
- *Boston, Stamford, and Lincolnshire Herald*, 24 December 1850
- *The Britannia*, 1 March 1851

The list is Payne's own, included in his letter to the Lord Mayor. It suggests a modern public relations savvy that Payne was keen to leverage (he was an elected official, after all). So too does it suggest the relative prominence of newspaper publicity compared to one lone government report. More generally, the list reveals how by the late 1840s newspapers of all persuasions—even the *Morning Post*—shared his interests, whether in expanding participatory governance, bringing arsonists to justice, supporting a regime of property and liability (unlisted above, the director of a fire insurance company also wrote in support of Payne in *The Times*), or more generally interrogating the urban-industrial uncertainties whose consequences were more materially and politically significant than ever.[82]

Payne's example suggests a mid-century moment of transition, an attempt to manage the uncertainties preoccupying several related domains, the coroner's inquest and the newspaper in particular. They share economic and conceptual investments in the apprehension of accident, explaining its causality, and reckoning with its consequences. They also demonstrate how accident becomes an important part of their own designs, whether in claiming broader political power for coroners and juries or in structuring the circulatory patterns and page formats of newspapers themselves. Inquests further reveal accidents as simultaneously factual and contingent forms, enabling generic hybrids which attempt to categorize what is consistently exceptional or individuated. Verdicts and their reports in newspapers are neither legal settlements, nor definitive answers about the causality of a dizzying array of accidents of modern (and especially metropolitan) life. They instead impose a being-in-uncertainty, like the narrative contingency of the inquest itself, or like the experience of regularized miscellaneity in a column like 'The Chapter of Accidents' or

---

[82] 'Inquests on Fires', *The Times* (London), 22 April 1850, 3.

'The Metropolis'. They formalize a causality that is not really causal at all. And significantly, they do so as an experience of print.

THE MARGINS OF CAUSALITY

This chapter proposes a triad of topics in which the Victorian newspaper made questions of causality conspicuous: accident and offences news, coroners' reports, and news of miscellaneous events or what Roland Barthes has called the *faits divers*.[83] This last category may be the most slippery, seemingly omnipresent in newspapers and ironically difficult to define, which probably contributes to its being so frequently dismissed as 'miscellaneous'. Barthes wrangles it into a trans-historical structuralism of the news, as we shall see. But the *fait divers* has a particular historical resonance, one that is best understood in terms of the nineteenth-century newspaper's transformation into an everyday court of inquiry, a public interrogator of causality in print.[84]

In 1836, *The Times* ran an article about a traffic fatality entitled 'Shocking Cab Accident': a custom-house employee was run over by 'a cab driven at an unnecessarily rapid rate'.[85] As the next chapter will show, accidents—and reports about them—were unfortunately common within the commercial passenger traffic of London in the 1830s and 1840s. To modern sensibilities, just as shocking as the accident might be, the abrupt transition to what immediately follows in *The Times*' column—a paragraph about a giant turnip: 'There was pulled on Monday last, in a field near to Jedburgh,...a turnip of the white Norfolk kind, of an unusual size.... The turnip was remarkably sound and well shaped'. No headline breaks the text between the shocking cab accident and the report of the 18 pound vegetable. The paragraph is simply credited to the *Dumfries Courier*—recalling Anthony Hewitson and his production of information commodities for circulation across metropolitan and provincial press networks. In this case, the source is surely John M'Diarmid, the editor

---

[83] Roland Barthes, 'Structure of the Fait-divers', in *Critical Essays*, trans. Richard Howard (Evanston, IL: Northwestern University Press, 1972), 185–96.

[84] Anne Humpherys almost takes it for granted that news tells stories to explain the world in terms of cause and effect: 'If I am puzzled by a series of events I witness on the street, I am likely to try to make sense of them by fitting them into familiar "narrative" patterns...a recognisable narration of events with a beginning, a middle and end, linked together through conventional patterns of cause and effect'. See Anne Humpherys, 'Popular Narrative and Political Discourse in *Reynolds's Weekly Newspaper*', in *Investigating Victorian Journalism*, ed. Laurel Brake and Aled Jones (New York: St. Martin's Press, 1990), 33.

[85] 'Shocking Cab Accident', *The Times* (London), 14 October 1836, 4.

of the *Dumfries Courier*, who, according to local history, was so well known for 'droll stories regarding prodigies in the earth, air, and waters, or in the fertile fancy of the editor, that the paper became famous for its wonderful paragraphs, and was eagerly read by all lovers of the marvelous', as well as eagerly copied by so many publishers of such news.[86] The prodigal, marvellous, miscellaneous: this was the cheap, readily available, and popular stuff of newspaper filler which so frequently inhabited the same columns and conceptual categories as accidents.

News of the marvellous was itself not new. For example, royal censorship in the seventeenth century attempted to restrict printed news to the 'relation', a short narrative focused on an event, which frequently took the form of 'Wonderful and Strange Newes'. John Trundle, a publisher of newsbooks at the time, was fond of printing stories about the supernatural and reimagining them as contemporary events.[87] Lorraine Daston and Katherine Park have outlined an alternative trajectory of 'wonder' against the rise of empiricism, and marvellous news suggests the persistence of wonder within the conventional trajectory of news into a discourse of journalistic objectivity or fact.[88] Wonder endured in contexts where its imaginative and cosmological possibilities had not been fully foreclosed. Including, in the nineteenth century, the newspaper, with its expanding appetite for news content in defiance of the predictable. As the old saying goes (variously attributed), 'When a dog bites a man, that ain't news. When a man bites a dog, that's news'.[89]

Wonder sells. Newspapers made ordinary information saleable, argues John Sommerville, and therefore had incentives to find information that seemed extraordinary.[90] However, increasingly distant from the earlier cosmological frameworks in which 'wonderful and strange newes' had signified, nineteenth-century newspapers had to cultivate it elsewhere, harvest it from the ordinary, reinvent wonder within a reading experience

---

[86] William McDowall, *History of the Burgh of Dumfries* (Edinburgh: Adam and Charles Black, 1867), 853, <http://books.google.com/books?id=D7QHAAAAQAAJ>.

[87] Clarke, *From Grub Street to Fleet Street*, 13–14.

[88] Lorraine Daston and Katherine Park, *Wonders and the Order of Nature, 1150–1750* (New York: Zone Books, 1998).

[89] By legend this was the response of *New York Sun* city editor John Bogart (1845–1921) to a cub reporter who, in the early 1880s, asked him to define 'news.' The author of a 1918 history of the *Sun* credited Bogart with this comment. It was recalled when he died in 1921. The observation has also been attributed to *Sun* editor Charles A. Dana; to its first managing editor, Amos Cummings; and to early-20th-century British press baron Lord Northcliffe (Alfred Harmsworth). Ralph Keyes, 'Who Said That?', *Bark Magazine*, August 2006, <http://www.ralphkeyes.com/quote/press-quote/>.

[90] Sommerville, *The News Revolution in England*, 4.

which periodically renewed itself, sometimes daily. According to Roland Barthes, this is the function of the marvellous stuff of the *faits divers*—his term for the shorter bits of newsy miscellany with which many papers filled their columns. Barthes argues that it represents far more than just saleable, miscellaneous journalistic filler. Instead, Barthes reads the *faits divers* as self-renewing interrogative experiences of 'Why?' We can situate Barthes' argument in the material context of nineteenth-century newspapers whose evolving coverage of accidents manifests just such persistent causal inquiries.

Barthes proposes that the *fait divers* is a self-contained, fragmentary hermeneutic that plays by different rules of causality. Because the laws of causality loosely define what we all already know or would expect, newspapers are more likely to report things in seeming defiance of those laws or what is 'remarkable'. Lightning strikes twice; massive marine animal strands itself on the beach; woman shot by husband—the police chief. The appeal of such news items begins where received notions of causality and social determination break down, and where notions of a 'slightly aberrant causality'—perhaps providential, perhaps aleatory—emerge instead.[91] As Sommerville interprets it, '[t]his miscellaneous stuff does not belong to any context that would give it "importance" or meaning' but generates its own interest 'by showing something incongruous, coincidental, or strange in their causation—qualities that seem to call for explanation but defy explanation at the same time'.[92] That tension or in-betweenness manifests a new species of wonder or perhaps carries forward a quasi-religious consciousness that converts news items into articles of faith.

But, as Barthes suggests, neither religion nor the marvellous really explains the interrogative signature of such news. Rather—and particularly in the nineteenth century—the *faits divers* is an experience of heterodox causality, of uncertainty about the role of chance within notions of probability. In the *fait divers*, 'causality remains "suspended" between the rational and the unknown... imbued with an alien force: chance'.[93] The *fait divers* produces its own species of wonder at a junction between two worlds and properly belongs to neither:

> we might say that the causality of the *fait-divers* is constantly subject to the temptation of coincidence and, inversely, that coincidence here is constantly fascinated by the order of causality. Aleatory causality, organized

---

[91] Barthes, 'Structure of the Fait-divers', 188.
[92] Sommerville, *The News Revolution in England*, 137.
[93] Barthes, 'Structure of the Fait-divers', 191.

coincidence—it is at the junction of these two movements that the *fait-divers* is constituted.[94]

What Barthes finds in the *fait divers* can translate into a longer story about Victorian probability thinking: the uneasy junction of paradigms when aleatory suspicions struggle with inherited orders of causality. Though Barthes does not use the term, this junction between the causal and the aleatory is the emerging concept of the accident. The accidental combines the suspicion of design with the suspicion of chance; it is the coincidence of these interpretive paradigms, ideas about what is designed and what is random. If, as critics like Ian Hacking have suggested, 'the probabilistic revolution' was accomplished by the nineteenth century, then we can see its public campaign in the marginalized contents of the Victorian newspaper.

This might be a grand thing to say about a turnip, no matter how huge. And is that not a marvel instead? A precise categorical definition of these news items may be beside the point. Barthes selects examples of the *faits divers* quite strictly. On the other hand, newspaper historians tend to dismiss them as merely miscellaneous and hence overlook their particular significance. I would emphasize a different interpretive frame. In the nineteenth century, the *faits divers* conspicuously overlaps with a set of other news items just as concerned with chance and causality, especially accident news and coroners' reports. Frequently, the 'faits divers' is not even distinguishable from such related news. These subgenres are thematically interpenetrating, just as their categorization in newspapers was so overlapping and inconsistent. For example, the 'Accidents and Occurrences' (and soon to be 'The Chapter of Accidents') column of *The Examiner* for 4 December 1858 includes reports of several serious railway and quotidian accidents. Included among these are 'Lost in the Woods' about a Reverend and his 'extraordinary adventure'; 'Another Accident from Wearing an Inflammable Dress' which adds another chapter to an awful domestic risk (beware crinoline); and 'A Story of Police Life' about a policeman at home: he gets off work, goes to bed, and his wife anxiously complains of 'indisposition' and requests some brandy. So he hurriedly puts on some nearby clothes, goes to the pub, reaches into his pocket, finds a lot of money, and realizes he has unknowingly dressed in another man's pants—with the obvious implications. If such an 'Occurrence' could have happened to anyone, not just anyone's story would have made it into the newspaper, which exploits the ironies of police detection at home for a piece of miscellaneous news. Thematically, it is

---

[94] Barthes, 'Structure of the Fait-divers', 194.

not miscellaneous at all, but coincident with the 'Accidents' on the page and with the causal inquiries they all perform.

Another example. The *Daily News* for 9 December 1858 offers abundant reports and letters about fires and a bad railway accident. Amid these items appears 'Fatal Accident to a Clown' describing how an ambitious performer attempted—and failed to complete—a triple somersault at a circus. The grim story has the elements of paradox of Barthes' *faits divers*. Were this a story of another circus performer, it would report the risks of a dangerous job. But we learn that this jump was not part of the clown's routine. He had proposed it on the spot, ad libbing gymnastics alongside his comic entertainments. High-flying absurdity turns deadly serious. The entertaining clown in the spotlight falls under the forensic gaze of a coroner's jury. The piece ends with an inquest and the verdict of accidental death. The report abuts and embodies the day's news of accidents and inquests, all working out questions of causality gone awry.

In this light we could return to the lists of 'miscellaneous' stories which Brown, Clarke, and Hobbs use as evidence for other claims and find the conspicuous presence of accident news in all of these three forms. Even Sommerville, who is sensitive to the *faits divers* and its mythological functions, suggests that 'the heart of the news does not lie in these fillers'.[95] He and other critics are primarily interested in the newspapers as an experience of suspended continuity. In a sense, they are right to marginalize these fillers, but wrong to understate their thematic importance. If not the 'heart of the news', these items feature as some of the most conspicuous elements in its circulation—and not only within newspapers, but between newspapers throughout the international–metropolitan–regional–local network. Accident news was especially conducive to circulate for economic, logistical, and thematic reasons. If marginal, it also suggests how newspapers developed marginality as a generic condition, making the improbable, criminal, or indeterminate, into the expected features of the news. If discontinuous, accident news suggests how newspapers engendered a faith in discontinuity or 'aberrant causality' as part of the reading experience. Considering the expansion of newspapers and such reports over the century as well as the penetration of newspapers into people's reading habits, the marginalized miscellany of accident news has an aggregate influence which has been seriously overlooked.[96]

---

[95] Sommerville, *The News Revolution in England*, 137.
[96] At the end of the century, Frank Taylor finds the power of the newspaper's influence in its own ubiquity: 'Perhaps the most vital part of that process is its perpetuity. The daily reiteration of the same argument, the daily presentation of the same aspect, the daily contact with the same mental and moral atmosphere, these things are like the dripping of water on a

Accidents and newspapers were reciprocally shaped, each providing the other 'virtual structures... through which the continuous flux of social life could be ordered and understood'.[97]

The kinds of accident news that I have highlighted will come up again in the chapters to follow which draw upon contemporary newspaper accounts as historical sources, including reports of omnibus and cab accidents, industrial fires, railway accidents, and others. The following chapters consider each of these contexts more closely, demonstrating how they shape particular forms of writing and how those written forms encode complicated ideas about the metropolis and probability. But newspapers are more than simply sources for many of these concerns: they also model the generic and conceptual transformations of accident within Victorian print culture. The newspaper was one of the more conspicuous public realms in which notions of accident were configured with material consequences for content, format, and circulation. Newspapers also challenged other genres to reckon with their growing prominence and representational protocols, especially (though not exclusively) as regards accidents.[98] Thus, while the Victorian newspaper suggests the increasing prominence of accidents in the attention of the reading public, it more importantly brings into focus the key conceptual relations that this book will emphasize: between material accidents, the print culture they inflect, and the conceptual career of probability in the nineteenth century.

---

rock'. See *The Newspaper Press as a Power in Both the Expression and Formation of Public Opinion* (Oxford: B. H. Blackwell, 1898), 17–19.

[97] Mussell, *The Nineteenth-Century Press in the Digital Age*, 52.

[98] Rubery suggests that 'Victorian novelists drew upon the news both as a means of formal innovation and as a countertext against which to define their own fictional discourse'; *The Novelty of Newspapers*, 12. Liddle argues the significance is even larger: 'the genre forms developed for and used in periodicals were the discursive competitors and companion forms of nearly all Victorian literature'; see *The Dynamics of Genre*, 158.

2

Dickens and the Traffic of Accidents

THE KNOWLEDGE OF LONDON

There is a familiar figure on the streetscape of contemporary London. He buzzes up a road and stops on the corner, looking down for a minute to the clipboard affixed behind the conspicuous red 'L' on his motorscooter's windscreen. His helmet comes up and scans the surroundings: buildings, parks, intersections, landmarks. A glance back at the clipboard, maybe a quick mark with a pen, and the scooter whines away to stop in another block or two. The process begins again. He tries to absorb places and routes and problems. He is studying to be a cab driver. He is meandering the streets in pursuit of 'the knowledge'.

Such is the formidable name of the licensing examination for London's cab drivers, in place since its original institution around 1850.[1] Before 'the knowledge' examination was formalized, hackney coachmen, cab drivers, and omnibus conductors were still subject to other modes of licensing. But this did not necessarily mean they knew where they were going—or even how to drive. Before the London Hackney Carriage Act of 1843, only the *proprietors* of the cab and omnibus companies had to be licensed and these licenses represented commercial privileges rather than geographical savvy or operational integrity.[2] Skills for driving were either assumed or learned on the job, which is to say on the streets. When, in 1832, a fourteen-year-old boy legally at the reins of his father's cab knocked down and killed Lady Caroline Barham, an uproar ensued, fuelled by class prejudice and drawing on general indignation with the seeming ubiquity of cab accidents in London.[3] In 1836, *The Times* reported that 'not fewer than two-thirds of the coroners' inquests which were held in London and Westminster arose from cab and omnibus accidents'.[4] A flurry of legislation

---

[1] Philip Warren, *The History of the London Cab Trade: From 1600 to the Present Day* (London: Taxi Trade Promotions, 1995), 97.
[2] Warren, *The History of the London Cab Trade*, 95.
[3] Trevor May, *Gondolas and Growlers: The History of the London Horse Cab* (Phoenix Mill, Gloucestershire: Alan Sutton, 1995), 35.
[4] 'Omnibus Conductors and Cab-Drivers', *The Times* (London), 2 September 1836, 4.

followed in the attempt to regulate street traffic. The Metropolitan Police Act of 1839 gave new public functions to the police 'including the regulation of omnibus routes during divine service; street obstruction and nuisances; and furious driving'.[5] The Hackney Carriage Act of 1843 finally required the licensing of drivers, at first by a Registrar of Metropolitan Public Carriages and after 1850 by the Metropolitan police.[6] In classic Foucauldian form, the 'knowledge' and disciplinary power were one, directing traffic on London's streets.

The problems of a shifting licensing authority were compounded by the influx in numbers and kinds of road vehicles—hackney carriages, two-wheeled cabriolets, four-wheeled cabs like growlers or broughams, and even larger omnibuses—as well as the swelling traffic of commerce, livestock, and pedestrians in a metropolis whose human population more than doubled in the 50 years from 1800. Just as regulatory power had not been settled, neither had forms of 'knowledge' about this increasingly large and complicated place. In terms of urban transport, for example, Paul Dobraszczyk points out '[t]he extraordinary range of graphic formats' of printed information for cab passengers. This information, he claims, 'also addressed a question that lies at the heart of much Victorian urban investigation: how to impose a sense of order on an increasingly complex and chaotic environment?'[7] As Dobraszczyk suggests, the methodological tools to deal with the uncertainties of urban transport 'also defined the development of other disciplines of knowledge in nineteenth-century London'.[8] Thus, at the dawn of the Victorian era, 'the knowledge of London' was as contested as the licensing practices that that examination would partly formalize. For cab drivers, passengers, as well as social demographers, freelancers, and writers of London guidebooks and narratives, it took various forms of meandering, looking, jockeying, sketching, cataloguing, and attempting to compile a representation of what ultimately might be beyond knowledge itself. And, like the vehicular melee in the streets, such knowledge seemed punctuated by accidents: by the seemingly random encounters in the city, by the collisions that collapsed social extremes, by the exceptions and oddities that constellated the urban cosmos.

The attempts to 'know' London flourished across diverse genres of printed texts, such as Pierce Egan's rollicking *Life in London* (1820–1), newspaper sketches of London life and places, tourist handbooks, guides

---

[5] May, *Gondolas and Growlers*, 76.   [6] May, *Gondolas and Growlers*, 35.

[7] Paul Dobraszczyk, 'Useful reading? Designing information for London's Victorian cab passengers', *Journal of Design History* 21, no. 2 (Summer 2008): 137, 138.

[8] Dobraszczyk, 'Useful Reading?', 138.

to 'fast' life and nightlife, transport guides including Edward Mogg's *Omnibus Guide* (1844) and William Mogg's *Ten Thousand Cab Fares* (1851), Parliamentary 'blue books', periodicals like the weekly *Bell's Life in London*, serial fictions like G. W. M. Reynolds's *Mysteries of London*, and disquisitions like Robert Mudie's *Babylon the Great: A Dissection of Men and Things in the British Capital* (1825).[9] These texts catered to citizens as well as visiting strangers and arm-chair tourists, all increasingly curious about the byways and sub-regions of a place so complex, so jumbled with persons and things, as to become a Babylon. Babylon's confusion and competing voices can equally describe the forum of early-nineteenth century writing about the metropolis. What distinguishes these years is how unsettled were the protocols of knowing and writing about London at all. Experimentation was the only license. Across an array of domains of cultural investigation, across a range of generic modes, the traffic of ideas was subject to plenty of collisions.

The 1830s were formative years for competing modes of urban representation, particularly in terms of what discourse could accommodate, according to Mudie, 'this discord of order and activity (if I may so name that which is inexpressible)'.[10] The attempts to order or at least describe metropolitan discord were coming from all disciplinary quarters.[11] London was the epicenter of a 'frenzy of state formation and cultural regulation' which took various forms of public management, commercial investment, and nascent disciplinary approaches including statistical

---

[9] Martha Vicinus, 'Dark London', *Indiana University Bookman* 12 (1977): 63–92.
[10] Robert Mudie, *Babylon the Great: A Dissection and Demonstration of Men and Things in the British Capital* (London: Charles Knight, 1825), 47. As Mary Poovey argues in *Making a Social Body: British Cultural Formation, 1830–1864* (Chicago, IL: University of Chicago Press, 1995), the political turbulence of the early nineteenth century had profoundly unsettled the enterprise of social classification, requiring notions of the encyclopaedic city to be reimagined through an array of mechanical and organic metaphors and classificatory schemes. Pierce Egan considers London 'a complete CYCLOPÆDIA' which his own book implicitly embodies; see 'Life in London', in *Unknown London: Early Modernist Visions of the Metropolis, 1815–45*, ed. John Marriot, Masaie Matsumura, and Judith R. Walkowitz (London: Pickering & Chatto, 2000), V, 23. By contrast, Mudie finds the metropolis conceptually overwhelming, a sprawling urban organism that prompts the medical metaphor of his book's subtitle, 'a dissection of men and things'. The emerging idioms of urban knowledge—dissection, classification, taxonomy—all attempt to manage the relations between part and whole, singular and general, component and system, within the labyrinthine logic of the early-Victorian metropolis.
[11] While London had long been a favourite site for enterprising taxonomists, by the 1830s the technologies of sorting and classification came into full bloom. Foucault locates the heyday of classification in the eighteenth century and its enthusiasm for Linnaean taxonomies; see *The Order of Things: An Archaeology of the Human Sciences* (New York: Pantheon Books, 1970), 125 ff. But I would suggest that, by the beginning of the nineteenth, the city became the premier cultural laboratory for taxonomic techniques and vocabularies.

demography and political economy.[12] A young Charles Dickens joins the fray with a series of pseudo-ethnographic essays that would be collected as *Sketches by Boz: Illustrative of Every-day Life and Every-day People*. The *Sketches* capitalize on a widespread curiosity about the proliferating persons, things, and relations in the capital city, as well as about the theories, classificatory schemes, and 'learned speculations' that were proliferating to explain them. In 'Our Next-door Neighbour', Boz sarcastically situates his 'theory' amid a spate of similar projects: 'This is a new theory, but we venture to launch it, nevertheless, as being quite as ingenious and infallible as many thousands of the learned speculations which are daily broached for public good and private fortune-making'.[13] This 'new theory' turns out to be an analogy between door knockers and the physiognomies of the tenants within; it is patently and purposely absurd. However, *Sketches by Boz* simultaneously invokes and mocks the strategies of urban taxonomy when a range of such epistemologies are in development and in doubt. If he lampoons 'many thousands of the learned speculations' about public life, Boz also harnesses their epistemophilia to drive the fictionalized jaunts he takes around town.

Sketches by Boz also reveals a fascinating intersection of two realms— urban classification and commercial transport—at a time when, for each, their protocols were still emerging and contested. The careening cabmen of London overlap with the cohort of urban chroniclers in several ways. In the most basic sense, they provided transport, materially facilitating a 'knowledge of London' which mapped its socio-geographic diversity onto its early sprawl and means of getting around. Additionally, the on-street competition between commercial operators and vehicles became one of the more visible aspects of public urban life. Omnibuses and cabs with their charismatic operators quickly became favourite subjects of London sketches and guides. Commercial transport also encapsulated one of the signature paradoxes of Victorian Babylon, as it simultaneously facilitated and blocked urban growth and circulation.[14] Its vehicles were a vital nuisance, calling attention to top-down urban planning to regulate the bottom-up traffic on the streets. Particularly in cases of fraud or misdirection or accidents, these vehicles provoked people to consider how to systematize transport well before London ever had a transport

[12] Elaine Freedgood, *Victorian Writing About Risk: Imagining a Safe England in a Dangerous World* (Cambridge; New York: Cambridge University Press, 2000), 83.
[13] Charles Dickens, *Sketches by Boz: Illustrative of Every-Day Life and Every-Day People* (London; New York: Oxford University Press, 1966), 41. Unless otherwise indicated, subsequent page numbers will be cited in-line, to this edition.
[14] Lynda Nead, *Victorian Babylon: People, Streets, and Images in Nineteenth-Century London* (New Haven, CT: Yale University Press, 2000), 16 ff.

system. Before the Metropolitan police instituted the 'knowledge' examination, assumed the authority to regulate traffic, and standardized fares, the competitions and vagaries of urban transport brought into focus the dynamics of unregulated development and systematization which, for so many Victorian observers, seemed to characterize the metropolis itself.

This chapter opens a window onto the dynamics of urban knowledge by looking to the conspicuous presence of vehicular urban transport within the publication history and recurring subjects of Dickens's *Sketches*. With its 'discord of order and activity', street traffic inspires the social theories that the *Sketches* do articulate, a dynamic of anarchy and systematization that is much more than a description of 'Every-day' London, but an innovative epistemological and generic practice. The *Sketches* enfold various genres and techniques of urban representation, including the ethnographic essay and the cab passenger's book of fares, in claiming their own unique 'knowledge of London'. They take particular inspiration from the accidents of urban transport, using them to mount a spirited defence against knowing London through the forms of arithmetical demography or proto-sociology on the rise. Dickens imagines the possibilities of the accidental within rigid schemes of measurement or classification and designs an 'omnibus genre'—the sketch—for the purpose. Boz's own traffic in accidents not only informs the sketch genre he pioneers, but also the lasting imaginative legacy of London that Dickens would bequeath.

BOZ ON THE BUS

Readers of the weekly periodical *Bell's Life in London* would have been interested but not surprised by an October 1835 article which opens:

> IF we had to make a classification of society, there is a particular kind of men whom we should immediately set down under the head of 'Old Boys;' and a column of most extensive dimensions the old boys would require. To what precise causes the rapid advance of old-boy population is to be traced, we are unable to determine. It would be an interesting and curious speculation.
>
> (244)

So begins the comical sketch 'Love and Oysters', one of twelve in a series of 'Scenes and Characters' published in *Bell's* by a writer signing himself 'Tibbs'.[15] The sketch announces its taxonomic interests from the start,

---

[15] Dickens published these twelve pieces under the pseudonym 'Tibbs'. This piece later reappeared in collected editions of *Sketches by Boz*, and was re-titled 'The Misplaced Attachment of Mr. John Dounce'. For details on the complex publication history of the

and we zoom in from 'a classification of society', to 'a particular kind of men', down to the very individual—introduced subsequently—Mr John Dounce, who typifies the species.[16] The population of this sociozoological oddity is conspicuously booming, like that of so many unfamiliar persons and classes within the early nineteenth-century metropolis. But why, no one can tell, least of all our humble narrator who fails to find the origin of this particular species. Instead, he offers an imaginative 'speculation'. Even as he declares his intent to classify society and scrutinize a specific type, the narrator hedges his bets: the 'precise causes' of this phenomenon he is 'unable to determine'. These few short lines oscillate between the determinacy of classification and the contingent social types sprouting on the urban landscape. They move from pronouncement to curious speculation, from taxonomic sorting to imaginative ramble.

In its mock-academic introduction and 'curious speculation', 'Love and Oysters' draws the pattern for Dickens's complex intervention into urban taxonomy that registers throughout the *Sketches*. But the series did not start this way. Dickens began them in the *Monthly Magazine* with 'A Dinner at Poplar Walk' (December 1833), which was later re-titled 'Mr. Minns and His Cousin' and published under the section 'Tales' in collected editions of the *Sketches*, the first in 1836. This trial balloon was followed by other such 'Tales', all published anonymously and all concerned with farcical, middle-class doings in the suburbs. *Sketches by Boz* did become a sensation, but it was not because of these initial stories which were mildly praised as 'amusing' or 'clever'.[17] Then Dickens made a big change, publishing instead in newspapers like the daily *Morning Chronicle* as well as its offshoot *Evening Chronicle*, signing his articles with a consistent pseudonym ('Boz'), and moving his subject matter from the suburbs to the downtown scenes and characters for which the *Sketches* would become famous. Under the *Morning Chronicle*'s heading of

---

Sketches, see John Butt and Kathleen Tillotson, 'Dickens as a Serial Novelist', in *Dickens at Work* (London: Methuen, 1957), 13–34; Richard Maxwell, 'Dickens, the Two Chronicles, and the Publication of *Sketches by Boz*', *Dickens Studies Annual* 9 (1981): 21–32; Paul Schlicke, '"Risen Like a Rocket": The Impact of *Sketches by Boz*', *Dickens Quarterly* 22, no. 1 (March 2005): 3–18.

[16] Virgil Grillo dismisses such introductions as 'undoubtedly the outgrowth of a schoolboy's exercises in classic definition whereby he offers first the *genus* and then the *differentia* of the object to be defined'; see *Charles Dickens' Sketches by Boz: End in the Beginning* (Boulder, CO: Colorado Associated University Press, 1975), 72. If the *Sketches* show amateur classificatory earnestness, that also characterizes the attempts to ground social types in some form of stable knowledge.

[17] Kathryn Chittick, *Dickens and the 1830s* (Cambridge; New York: Cambridge University Press, 1990), 47–9; Schlicke, 'Risen Like a Rocket', 8.

'Street Sketches', it all began with a piece called 'Omnibuses' (26 September 1834).

'Omnibuses' marks a crucial pivot in Dickens's career and turns the *Sketches* toward a continuing interest in vehicular urban transport and its operators. The first in the *Evening Chronicle*'s 'Street Sketches of London' series was 'Hackney-coach Stands' (31 January 1835). Related sketches would include 'The Steam Excursion' (October 1834), 'Early Coaches' (19 February 1835), 'The River' (6 June 1835), 'The Prisoner's Van' (29 November 1835), 'Some Account of an Omnibus Cad' (1 November 1835), and 'Hackney-cabs, and Their Drivers' (17 September 1836)—the latter two sketches revised and combined in collected editions as 'The Last Cab-driver, and the First Omnibus Cad'.[18] In addition to the sketches so explicitly concerned, urban transport also textures a number of the other essays. In highlighting these sketches, I am not proposing a dominant interpretive pattern, but instead suggesting an alternative context in which to consider the *Sketches*' classificatory and generic projects.

With these sketches, Boz turned away from 'Tales' to what Kathryn Chittick calls 'the recording simply of his great knowledge of London' or, in Michael Slater's words, 'the writer's astonishing knowledge of London'.[19] Reviews changed their emphasis to praise the 'acuteness' of Boz's observations of the town.[20] The ballyhoo over Boz's 'close and accurate' reportage was, in some ways, Dickens's reward for good timing, seizing upon the growing fascination with London and the classificatory modes by which it was popularly described. Partly as a result, Dickens has also earned strong criticism for indulging an epistemological fantasy, joining what Judith Walkowitz calls 'a throng of missionaries and explorers', men who tried to read the "illegible" city, transforming what appeared to be a

---

[18] Grillo argues that, considering the publication patterns of these transport sketches, Boz is just recycling content for different audiences in different periodicals: 'Omnibuses' appears in the *Morning Chronicle*, 'Hackney-coach Stands' in the *Evening Chronicle*, 'Some Account of an Omnibus Cad' in *Bell's Life*, and 'Hackney-cabs, and Their Drivers' in the *Calton Chronicle*, and 'The Last Cab-Driver and the First Omnibus Cad' in collected editions of *Sketches by Boz*. See *End in the Beginning*, 92. In Grillo's view, Dickens is less preoccupied with transport than it would seem. Even granting this argument, Dickens is still exploiting the circulatory networks of periodicals that, as demonstrated in Chapter 1, keeps accidents very much in the public eye.

[19] Chittick, *Dickens and the 1830s*, 48; Michael Slater, *Charles Dickens* (New Haven, CT: Yale University Press, 2009), 41.

[20] Chittick, *Dickens and the 1830s*, 49. Unlike the monthly tales, the street sketches were not initially reviewed because they appeared in newspapers. Chittick claims that the praise for newspaper sketches came after they were collected. But Forster suggests that the original periodical sketches 'were talked of outside as well as in the world of newspapers'. See *The Life of Charles Dickens* (Philadelphia, PA: J. B. Lippincott & Co., 1872), 106, <http://books.google.com/books?id=r00YAAAAYAAJ>.

chaotic, haphazard environment into a social text that was 'integrated, knowable, and ordered'.[21] From this perspective, the 'knowledge of London' overlays an asymmetrical cultural geography based on gender and class. What Boz describes as his 'amateur vagrancy' also seems to anticipate the *flâneur*, an exploitative masquerade of sexual and commercial consumption which privileges the male gaze at the expense of marginalized social actors.[22] These angles have generated robust criticism on Dickens, Boz, and the *Sketches*. But that criticism has also, in a sense, missed the bus. I want to shift the context for Boz's peregrinations and consider the 'knowledge of London' less as a dream of power and instead as a specific engagement with the material practices of knowing London in the 1830s.

Ana Parejo Vadillo has argued that scholarship on urban modernity—including critiques of the *flâneur*—has privileged 'an urban epistemology that gives primacy to walking over any other form of urban mobility'.[23]

---

[21] *City of Dreadful Delight: Narratives of Sexual Danger in Late-Victorian London* (Chicago, IL: University of Chicago Press, 1992), 18.

[22] In the sketch 'The Prisoner's Van' as originally published, Boz confesses:

> We have a most extraordinary partiality for lounging about the streets. Whenever we have an hour to spare, there is nothing that we enjoy more than a little amateur vagrancy—walking up one street and down another, and staring into shop windows, and gazing about us if . . . the whole were an unknown region to our wondering mind.
>
> (Quoted in Slater, *Charles Dickens*, 53)

For a sample of the extensive critique of Victorian urban exploration and *flâneurism*, see Walkowitz, *City of Dreadful Delight*; Deborah Epstein Nord, *Walking the Victorian Streets: Women, Representation, and the City* (Ithaca, NY: Cornell University Press, 1995); Deborah L. Parsons, *Streetwalking the Metropolis: Women, the City, and Modernity* (Oxford; New York: Oxford University Press, 2000); Amanda Anderson, *Tainted Souls and Painted Faces: The Rhetoric of Fallenness in Victorian Culture* (Ithaca, NY: Cornell University Press, 1993); Regenia Gagnier, *Subjectivities: A History of Self-Representation in Britain, 1832–1920* (New York: Oxford University Press, 1991). Other critics have taken issue with the characterization of Dickens as a *flâneur*. Michael Hollington argues that Boz strategically adapts *flâneurism* as a mediating principle between purposive and non-purposive activity, solitude and multitude, psychological and public spaces, the familiar and fantastic; see 'Dickens the Flâneur', *Dickensian* 77, no. 2 (Summer 1981): 71–87. For Alan Robinson, Boz is not a *flâneur* because the narrative geography of the *Sketches* 'belongs to the complacent Regency convention of London "contrasts" rather than the Victorian convention of the traveller, like Mayhew, into "the undiscovered country of the poor" or the explorer of the Dark Continent of the East End'; *Imagining London, 1770–1900* (Basingstoke, Hampshire; Hampshire NY: Palgrave Macmillan, 2004), 82. Geoffrey Hemestedt suggests that *flâneurism* consigns Boz into critical frame about middle-class anxieties and does not account for his sustained engagement with the marginalized social subjects of his sketches; see 'Inventing Social Identity: Sketches by Boz', in *Victorian Identities: Social and Cultural Formations in Nineteenth-Century Literature*, ed. Ruth Robbins and Julian Wolfreys (Basingstoke Hampshire: Macmillan, 1996), 215–29. Chittick points out that, without an hour to spare, the young Dickens simply could not afford to idle; *Dickens and the 1830s*, 45.

[23] Ana Parejo Vadillo, *Women Poets and Urban Aestheticism: Passengers of Modernity* (Basingstoke, Hampshire; New York: Palgrave Macmillan, 2005), 3.

While her project is to explore 'the importance of the late-Victorian aesthetics of transport in the development of a new urban epistemology', earlier Victorian engagements with transport are also suggestive of new urban epistemologies.[24] These were not articulated as aesthetics per se, but emerged within a variegated print culture focused on urban scenes, characters, and networks in which Boz was very much involved. The 'Street Sketches' did inaugurate Dickens's legacy among Victorian London's greatest pedestrians.[25] But Dickens did not set forth on foot. He launched his new thematic concerns with 'Omnibuses'—at once the topic and vehicle by which he moved his enterprise from suburbia to the centre. Simultaneously appearing with the bus sketch was 'Boz'—the coincidental consonance suggests that Boz was built as a metaphorical vehicle for urban exploration. Born(e) on the omnibus, Boz the street sketcher adopts the conditions of transport into his signature genre.

Moving Boz's sketches into the domain of commercial transport may help resolve some critical extremes about the consequences of urban representation. Michel de Certeau suggests two primary approaches to knowing the city, as Nead lucidly explains:

> the panoptic, aerial viewpoint of the mapmakers and city-planners and the perception of the walker at ground level. The aerial viewpoint articulates a totalising mastery of space; it renders the city legible and comprehensible. At street level, however, space cannot be controlled in a single gaze, but is apprehended through a rhetoric of walking and its associated symbolic mechanisms of dreams, memories and fables. The poetic space of the pedestrian is, for de Certeau, a space of resistance, which defies the attempts of the planners and improvers to discipline the contingencies of everyday life.[26]

Boz inhabits both the aerial and the asphalt, the panoramic and the particular. He takes the totalizing survey and closely attends to specifics, details, particulars which might—or might not—aggregate into encyclopaedic knowledge.[27] And his model for doing this is the transport system.

---

[24] Vadillo, *Women Poets and Urban Aestheticism*, 25.
[25] See Jeremy Tambling, *Going Astray: Dickens and London* (Harlow, Essex: Pearson Longman, 2009), for example, as only the most recent of a long line of books about Dickens and his London.
[26] Nead, *Victorian Babylon*, 7.
[27] Christopher Ferguson uses de Certeau's phenomenology as a framework to investigate Victorian print culture and argue that knowledge of early nineteenth-century cities only seemed possible in these two frames; see 'Inventing the Modern City: Urban Culture and Ideas in Britain, 1780–1880' (Ph.D. Dissertation, Indiana University, 2008). Martina Lauster slightly changes these terms to 'panoptic' and 'encyclopedic' knowledge of the city comprised in sketches; see *Sketches of the Nineteenth Century: European Journalism and Its Physiologies, 1830–50* (Basingstoke, Hampshire; New York: Palgrave Macmillan, 2007).

Urban transport offers Boz a material context in which to imagine the connections of the pedestrian and panoptic as well as to model the development of complex systems. In his recent work, Jonathan Grossman identifies the stagecoach network and Dickens's subsequent novels (beginning with *The Pickwick Papers*) as generating such systemic awareness. I turn to earlier metropolitan contexts of commercial transport to elaborate the generic properties of the sketch rather than the novel. Departing from Grossman, my focus on metropolitan accidents suggests the unique contingencies within the genre as well as within Dickens's representation of systems more broadly. Those contingencies help Dickens shape his discursive goals by framing 'the knowledge of London' in different terms.[28]

As that sketch 'Omnibuses' explains right away, the omnibus is 'the machine in which we make our daily peregrination from the top of Oxford-street to the city' (139). For Boz, 'peregrination' is not synonymous with walking, but encompasses a broadening range of transport modes and routes. Critics have rightly noted Dickens's attention to urban byways, antiquated streets, and roads less taken, but that should not obscure how new vehicles, operators, and passengers made even primary routes seem like unfamiliar places or carnivalesque zones of contact unique to the metropolis and ripe for reportage. On his 'daily' route to town, Boz turns his attention to the new everyday, to the curious and extraordinary facets of the routine. As John Stokes points out, 'the urban journey is an everyday event whose semi-regularized nature... conceals its important function within the overall life of the city'.[29] In the spirit of revealing those functions, Boz claims that on an omnibus, 'sameness there can never be' (139). In de Certeau's framework, commercial bus routes seem more closely allied to the totalizing structures of planning and metropolitan improvement than to the imaginative 'poetic space of the pedestrian'. However, Boz turns to urban transport for precisely that tension: its planned, commercial routines nonetheless enfold the insurgent and accidental into its systemic properties. The early omnibus was 'semi-regularized' at best.

'It is very generally allowed that public conveyances afford an extensive field for amusement and observation', Boz begins, deciding subsequently

---

Simon Parker traces his history of urban theory to exactly this split between modes of philosophical and empirical investigation in *Urban Theory and the Urban Experience: Encountering the City* (Abingdon, Oxfordshire; New York: Routledge, 2004).

[28] Jonathan H. Grossman, *Charles Dickens's Networks: Public Transport and the Novel* (Oxford; New York: Oxford University Press, 2012).

[29] John Stokes, '"Encabsulation": Horse-Drawn Journeys in Late-Victorian Literature', *Journal of Victorian Culture* 15, no. 2 (August 2010): 245.

that 'of all known vehicles... there is nothing like an omnibus' (138, 139). There was nothing like an omnibus until 1829 when they arrived in London and, along with the two-wheeled cabriolet or 'cab', began to seriously challenge the dominance of the hackney coach. The omnibus added to the competition—and the traffic—of commercial transport on London roads and waterways. As Gavin Weightman and Steven Humphries argue, '[t]he real revolution in London transport' was the omnibus; the resulting 'bus mania' in the 1830s was comparable to the 'railway mania' in the decade to follow.[30] The omnibus was capturing passengers, entrepreneurial ambitions, and attention in print.[31] As Boz elsewhere quips, 'the appearance of the first omnibus caused the public mind to go in a new direction, and prevented a great many hackney-coaches from going in any direction at all' (148). In the broadest sense, they prompted greater public attention to what Boz calls 'the progress of the system of which the first omnibus was a part', through novelty and nuisance alike (148). The omnibus—and 'Omnibuses' too—brings with it a general awareness of the changing landscape of London's transport infrastructure and its impact on the metropolitan 'every-day' (in the *Sketches*' subtitle) for so many un/commercial travellers. In related ways, they prompt our attention to the progress of the sketches of which 'Omnibuses' was the first part. The near-chaos of post-omnibus urban transport coincides with *Sketches*' development into a classificatory system or a descriptive catalogue aiming at the very 'knowledge of London' which drivers would soon be required to demonstrate.

The larger turn the *Sketches* make to urban scenes and characters happens in microcosm on this inaugural bus ride. As Boz (139) explains, '[t]he passengers change as often in the course of one journey as the figures in a kaleidoscope, and though not so glittering, are far more amusing... As to long stories, would any man venture to tell a long story in an omnibus?' Gone are the narratives which, however brief, shaped the early 'Tales'. In their place are the brief, fractured experiences that encourage many critics to credit the *Sketches* for exposing a quintessentially modern urban condition, reflected in their kaleidoscopic or visual form as well as in the unpredictable encounters they dramatize in urban space.[32] As

[30] Gavin Weightman and Steven Humphries, *The Making of Modern London, 1815–1914* (London: Sidgwick & Jackson, 1983), 102–3.
[31] For useful background on the appeal and changing accessibility of the omnibus for London's socio-economic classes, see Parejo Vadillo, *Passengers of Modernity*, 18–21.
[32] For an example of such urban essentialism, see Frederic Schwarzbach, '*Sketches by Boz*: Fiction for the Metropolis', *Dickensian* 72 (13–20): 1976. By contrast, Vadillo makes a wonderful point about the omnibus in relation to the now-standard critical narrative about the transformation of vision in the nineteenth century:

Amanpal Garcha claims, 'cities seemed to exist in a state of constant flux... [and] urban life appeared to be a subject that might only be represented with a quick, ready hand'.[33] Efraim Sicher argues that the *Sketches* 'adapt narrative sequence to the labyrinthine interconnections of city life, the mysteries of identity, the confusion and variety'.[34] However, these perspectives represent a tendency to mythologize urban modernity, taking as given the tropes writers like Dickens imparted to London as a Victorian Babylon: labyrinthine, illegible, mysterious. They also overlook the specific histories, the particular routines, by which the metropolis comes into being—and which Dickens is quite careful to elucidate, in however seemingly fractured a manner.

De Certeau recommends closer attention to the tactics and texts of urban navigation. He links the terms vehicle and metaphor in an especially useful way for considering 'Omnibuses': 'In modern Athens, the vehicles of mass transportation are called *metaphorai*. To go to work or come home, one takes a "metaphor"—a bus or a train. Stories [are also] spatial trajectories.... Every story is a travel story—a spatial practice'.[35] We do not have to route through modern Athens to make these connections to early Victorian London, where 'the knowledge' was contested by texts and taxis alike. De Certeau's notion of 'spatial practices' helps connect the metaphorical and historical vehicles of Boz's sketches. The omnibus offers a particular means of accessing the city—from Oxford Street to the Bank. For Boz's readers, it also embodies the prevailing themes of the *Sketches*' new metropolitan focus. The omnibus is a moving heterotopia, blurring the thresholds of citizen and crowd, private and public, routine and disruption, law and disorder. For example, the conductor in 'Omnibuses' has a 'somewhat intemperate zeal on behalf of his employers, [which] is constantly getting him into trouble, and occasionally into the house of correction. He is no sooner emancipated, however, than he resumes the duties of his profession with unabated ardour' (139). The conductor seems bipolar, oscillating between public and commercial institutions, 'house' and omnibus,

---

It is no coincidence that Jonathan Crary situates the appearance of a new observer in or around the 1820s, the decade in which omnibuses appeared in the metropolis, although he never actually makes that connection.... It is this 'uprooting' of vision that seems to me to suggest that the advancement of mass transport was crucial in this reorganization.

See *Passengers of Modernity*, 33.

[33] Amanpal Garcha, *From Sketch to Novel: The Development of Victorian Fiction* (Cambridge; New York: Cambridge University Press, 2009), 113.

[34] Efraim Sicher, *Rereading the City, Rereading Dickens: Representation, the Novel, and Urban Realism* (New York: AMS Press, 2003), 41.

[35] Michel de Certeau, *The Practice of Everyday Life*, trans. Steven Rendall (Berkeley, CA: University of California Press, 1984), 115.

discipline and zealous prosecution of his own disruptive work. He inevitably declares to any inquiring passenger on the street that there's 'Plenty o' room, sir' (139). That passenger is then stuffed into an already-packed bus, thrust into an immobile crowd on the move. As Stokes explains, urban transport offers 'a variable interface between inner space and the outer world'.[36] The omnibus becomes a permeable zone that warps the contours of the new everyday. If it offers a kaleidoscopic metaphor for metropolitan modernity, then it also has cultural specificities with particular relations and resistance to such larger narratives.

Boz is intensely curious about 'the first omnibus [which] caused the public mind to go in a new direction' as well as about the roads or routes it bypassed, about what existing forms are being displaced in 'the progress of the system of which the first omnibus was a part'. The sketch 'Hackney-coach Stands' considers the soon-to-be antiquated vehicles that had heretofore dominated London commercial passenger traffic. From 1662, the Hackney Coach Office had essentially managed all of London's passenger vehicles on public roads, but it was shuttered in the 1830s when its licensing monopoly was broken and commercial licenses became available for cabriolet, stagecoach, and omnibus drivers.[37] Hackney coaches were soon 'swamped by cabs and omnibuses', as Boz explains (81–2), and went into decline. But the hackney coach in Boz's essay is more than an aspect of a transport system. It becomes a character to sketch in its own right: a unique, eccentric, and shabby inhabitant of London itself. Boz acknowledges that hackney coaches populate other cities, but only to 'maintain that hackney-coaches, properly so called, belong solely to the metropolis' (81). They represent a class of vehicles which Boz would systematize into his metropolitan taxonomy.

For Boz, the hackney coach represents more than a rickety and slow vehicle: it is also a synecdoche for the operators, horses, routes, and shilling-a-mile fares that constitute a certain metropolitan network with which Boz is very familiar:

> Our acquaintance with hackney-coach stands is of long standing. We are a walking book of fares, feeling ourselves, half bound, as it were, to be always in the right on contested points. We know all the regular watermen within three miles of Covent-garden by sight, and should be almost tempted to believe that all the hackney-coach horses in that district knew us by sight too, if one-half of them were not blind.
>
> (82)

---

[36] Stokes, 'Encabsulation', 239–40. [37] May, *Gondolas and Growlers*, 33.

The reference to 'three miles of Covent-garden' is telling, in that recent legislation for commercial privileges and fares had used such a set radius. The territory for licensed hackney coaches was traditionally the region covered by London's Bills of Mortality—a somewhat chilling overlap with the fatalities that increasingly indexed London's traffic. From 1828 to 1853, that coverage was redrawn, encircled by a three-mile radius from the General Post Office, St. Martin's-le-Grand.[38] An 1853 licensing act described a four-mile radius around Charing Cross station. In each scheme, few cab journeys were made beyond the legislated boundary. The licensed territory essentially circumscribes a metropolis by its network of commercial passenger traffic. So too does it circumscribe the boundaries of a 'knowledge of London' which an aspiring driver would have to know.

The *Monthly Review* sneered that such a metropolitan horizon profoundly limited Boz's capacities as a writer: 'he may never have been twenty miles from Temple Bar, which indeed is not unlikely, if one is to judge from these "Sketches"'.[39] But that zone is precisely where Boz intervenes, hijacking the operating networks which produce the knowledge of London. Though he became one of London's most famous pedestrians, Dickens would have made a great cab driver. He was famous in his day for an encyclopaedic command of London geography. Like Sam Weller (whose father Tony was a coach driver) in *The Pickwick Papers*, his 'knowledge of London was extensive and peculiar'.[40] Dickens would have passed the 'knowledge' examination on the first try. Or at least Boz would have: he is 'a walking book of fares'. In the longer quote above, Boz uses his 'book' to defend against fraud, commonly suspected of drivers whose very conditions of employment, as Moore points out, were 'calculated to encourage extortion'.[41] This 'book' is not just a figure of speech: actual fare books were part of 'the extraordinary range of information designed for London's cab passengers in the nineteenth century, [including] fare books, lists, posters and maps'.[42] These texts and visual aids were intended to help passengers negotiate with drivers, plotting their own routes against given rates and thus resolving 'the uncertainty at the root of passengers' experience of cabs'.[43] Many popular guides, beginning with John Carey's

---

[38] Henry Charles Moore, *Omnibuses and Cabs: Their Origin and History* (London: Chapman & Hall, 1902), 233, <http://books.google.com/books?id=i33tAAAAMAAJ>.
[39] 'Rev. of Sketches by "Boz," Illustrative of Every-day Life and Every-day People', *Monthly Review*, March 1836, 357.
[40] Charles Dickens, *The Posthumous Papers of the Pickwick Club*, Oxford Illustrated Dickens (Oxford; New York: Oxford University Press, 1987), 269. Interestingly, Michael Slater describes Sam Weller as 'a racier, fully characterised, successor to Boz in Dickens's oeuvre'; see Slater, *Charles Dickens*, 76.
[41] Moore, *Omnibuses and Cabs*, 238.   [42] Dobraszczyk, 'Useful Reading?', 121.
[43] Dobraszczyk, 'Useful Reading?', 122.

New Guide for Ascertaining Hackney Coach Fares (1801), claimed to have actually measured the streets and offered passengers personal notes and diagrams that reveal such texts as fascinating generic experiments.

Boz's 'walking book' is a similar hybrid of written genres and modes of visual and textual representation. With them, he fashions a mental map of metropolitan routes comprising pedestrian, vehicular, and textual experiences. *Sketches by Boz*, in addition to being recognizable as an exercise in urban classification, also registers as part of the diverse print culture competing to inform urban travellers.[44] As a 'book of fares', *Sketches* joins this array of printed information, converting the social uncertainties and visual phantasmagoria of urban transport into a textual experience. These were not just books about transport but also books, pamphlets, and papers aboard it. In 1851, observing 'the introduction of books and newspapers into some of the metropolitan omnibuses', *Punch* quips that these texts 'turn every omnibus into a vehicle for knowledge'.[45] Years earlier, Boz was already exploiting this collapsing metaphor, using the omnibus to fashion his generic vehicles, writing about and for the transport economy itself.

Not only in the business of books and newspapers, Boz implicitly competes within a transit system of 'knowing' and navigating London. Boz represents, like the omnibus, the replacement of the hackney coach: his vision bests the blind horses pulling the vehicles; he celebrates the omnibus; and he writes the *Sketches* as itself a 'walking book of fares'—an extensive, peculiar, and wide-eyed survey. It becomes a mode of imaginative transit claiming to be a licensed form of knowing the metropolitan radius. Boz was charging fares, too: unlike his earlier tales for the *Monthly Magazine*, the street sketches in the *Morning Chronicle* were the first for which Dickens was actually paid. Dickens sold them not as literary fiction but as 'essays'—excursions which many readers praised as a fair guide to London's social topography.[46]

Then again, maybe he would not have made a great driver, as Boz confesses himself accident prone: 'We take great interest in hackney-coaches, but we seldom drive, having a knack of turning ourselves over when we attempt to do so' (82). Considering how Boz describes the qualifications and professional habits of employed drivers, this probably would not disqualify him from taking the reins. Accidents, collisions, and

---

[44] For the fascinating range of graphical and textual attempts to represent this zone and its routes to passengers in print, see Dobraszczyk, 'Useful Reading?'.
[45] 'Riding and Reading', *Punch*, 1851, 241.
[46] Chittick, *Dickens and the 1830s*, 48.

tactical jostling seem as ubiquitous as the vehicles themselves.[47] For example, near the end of 'Hackney-coach Stands', Boz notes the interminable slowness of these vehicles, but ironically declines to take a cab instead: 'Talk of cabs! Cabs are all very well in cases of expedition, when it's a matter of neck or nothing, life or death, your temporary home or your long one' (84). Omnibuses too—their routes seemingly prescribed and undeviating—are similarly subject to accidents and collisions, especially considering their enterprising drivers and conductors who were so frequently depicted as having a colourful, if not criminal, past.

Accidents and the dangers of street traffic were certainly on the public mind, parliamentary agenda, and pages of newspapers. While those concerns relate to the chaos and competition within new forms of passenger and commercial traffic, they also expose anxieties about insurgency or criminality in the urban male population of the lower classes. Boz claims to sketch representative examples in the guises of drivers, watermen, and conductors or 'cads', but his fascination with their comic, carnivalesque, and sometimes dangerous behaviour should be qualified. For Regenia Gagnier, it is symptomatic of a bourgeois fantasy about working-class masculinity, at once exoticized and exploited by 'popular fictive and semifictive representations of London "lowlife" that romanticized the "freedom" of streetfolk and sensationalized their "violence".'[48] There is much to agree with here, but Boz also exploits such 'freedom' and 'violence' to other ends: not simply to fantasize the working class, but to intervene in disciplines of which would circumscribe their agency, including traffic policing and social classification.[49]

In attending to the mishaps of traffic, the transport sketches emphasize the presence of accidents within the system whose 'progress' Boz ironically charts. In a basic sense, a traffic 'accident' refers to the unintentional collisions of material bodies, whether vehicles, persons, and/or things. In Boz's sketches, accident also ironically signals the intentional disruptions by which drivers and conductors compete with other operators and manipulate their customers or 'fares'. And it can also suggest the haphazardness of a dynamic system of routes and deviations, routines and chance

---

[47] In general, urban horse traffic had a poor accident record, as Lay argues, as 'the behavior of horse traffic was much less disciplined and less predictable than that of modern car traffic'. See M. G. Lay, *The Ways of the Road: A History of the World's Roads and of the Vehicles That Used Them* (New Brunswick, NJ: Rutgers University Press, 1992), 184.
[48] Gagnier, *Subjectivities*, 88.
[49] For Garcha, the cad embodies 'the hurried, irrepressible energy of London's modern, market culture' and 'shows the doubleness of modern, capitalist spatial and temporal motion: it inflicts psychic and physical damage, even to the point of death, but it also unleashes new, unprecedented amounts of energy'. See *From Sketch to Novel*, 136.

events, insurgent operators and the police. *Sketches by Boz* uses these overlapping significations of accident to characterize an emerging transport 'system' as well as to unsettle and ironize its own claims to systemic or classificatory understanding.

THE TRAFFIC OF ACCIDENTS

The sketches 'Hackney-cabs, and Their Drivers' and 'Some Account of an Omnibus Cad' each consider the newly popular vehicles rapidly displacing the hackney coach—vehicles which seem 'ubiquitous' and 'omnipresent' to Boz's eye (144). Each sketch—particularly revealed by their revised, conjoined version 'The Last Cab-Driver, and the First Omnibus Cad'—is also concerned with charismatic operators, whom Boz claimed might actually be related by kinship but certainly belong to the same 'class of men' (151). So used, 'class' simultaneously evokes the socio-economic difference that Gagnier cites as well as a classificatory grouping within Boz's loose taxonomy. What distinguishes these sketches is their attention to the relations between individual and categorical class, drawn in several ways: as the effects of a single vehicle upon the 'progress of the system' of which it is a part; as the ironic attempt to classify an 'eccentric' character who by definition breaks taxonomic logic; and as the comic mutual dependency of the rogue and the regulatory police. 'Accident' (in its various senses) is the mediating principle in each context. Boz makes accident the exception, which time and again proves the unruly.

After the licensing monopoly of hackney carriages was broken, cabs proliferated in London, most of them 'painted in the most startling and conflicting colours' to better attract the attention of fares.[50] One such cab catches Boz's roving eye again and again:

> wherever we went, City or West End, Paddington or Holloway, North, East, West, or South, there was the red cab, bumping up against the posts at the street corners, and turning in and out, among hackney-coaches, and drays, and carts, and waggons, and omnibuses, and contriving by some strange means or other, to get out of places which no other vehicle but the red cab could ever by any possibility have contrived to get into at all.
>
> (142)

Cabriolets were smaller, lighter, and fleeter than their fellow vehicles on the streets, and drivers apparently took advantage, trying to shoulder out the competition. For Boz, what makes the 'red cab' unique is its coexistence as a singular and general phenomenon. The red cab contrives to

[50] Moore, *Omnibuses and Cabs*, 227.

occupy all of the interstices of street traffic, 'wherever' Boz might go. In the sketch, the red cab's 'ubiquity' also means the ubiquity of its accidents: collisions of chance as well as contrivance. To board a cab is to 'trust to chance' and submit to its 'strange means': as Boz explains, getting into a cab is difficult, but getting out is harder: 'we think the best way is, to throw yourself out, and trust to chance for alighting on your feet' (143).[51] Or aim for the driver, who might break your fall. Even a passenger hesitant to make such an uncertain exit might find themselves ejected by accident. According to Moore, cab drivers were 'fond of showing their superior speed' and vehicular dexterity, but 'while doing so frequently ran against street posts or collided with other vehicles; and when either of these things happened, or the horse fell, the "fare" was usually pitched forward into the road'.[52] Boz animates just such an episode:

> the red cab; it was omnipresent. You had but to walk down Holborn, or Fleet-street, or any of the principal thoroughfares in which there is a great deal of traffic, and judge for yourself. You had hardly turned into the street, when you saw a trunk or two, lying on the ground: an uprooted post, a hat-box, a portmanteau, and a carpet-bag, strewed about in a very picturesque manner: a horse in a cab standing by, looking about him with great unconcern; and a crowd, shouting and screaming with delight, cooling their flushed faces against the glass windows of a chemist's shop.—'What's the matter here, can you tell me?'—'O'ny a cab, sir.'—'Anybody hurt, do you know?'—'O'ny the fare, sir.'
>
> (144)

The reckless red cab transforms the streetscape from the inside out. It is an integral and disruptive element in the traffic it newly characterizes, 'omnipresent' in 'the principal thoroughfares' and in 'traffic'. The 'picturesque', ironically invoked here, similarly integrates disorder into a governing aesthetic, ready-made for a sketch artist of urban disarray.[53] This accident

---

[51] Getting in and out of early cabriolets was indeed difficult, and many passengers—particularly the elderly or anyone unwilling to 'trust to chance'—welcomed the introduction after 1840 of the four-wheeled cab, whose most popular version was the brougham. Moore, *Omnibuses and Cabs*, 225.

[52] Moore, *Omnibuses and Cabs*, 208.

[53] Garcha offers useful perspectives of the relations between the sketch, the picturesque, and the modern city:

> As the sites where new goods entered the marketplace, new technology and new printed works first appeared, and new modes of creating and consuming money arose, cities seemed to exist in a state of constant flux. . . . Like the continually transforming landscapes that William Gilpin asserts can only be captured by extemporaneous, unfinished pencil sketching, urban life appeared to be a subject that might only be represented with a quick, ready hand.

See *From Sketch to Novel*, 113.

immediately provokes questions from the narrator, an implied accident reporter or 'penny-a-liner' on the scene.[54] What is the source of this massive upheaval? Only a cab.

The 'red cab's licensed driver' is missing. Until he coolly walks out of the shop, takes the reins again, and starts off 'at full gallop', spreading his particular mayhem into the general traffic (144). Boz says 'the influence it exercised' also extends to the courts of justice. When the driver does get 'pulled up' in court, the Lord Mayor, the constables, and police offers are so taken with the driver's irrepressible comedy as to release him again at 'full gallop...to impose on somebody else' (144). The police, the crowd 'screaming with delight', and Boz himself are all too pleased with the red cab's insurgent potential, transforming commercial traffic into entertainment for public view and published sketch. While it is possible to argue, as does Gagnier, that the sketch popularizes and sensationalizes the violence of this character, effectively delimiting the agency which might be available to him, Boz has larger designs in sketching his accident-prone drivers.

The original sketch does conclude with the red cab driver's eventual incarceration. In the revised and combined sketch, 'The Last Cab-Driver, and the First Omnibus Cad', Boz extends the driver's influence, proposing a genealogy of sketchy operators who spread discord throughout London's traffic. Originally published as 'Some Account of an Omnibus Cad', the appended sketch offers a complementary take of the accidents on an omnibus.[55] This particular bus takes a downtown route via Oxford Street, recalling Boz's daily commute in the earlier sketch 'Omnibuses'. However, 'Some Account of an Omnibus Cad' does not strongly distinguish the bus from other public conveyances. Its operators have done all the rounds. The omnibus has two working employees: first, a driver who was formerly an 'enterprising young cabman, of established reputation as a dashing whip—for he had compromised with the parents of three scrunched children, and just "worked out" his fine for knocking down an old lady' (149). And second, a conductor, one Mr William Barker who is hired because of his 'qualifications' (149)—including having been transported for seven years to a penal colony and his subsequent job watering horses at

---

[54] In his youth, Dickens was paid as a 'penny-a-liner' by the short-lived *British Press* for 'bringing to the paper voluntary reports of accidents or fires not covered by the paper's regular reporters'. See Slater, *Charles Dickens*, 27.

[55] Though larger and running on prescribed routes, omnibuses sometimes raced and careened in traffic with the same abandon as cabriolets. Citing one set of early omnibus competitors—whose racing was sometimes encouraged by passengers—Moore points out that 'the accidents which they caused in their wild career became so appallingly numerous' as to incite governmental rewards for whistleblowers. See Moore, *Omnibuses and Cabs*, 49–50.

a hackney coach stand. The term 'transport' here combines criminal deportation with work on passenger vehicles. As Boz speculates, he is transported back to London for a reason: 'the British Government required Mr. Barker's presence here', putting him to work at a hackney coach stand 'with a brass plate and number suspended round his neck by a massive chain' (148). Barker is not paroled, but subject to the discipline of a new form of 'transportation'—licensed commercial traffic. But it is here that Barker escapes.

The omnibus has a reckless driver at the wheel, but Boz focuses more on Barker for his disruptive potentials. Like his predecessor, the 'red cab's licensed driver', Barker makes mayhem and spreads it widely into notions of systems and governance. Like the former cabman now driving the omnibus, Barker sees the coming change in the economy of urban transport, and he is too smart to be left holding the reins: 'The genius of Mr. Barker at once perceived the whole extent of the injury that would be eventually inflicted on cab and coach stands, and, by consequence, on watermen also, by the progress of the system' (148). That systemic change gets characterized as an inflicted injury, an ironic form of 'progress' which literalizes the collision of competing forms of traffic. In this same injurious spirit, Mr Barker embarks 'on a new sphere of action' (149). His 'genius' contrasts with 'the public mind', suggesting that if the latter goes 'in a new direction', Mr Barker contrives to direct and disrupt its route.

By ironically electing Mr Barker as a 'genius' and 'the first omnibus cad', Boz imagines him as the driver of systemic change, or at least the inaugurator of an emerging class of conductors who, because of the impertinences for which Barker is famous, became known as 'cads'. Here as elsewhere, Boz claims to be drawing from everyday life. In the 1830s, the omnibus 'cad' had already become a public nuisance, prompting *The Times* to classify its type: the 'Ill-conducted Conductor' as opposed to the 'Well-conducted Conductor'.[56] (Moore offers a useful caveat that omnibus passengers were just as unruly; *The Times* also published a guide to 'Omnibus Law' in 1836, essentially a guide for proper passenger behaviour, which was also apparently in short supply.[57]) Boz is drawn to the 'cad' for precisely the conceptual tension in *The Times*' sobriquet: the 'Ill-conducted Conductor' who might be the professional embodiment of the 'discord of order' that Mudie perceives as a new metropolitan condition.

---

[56] 'Omnibus Conductors', *The Times* (London), 29 January 1841, 5. For additional background on the 'cad', see Moore, *Omnibuses and Cabs*, 51–8.
[57] 'Omnibus Law', *The Times*, 30 January 1836, 3.

'The First Omnibus Cad' has also attracted attention from critics who want to rescue the *Sketches* from its imputed policing functions, romanticization of low life, or displacement of middle-class anxieties. Ian Wilkinson emphasizes the fluidity of identities among the underclass in the *Sketches*, as figures like Barker use the carnivalesque to upend social functions and types.[58] Geoffrey Hemestedt similarly argues that Barker disturbs the socioeconomic classification of selfhood that Boz means to critique: 'For Boz the phenomena of the city proclaim a crisis of classification that cannot be resolved by such a word, a fall-back category to which we are invited to consign those citizens who do not fit into the dominant order'.[59] In this sense, Boz does not seek to classify at all, but to show its failure to accommodate second-order economies, to imagine collective social identities made possible by the dynamics outside the mainstream of capital. Thus, Barker encapsulates the overall project of the *Sketches* to challenge taxonomic coherence and dispute the emerging discourses of social classification.

Mr Barker is quite a character, which is to say that—like John Dounce of 'Love and Oysters' in the sketch immediately preceding—he is an eccentric.[60] As Amanda Anderson suggests, Dickens's 'gallery of eccentric caricatures reflects a profound fascination with the forces of social determination' and the personae who may escape its field.[61] In the sketch as first published, Dickens writes a comic faith in destiny directly into Barker's character, describing him in the final paragraph '[l]ike many other great men' as 'a rigid predestinarian'. Boz roundly mocks what he calls this 'logical mode of reasoning' through Barker's vernacular after the cad roughs up an impertinent customer who threatens to report him to the cops: 'If I am to get into trouble for this 'ere consarn, I may as vell get into trouble for somethink as for nothink'. At a glance, Barker seems like a working-class clown performing a gag on philosophical necessitarianism. But Barker is anything but subject to a deterministic logic. Though tangled in petty crime and in trouble with the police, he escapes discipline as easily as the red cab driver avoids a traffic jam. As Boz describes, '[h]is feverish attachment to change and variety nothing could repress; his native daring no punishment could subdue' (147). The paradox of 'a rigid predestinarian' who is also feverishly committed to 'change and variety' establishes the dynamic of determinism/liberty or fatality/accident by which the sketch operates.

[58] 'Performance and Control: The Carnivalesque City and Its People in Charles Dickens's *Sketches by Boz*', *Dickens Studies Annual* 35 (2005): 1–19.
[59] Hemestedt, 'Inventing Social Identity', 226.
[60] Slater claims that '[t]he sprightly cad described in "Omnibuses"... has some claim to be considered the first original "Dickens character".' *Charles Dickens*, 44.
[61] Anderson, *Tainted Souls and Painted Faces*, 66.

Boz conveys the story of William Barker through a sequence of increasingly specific anecdotes, moving from the commercial type—'a waterman of our acquaintance, who, on one occasion, [we met] when we were passing the coach-stand over which he presides' (146)—to the man himself: 'The identical waterman afterwards attained a very prominent station in society;... we know something of his life' (147). As Wilkinson argues, because of Barker's carnivalesque agency, this 'waterman' of acquaintance evolves from the 'identical waterman' to 'Mr. William Barker', to 'Bill Boorker', and to 'Aggerawatin Bill': he breaks the subjective mold of self-identical routinized labour. The 'prominent station' he attains is equally unstable. The process of his transformations remains inscrutable: 'We at once avow a similar inability to record at what precise period, or by what particular process, this gentleman's patronymic, of William Barker, became corrupted' (147). Since he cannot 'record', Boz will instead 'remark' the dynamics of Barker's personae, which change thanks to 'remarkable' incidents. These keywords occur throughout the *Sketches*. Like the city, Barker is a palimpsest upon which to re-mark and re-classify, tracing the ordinary from extraordinary moments. His otherwise marginalized identity is neither indelible nor interiorized but contingent, taking shape amid the traffic of urban accidents.

The introduction of the 'identical waterman' heads a remarkable sequence of how Boz ironizes the connections between his man-on-the-street experience and his narratives. Especially fascinating about this passage is how Boz works through the language of probability, which, when coupled with the 'logical mode of reasoning' of Barker's ironic predestinarianism, brings into focus the epistemological contests in the *Sketches*. From his previous, generalized experiences with the waterman, Boz introduces 'Mr. William Barker' as a representative example to support his claims about the omnibus cad:

> as we know something of his life, and have often thought of telling what we do know, perhaps we shall never have a better opportunity than the present.
> Mr. William Barker, then, for that was the gentleman's name, Mr. William Barker was born—but why need we relate where Mr. William Barker was born, or when? Why scrutinise the entries in parochial ledgers, or seek to penetrate the Lucinian mysteries of lying-in hospitals? Mr. William Barker *was* born, or he had never been. There is a son—there was a father. There is an effect—there was a cause. Surely this is sufficient information for the most Fatima-like curiosity; and, if it be not, we regret our inability to supply any further evidence on the point. Can there be a more satisfactory, or more strictly parliamentary course? Impossible.
> (147, original emphasis)

At the moment Boz embarks on Barker's biography, he summarily discards as ridiculous all the conventional forms of documenting such a life.[62] Boz plays with the dissonance of, on the one hand, the classificatory evidence of archives and human memory, and, on the other, the irrepressible, singular persona that constantly escapes such scrutiny. Where does he come from, what does he do, who is responsible for Mr William Barker? In classifying 'the first omnibus cad', the model of the type, Dickens wants us to recognize that his primary evidence, Barker, is, in all probability, made up. He wants us to accept the fabulistic as parliamentary-grade proof of Barker's identity. Our 'Fatima-like curiosity' must be satisfied; do not go looking any further. As she peeks into Bluebeard's closet and discovers the corpses of her predecessors, Fatima is shocked to realize that she, too, is potentially another one in the series, not individuated as the singular beloved as Bluebeard would have her believe. The skeleton in Boz's closet, which he alternately showcases and stashes away, is his complicity with rendering individuals into dehumanized types.

Boz occupies a problematic position both within and outside the discipline of social classification, metaphorically wanting both to float over the rooftops and saunter down any given byway, as Audrey Jaffe has argued.[63] But the 'Omnibus Cad' suggests these impulses may not be contradictory. The sketch uses Barker to dramatize the instabilities of any approach to classification. His satire is equal-opportunity: he puts all forms of documenting identity, discourses of fact, or 'logical mode[s] of reasoning' on the level of his street fable or Lucinian mystery.[64] As J. Hillis Miller famously pointed out, the *Sketches* time and again make conspicuous their own fictionality, and yet were still credited—and in some places still are—as 'close and accurate' reflections of the Victorian city.[65] In Miller's deconstructionist reading, Boz reveals the fabulistic at the heart of codes of the real: ledgers, history, parliaments, and urban sketches too. All depend on a myth of stable causality to determine the social. In the

---

[62] As Grillo points out, the sentence 'Mr. William Barker was born—' was the opening line of the originally separate sketch 'Some Account of an Omnibus Cad'. See *End in the Beginning*, 104.

[63] Audrey Jaffe, *Vanishing Points: Dickens, Narrative, and the Subject of Omniscience* (Berkeley, CA: University of California Press, 1991), 35.

[64] In her magisterial *A History of the Modern Fact: Problems of Knowledge in the Sciences of Wealth and Society* (Chicago, IL: University of Chicago Press, 1998), Poovey explains the rhetorical structures by which discourses of fact validated themselves, offering a compelling interpretive model for how Boz's sketches—claiming a transparency that is the sketch's generic privilege—were subsequently received.

[65] J. Hillis Miller, 'The Fiction of Realism: Sketches by Boz, Oliver Twist, and Cruikshank's Illustrations', in *Charles Dickens and George Cruikshank: Papers Read at a Clark Library Seminar on May 9, 1970* (Los Angeles, CA: William Andrews Clark Memorial Library, University of California, 1971), 1–69.

Sketches, Dickens offers instead a faith in paradox, in accidental and strange conjunctions, which enables the art of reimagining the city, its social types, and the individual agents who animate them.

Boz shifts from singularity to generality and back again. At first, Boz asserts of Barker that he really knows 'something of his life' and right now is the time to tell; from the social type of 'waterman' we get the proper name 'Mr. William Barker'. But then the narrator interrupts at the precise moment of individual explication: 'Mr. William Barker was born—but. . . ' If Barker continually defies types, so this sketch swerves at the threshold of its own generic type: the biographical history, in which so and so was born, and so forth. The sketch veers from the past tense and back to the 'opportunity' of the 'present', which is the moment of reading 'Some Account of an Omnibus Cad'. Boz gives up probing the archives of civic institutions from which a biographer might extrapolate someone's character. 'Mr. William Barker' may have appeared in parochial ledgers and hospitals, but, like the line of the dash that interrupts his documented history, 'Mr. William Barker' becomes merely a trace, a ghost in the archives of generalized knowledge, and a phantasm of the deductive logic that underwrites civic administration and parliamentary procedures. Barker must have been born: sons have fathers, effects have causes. But the dashes in this passage suggest that Boz gives up on the so-called problem of induction: 'There is an effect—there was a cause'. The connection between cause and effect, in that dash, is either broken or an unprovable article of faith, à la David Hume. According to Hume, we solve the induction problem by going about our daily business. Likewise does Dickens cashier the expected causal patterns of social determination for the emergent self-making that Barker performs in traffic. Dickens relocates the authoritative source of this person's identity not in bureaucratic demonstration, not in generic biographical claims, but in the irreducible vitality of his comic enterprise.

Dickens stakes the sketch's documentary status on its very irony. The paradox comes home in the sentence 'Mr. William Barker *was* born, or he had never been'. On the one hand, such a claim mocks the procedural pomposity of parliamentary proof, which also fuels the comedy of sketches like 'The Parlour Orator'. On the other, the statement gets comic energy from the darker side of the blatantly obvious: it plays with the representational uncertainty of the 'or': Barker is real, he is made up, it does not matter which. In other words, here is this particular person who might have never been born and upon whom the structure of social classification depends. The entire passage ends with 'Impossible', the punch line to the jokes about causal certainties. 'Impossible' is also a fabulist's confession, which closes the logic of the joke into a kind of hermeneutic. The joke establishes its own insider logic while taking apart the prevailing logic of its targets: civic archives, parliamentary proceedings, readers' everyday experiences. 'Impossible' becomes, impossibly, the stable logical ground by which the story of Mr William Barker can now proceed. As against the perpetually fraught discourses of factual validation, Dickens claims that self-contradiction, whimsy, and play are functions of classification.

Barker is not simply a romanticized stereotype of the criminal class or unrepressed desire, but a 'rogue' in the sense of a free radical, Maxwell's demon operating in the flesh in the city. On the streets and within the discourse of social classification that would neatly pin him down as a specimen, Barker is a vital force of accident and tactical social insurgency. And yet as the 'omnibus cad', Barker still shines in the constellation of urban social types that Boz charts. In this double role, Barker warps the gravity of Boz's social classification just as he changes the traffic network of which he is both a professional and criminal operator. In a stunning paragraph towards the end of the essay, Dickens sketches out an influence model for Barker's impact:

> To recapitulate all the improvements introduced by this extraordinary man into the omnibus system—gradually, indeed, but surely—would occupy a far greater space than we are enabled to devote to this imperfect memoir. To him is universally assigned the original suggestion of the practice which afterwards became so general—of the driver of a second bus keeping constantly behind the first one, and driving the pole of his vehicle either into the door of the other, every time it was opened, or through the body of any lady or gentleman who might make an attempt to get into it; a humorous and pleasant invention, exhibiting all that originality of idea, and fine, bold flow of spirits, so conspicuous in every action of this great man.
>
> (149)

Boz calls his sketch an 'imperfect memoir'. It might justifiably be read as a memoir of imperfections, not necessarily of a biographical subject, but an omnibus one, so to speak. Barker drives the haphazard transformations of the sketch genre and transportation system alike by imperfections, by accidents. In this sense, Barker hints at the evolution of character, narrative, or systemic understanding through mutation. Unlike biological science which came to formalize such a development hypothesis, Dickens makes no attempt to stabilize the process in an objective discourse that pretends to stand outside of it. Instead, his sketches gleefully embrace their own status as an imperfect and evolving genre.

This passage, in all its comic irony, outlines these developmental principles at work. Boz, with tongue firmly in cheek, credits Barker nonetheless with specific innovations to a general system. Barker is the 'extraordinary' source of the ordinary textures of public experience. Consider the diction in this passage of *universal, original, general*: Barker introduces a paradigm shift in omnibus behaviour that works from the ground up, rather than from the top down. In other words, the exception rewrites the rules of systemic change. Pattern-breaking singularity and bone-breaking accident get incorporated—'gradually, indeed, but surely'— into a system of urban exchange and a conception of metropolitan life. In the background are echoes of catastrophism and gradualism and their political associations with models of radical and conservative change. Barker enables the mixing of both. He is so thoroughly a part of the 'omnibus system' as to define it: the very phrase 'omnibus system' contradicts its would-be systemic totality. Whatever system this is—bus routes, the social body, London—it works as a carnivalesque counter-narrative to metropolitan improvement and a process of development that is gradual and sure.

That strange process reappears in the ending of 'The Last Cab-driver, and the First Omnibus Cad' when Boz sarcastically laments the disappearance of these figures:

> Improvement has peered beneath the aprons of our cabs, and penetrated to the very innermost recesses of our omnibuses. Dirt and fustian will vanish before cleanliness and livery. Slang will be forgotten when civility becomes general: and that enlightened, eloquent, sage, and profound body, the Magistracy of London, will be deprived of half their amusement, and half their occupation.
>
> (151)

This series of contrasts quickly sketches the metropolitan dialectics to which this 'class of men' makes a material contribution. 'Magistracy' depends upon insurgency, civilization upon its perception of barbarism, 'general' civility upon the singularities of slang. Barker and company seem to embody the second half of those equations, while the *Sketches* as a classificatory enterprise would represent the first. But, as Nead so thoroughly demonstrates, any metropolitan improvements or regulatory forms are bound to their opposites. Even London's first traffic light created as much mayhem as direction, frightening an otherwise-well-regulated troop of cavalry into confusion, causing the deaths of policemen, and in 1869 exploding and killing the operator attempting to light it.[66]

In a similar way, Barker represents the radical irruption of accidents into a system or into the social fabric; he becomes 'a man in public life' (149). That fabric is threaded with or torn by the traffic accidents that are

---

[66] Lay, *Ways of the Road*, 184.

his signature. Accident here literally means the collision of busses and passengers. But this kind of accident also stages the collision of interpretive paradigms. Behind every accident are questions of its intention or design and also questions about its possible randomness. With Barker, Dickens drags that collision into the middle of the street. Barker is at once the intention behind these accidents and the chameleonic specimen who is beyond capture, who disrupts traffic patterns and social systems alike by introducing randomness, spontaneous incident. He is an agent of accident with, as we might venture to call it, an accidental or omnibus agency: a masculine working-class subjectivity with various performances of type, with an omnibus potentiality. With Barker, Dickens elaborates what Sandra MacPherson calls 'a liberal countertradition focusing on harms rather than rights, accident rather than will'.[67] On an alternate trajectory of the modern liberal subject, MacPherson proposes that flat, typed, or thing-like characters ethically engage with a world of things. In this world, moral exemplarity is less useful than a sense of integrated responsibility. MacPherson traces this to the realist novel's 'formal and sociological interest in accidents'—an idea I elaborate in the following chapter, but her framework also helps recover Barker, Boz, and the urban sketch for Dickens's intervention into sociology.[68]

Far from rejecting the impulse to classify, generalize, and type, Dickens sets out to do so while allowing the tropes of accident to effloresce into what forms they may. In *Sketches by Boz*, Dickens leverages accident against the determinism of social type, even while obviously and exuberantly engaging in the practices of social typing. Dickens does not merely reinscribe a static taxonomic order of society in different ink, but animates the deep ambiguities if not contradictions of discourses which would theorize urban or systemic development. Those ambiguities manifest not only in the subjects that our enterprising taxonomist sets out to classify, but also in the particular generic conventions he employs for the work.

THE OMNIBUS GENRE

Boz's attention to urban transport makes conspicuous how accidents are at once integral and disruptive. They are part and parcel of the experience of 'fares' and they are inscribed within Boz's 'walking book' as a condition of urban knowledge. That dynamic extends throughout *Sketches by Boz*

---

[67] Sandra MacPherson, *Harm's Way: Tragic Responsibility and the Novel Form* (Baltimore, MD: Johns Hopkins University Press, 2010), 4.
[68] MacPherson, *Harm's Way*, 190.

which licenses 'accidental' notions of causality through generic and narrative conceits. Dickens's readers have credited the sketch genre as a 'close and accurate' description, a frame for social classification, and a textual encounter whose fragmentation and chance encounters seem finely tuned to an emerging metropolitan modernity. But *Sketches by Boz* does not merely indicate the changing social and phenomenal experiences of life in early-Victorian London. Instead, it imagines that experience on its own terms. And the vehicle for its 'knowledge of London' is genre. Boz pioneers a sketch genre that is at once interested in and structured by alternative notions of causality. Lukács named the novel as 'the most hazardous genre', but the street sketch might make a fair claim in its own reckoning with accident and metropolitan haphazardness.[69] The legacy of Dickens's London, or its apparent disclosure of an emerging urban modernity, is shaped by his accidental sketches.

Singular circumstances, providential encounters, eccentric persons, extraordinary happenings—these are keywords in writing the city as an accidental place. They are also telltales for how writers adapt urban randomness to narrative. Alexander Welsh underscores the incentives to associate the city with randomness, especially for writers like the young Dickens breaking into the narrative and anecdote business.[70] Julian Wolfreys claims that 'the city is performed through the chance viewing of its random elements which jumble together'.[71] A city of accidents and the unexpected licenses haphazard compositions of all sorts. Thus, the city time and again shows up in literary representations as a great gathering of incidents and the unexpected, which aspiring writers translated into professional capital.[72] For Wolfreys, such random jumbling is also symptomatic of blocked desires for classificatory order. In other words, the city reveals the dialectic between classificatory desires and the impossibility of their fulfilment.[73] That dynamic, between form and fragmentation, is likewise a signature of the sketch genre.

---

[69] György Lukács, *The Theory of the Novel; A Historico-Philosophical Essay on the Forms of Great Epic Literature*, trans. Anna Bostock (Cambridge, MA: MIT Press, 1971), 74.
[70] Alexander Welsh, *The City of Dickens* (London: Clarendon, 1971), 6.
[71] Julian Wolfreys, *Writing London: The Trace of the Urban Text from Blake to Dickens* (Basingstoke, Hampshire: Macmillan, 1998), 88.
[72] The narrator of *Life in London* makes this marketing strategy explicit: 'There is not a *street* in London but what may be compared to a large or small volume of intelligence, abounding with anecdote, incident, and peculiarities. A *court* or *alley* must be obscure indeed, if it does not afford some remarks.' The city is text, rich with unexpected incident enough to 'afford' a writer, newly speculating in fiction, to make his living. See Egan, 'Life in London', 25.
[73] This results from, in Wolfrey's Derridean view, deconstructive facets of language, the sheer proliferation of persons and things which exceed ordering, and the unknown chaotic energies of chance that consistently erupt within any system.

The sketch form enjoys a generic privilege of incompleteness and self-contradiction that, not unlike contemporaneous representations of London, seems to have its own accidental coherence.[74] Edgar Poe, reviewing a collected edition of *Sketches by Boz* in 1836, argues that the very fragmentation of the sketch gives it a 'unity of effect' which Poe ironically opposes to 'the common novel'.[75] Poe's defence of the sketch genre is part of an aesthetics of the tale or short story which he was so integral in theorizing.[76] There is another logic at work here, too. Poe, fascinated with the perverse, inverts the logic of accident/design as commonly mapped onto the sketch/novel. The brief sketch can achieve 'a quality not easily appreciated by an ordinary mind', but is nonetheless essential to its goals. Poe wants us to experience contingency as unity, fragmentation as generic success. But Dickens became less comfortable with fragmentation and increasingly tried to emphasize the premeditated design and 'unity of effect' in his subsequent novels, responding to the kind of critique levelled by R. H. Horne: 'Dickens evidently works upon no plan; he has a leading idea, but no design at all'.[77]

Where then do the sketches fit? Critics have varying perspectives about the relation of sketch and novel in Dickens's career. For example, Tim Killick argues that British writers of short fiction realized in sketches and collections a publication opportunity to compete with the novel.[78] Garcha is only the most recent to consider such sketches as 'literary apprenticeships' for the real (and realist) work of British novelists to come.[79] But the *literary* heritage of the sketch limits the horizon of its cultural engagements.[80] Certainly in Boz's hands, the sketch genre engages the broad interdisciplinary and intercommercial production of the knowledge of London. It joins an incredible array of textual forms and material practices

---

[74] From its long history in character sketches, a 'sketch' in eighteenth-century examples more typically marks out generalities or ideas. With young Dickens, as with his imitators, the sketch evolves into a study of the singular, from which general conclusions were often extracted, but with a focus on particularly, certain individuals, and specific places nonetheless. By 1840, the term 'sketchability' has arrived, being a property of particular objects. 'sketchability, *n.*', *Oxford English Dictionary* (Oxford University Press, 2012), <http://www.oed.com.proxy.lib.fsu.edu/view/Entry/180768?>.
[75] Edgar Poe, *Essays and Reviews* (New York: Library of America, 1984), 205.
[76] In *British Short Fiction in the Early Nineteenth Century: The Rise of the Tale* (Aldershot, Hampshire; Burlington, VT: Ashgate, 2008), Killick provides thorough background on the genre and its trans-Atlantic fortunes.
[77] Quoted in Peter Ackroyd, 'London Luminaries and Cockney Visionaries', in *The Collection* (London: Chatto & Windus, 2001), 424.
[78] Killick, *British Short Fiction in the Early Nineteenth Century*.
[79] Garcha, *From Sketch to Novel*, 27.
[80] So too its Anglophone heritage might be limiting—a horizon which Lauster deftly expands in her survey of European writers and sketch artists; see *Sketches of the Nineteenth Century*.

involved in knowing and navigating the metropolis, at a time when it too seems to have, to borrow Horne's phrase, 'no plan... no design at all'. As Marjorie Levinson has argued, the fragmentary sketch is symptomatic of a broader cultural fascination with imperfection and indeterminacy.[81] With its generic privilege of improbability, the sketch is uniquely suited to explore the margins of causality and order and the unstable metropolitan centre offered the perfect place for the job.

The *Sketches* have also been related to contemporary journalism. Sicher places the *Sketches* amid a new journalistic interest in particulars and quotidian events: 'The turn to a more pictorial journalism associated with... the *Morning Chronicle* offered imaginative illustrations of everyday incidents, of which Dickens's *Sketches by Boz* became a prime example and model'.[82] That these sketches illustrate and imaginatively transform the everyday are among their most enduring legacies. This city seems sensational, improbable, and episodic—like a newspaper, as Walter Bagehot famously suggested: 'Mr. Dickens's genius is especially suited to the delineation of city life. London is like a newspaper. Every thing is there, and every thing is disconnected'.[83] In some ways, *Sketches by Boz* does not pretend be anything else. Indeed, the 'Street Sketches' originally appeared in the columns of a daily paper. Not merely a model for 'imaginative illustrations of everyday incidents', the *Sketches* participate in the periodical development of news, especially the reporting of accidents and extraordinary things. Killick notes the 'proximity and free exchange' between tales, sketches, essays, and short stories in magazines.[84] That generic flexibility can also extend beyond literary forms; it typifies the fluidity of content within newspapers and the intertextuality of Boz's essays so published.

In this context, the literary sketch can be usefully related to the forms and functions of accident news identified in the previous chapter. Consider some of the publication circumstances surrounding Boz's sketches. On 16 September 1834, the *Morning Chronicle* published 'Omnibuses and Cabs'—proceedings from the police committee on '[t]he nuisances arising from omnibuses and cabs [which] increase in the city daily'. On 19 September, a letter to the editor 'On Preventing Accidents from Cabs, Omnibuses, &c.' made a suggestion about 'the numerous accidents which are continually occurring from the over-driving of cabs, omnibuses, &c.'

---

[81] Marjorie Levinson, *The Romantic Fragment Poem: A Critique of a Form* (Chapel Hill, NC: University of North Carolina Press, 1986), 9.
[82] Sicher, *Rereading the City, Rereading Dickens*, 1.
[83] Walter Bagehot, 'Charles Dickens', *The National Review* 7 (October 1858): 468.
[84] Killick, *Rise of the Tale*, 19.

On 26 September appeared 'Street Sketches—No. I.' subtitled 'Omnibuses' and signed by Boz. The second instalment of street sketches, 'Shops and Their Tenants' (10 October), occupies almost an entire column—but not quite. Boz has just explained that '[o]ne of our principal amusements is to watch the gradual progress—the rise or fall—of particular shops' (59). In the small space below is a paragraph on a catastrophic 'Destructive Fire' at a paint warehouse. In the column adjacent are entries on how 'Prince Augustus fell from his horse at Berlin on the 18th, and broke his leg' and titled 'Fatal Accident from Foul Air', a report on a labourer in Westminster who succumbed to miasma and fell while descending a well. The third street sketch (23 October) abuts a column headed 'The Late Calamitous Fire' at Parliament, reporting on fruitless inquiries at the House of Lords and Commons and the problematic curiosity of the public who want to see the ruins and take souvenirs. In the next column appears a coroner's inquest and a verdict of wilful murder. The fifth instalment of street sketches (15 December) is printed on the same page as 'Police Report Extraordinary' and 'City Improvements' concerning the 'skeletons' of several houses under construction.

While not the exhaustive contents of those issues, such news echoes the *Sketches*' interests in the motives, chances, inquiries, and objects comprising the mediated experience of the metropolitan everyday. If, as Poe argues, the sketch produces a 'unity of effect' by its very fragmentation, the newspaper produces similar effects of unity through miscellaneity. In the context of accident news—a category in which many of Boz's street sketches might comfortably fit—that 'unity of effect' is the suspension of causality. As Barthes argues of the *faits divers*, such news puts causality in 'suspension' between the rational and the unknown, and Boz's sketches operate on the same terrain.[85] With a hybrid of coincidence and causality, Dickens reveals the fallacies of urban sociology and suggests another vehicle for knowing London: the sketch genre, a textual *metaphorai* for getting around town, a hybrid of the newspaper and a walking book of fares.

Alison Byerly points out that literary sketches, 'while carefully contrived, maintain the feeling that we are accidentally glimpsing a momentary event'.[86] And Dickens 'repeatedly emphasizes the accidental origin' of his literary illustrations.[87] Considering the prominence of actual accidents

---

[85] Roland Barthes, 'Structure of the Fait-divers', in *Critical Essays*, trans. Richard Howard (Evanston, IL: Northwestern University Press, 1972), 194.

[86] Alison Byerly, 'Effortless Art: The Sketch in Nineteenth-Century Painting and Literature', *Criticism* 41, no. 3 (Summer 1999): 351.

[87] Byerly, 'Effortless Art', 355.

in these sketches as well as their proximity to related subjects in newspapers, I would modify Byerly's claim: Dickens uses the sketch to momentarily glimpse an *accidental* event.[88] In so doing, they take as their subject matter the paradox of causality that Barthes identifies. Dickens's sketches, so insistently accidental and part of a wave of everyday journalism, are immediately concerned with the phenomena of the ordinary, the remarkable particulars of urban experience and how they got that way. The spectacle and suspicion of coincidences, the tenuous meeting of the ordered and the aleatory, come home in his representations of the metropolis. Dickens puts this tenuous collision front and centre in his urban sketches: not merely to characterize the urban streets or to ironically suggest his own authorial design of what Boz claims to merely see. Instead, Dickens uses the sketch to dramatize the complicated work of social understanding in which the accidental reveals a dialectic beyond control. Thus, *Sketches by Boz* exposes the Victorian classificatory urge as a question of narrative. It offers itself as the experience of coming to grips not with the material, historical London, but with the expository practices of understanding it, which are anything but certain.

The sketch imagines itself as a window onto the instantaneous dynamics of urban masses and classes, for whom the sketch actually contrives social and narrative encounters. In Dickens's hands, the sketch is a tool to arrange chance compositions, an urban supercollider used to create the experimental conditions in which competing efforts to 'know London' take shape. It is an 'omnibus genre'—for its topical and discursive inclusiveness, certainly. But also because of its debts to commercial passenger traffic and its competitive ambitions to inscribe a 'knowledge of London' within its own generic vehicle. Moreover, like the 'omnibus system' which inaugurates Boz's metropolitan scenes and characters, his sketches absorb the accidental into their own systemic properties, in several senses. As a genre dynamically linked to the newspaper in which it flourished. As a literary commodity designed for collection in bound form with a unifying title—an 'omnibus title' according to Grillo.[89] As a supposed form of literary apprenticeship which informs the designs of more coherent novels. And as a text cited as evidence for disparate critical projects, from literary biography to formalism to historicism to deconstruction and back again. Grillo unintentionally suggests as much: 'Either by accident

---

[88] In this sense, George Cruikshank made an ideal illustrator for the *Sketches*: 'In each such picture Cruikshank catches a moment in which people are driven by the violence of their reactions to adopt without hindsight or foresight a gesture or pose that could only last an instant and then would pass, never to return.' See J. Hillis Miller, *Victorian Subjects* (Durham, NC: Duke University Press, 1991), 163.

[89] Grillo, *End in the Beginning*, 13.

or intention Dickens had hit upon a device for presenting a much more complicated picture of reality, and a form that could contain varying attitudes toward it while eliciting very different rhetorical responses'.[90] Grillo may miss the point about whether or not to credit Dickens for such an innovative form. Did he design it? Did it happen by accident? The play between 'accident or intention' is the very success of Dickens's project in the *Sketches*. That dynamo powers its classificatory intervention, its hybrid genre, and the knowledge of London that it bequeaths.

[90] Grillo, *End in the Beginning*, 73.

3

Industrial Accidents and Novel Insurances

> 'Something's up,' said Mary. She went to the door, and stopping the first person she saw, inquired the cause of the commotion.
> 'Eh, wench! donna ye see the fire-light? Carsons' mill is blazing away like fun;' and away her informant ran.
> 'Come, Margaret, on wi' your bonnet, and let's go to see Carsons' mill; it's afire, and they say a burning mill is such a grand sight.'
>
> Elizabeth Cleghorn Gaskell, *Mary Barton*

Early in Elizabeth Gaskell's 1848 novel *Mary Barton: A Tale of Manchester Life*, a cotton mill catches fire in the old business district of downtown Manchester and draws a huge, excited crowd to watch it burn.[1] Mary seems thrilled by the spectacle, which she hasn't before witnessed, though 'they say a burning mill is such a grand sight'. Fires in the city loomed large in the popular imagination as ready metaphors for the frenzy of England's urban-industrial growth in the first half of the nineteenth century. Because fires were frequent and very public catastrophes they provoked onlookers, property owners, journalists, novelists, Parliamentarians, and commercial parties like insurance directors to consider such accidents from various angles: scrutiny of their causes, worry over their frequency and damages, and development of financial and emotional structures to hedge against their recurrence.[2] Fires were part of a broader cultural negotiation of an emerging concept of risk, but they also seemed surprisingly resistant to prediction and forensic analysis. As dramatized by the draw of the burning factory in *Mary Barton*, these fires blazed away with the spectacle of risk unmanaged.

---

[1] In 1844 Henry Winkworth—silk manufacturer and father to Gaskell's friends Catherine and Selina—suffered a factory fire which may have inspired this episode in *Mary Barton*; see Graham Handley, *An Elizabeth Gaskell Chronology* (Basingstoke, Hampshire; New York: Palgrave Macmillan, 2004), 43.

[2] For a brief list of eye-catching fires across England in the first half of the Victorian period, see Clive Trebilcock, *Phoenix Assurance and the Development of British Insurance*, (Cambridge: Cambridge University Press, 1985), I, 424–5.

Fire had always posed infamous threats to urban life in England, though by the 1840s, it brought into focus other problems for which vocabularies and concepts were still developing. The disturbing prevalence of urban-industrial fires and the interesting array of responses to them provide the context for how 'accident' conceptually shifts into a risk to manage, into the domains of insurance and property and professional measurement. And even—for a brief period of time—into the domain of the coroner, as the first chapter has explained of William Payne. Payne's contested practice of adjudicating the causes of fires suggests how the coroner's legal horizon, the inquest into fatalities accidental or designed, was stretched to accommodate a problem for which other responses seemed inadequate. This chapter examines two other nascent forms of response which, like Payne's, stretched their own practices to accommodate the troubling causalities of the industrial metropolis: the fire insurance industry and the industrial novel. Sharing a preoccupation with urban-industrial calamities, they both accommodated accident's unsettled causalities with new strategies of written description.

As Eric Wertheimer has argued, unsettled concepts of risk, loss, and compensation formed a terrain of underwriting shared by the insurance and literary domains.[3] He claims that insurance is a writing business and that, next to literary endeavours, it is perhaps the most significant nineteenth-century business of figuring the representational fidelity of language. These insights can be linked to the broader discursive operations of risk management which, as Mary Poovey explains of the British financial system at large, involves representations from all sorts of mutually impinging cultural domains. Uniquely responsive to how professionals and publics depicted it, the financial system can hardly be distinguished from the practices of its representation. Thus, Poovey insists that financial instruments and writing 'need to be read as *interpretive descriptions*'.[4] As this chapter endeavours to show, responses to urban-industrial fires exemplify the ways that risk management imaginatively expanded its descriptive practices, reshaping concepts of probability in the process. In their writing about fires, both fire insurance and the industrial novel

---

[3] Eric Wertheimer, *Underwriting: The Poetics of Insurance in America, 1722–1872* (Palo Alto, CA: Stanford University Press, 2006). Stephen Arata in *Fictions of Loss in the Victorian Fin de Siècle* (Cambridge: Cambridge University Press, 1996) argues that 'fictions of loss' always concerned a related set of concepts in *fin de siècle* discourse about degeneracy: body, art, and nation. I use Wertheimer's study to argue that the 'writing of loss' similarly invokes a set of concepts—risk, loss, and compensation—that were active in early Victorian discourse about probability.

[4] Mary Poovey, ed., *The Financial System in Nineteenth-Century Britain* (New York: Oxford University Press, 2003), 5. Original emphasis.

intermingled strategies, contesting the interpretation of risk and compensation in ways that have lasting effects upon their institutions and genres.

As a genre, the Victorian industrial novel worked with and strained against the domain of insurance, which rivalled it as a conspicuous form of writing about risk and loss. Such crossover had been vital to the development of each, as Ian Baucom has suggested by comparing the 'novelizing protocols' of eighteenth-century insurance to the 'actuarial historicism' of the preromantic novel.[5] I am suggesting that the Victorian industrial novel and fire insurance present a unique case, updated for the problems of the nineteenth-century's accidental city and the forms of description it engendered. *Mary Barton* offers an ideal opportunity to scrutinize the interdependence of these writing practices and to see how the novel leverages its own heuristic practices against the frameworks of commercialized insurance on the rise. By the light of Gaskell's fictionalized accidents, we can see the interconnections of her novel with the emerging discourse of risk management and its particular struggle with fires. Lacking the coherent statistical approach that stabilized other types of insurance, fire insurers entertained a variety of evidentiary approaches to fire prediction, including descriptive, narrative, and tabular forms. In their reports and marketing, agents also relied upon scribal and sensational strategies more commonly associated with their literary contemporaries. For their part, novelists such as Gaskell shared certain concerns and writing practices by which fire insurers attempted, imperfectly, to contain the unprecedented risks of the industrial city. At stake were concepts of risk, loss, and compensation that defined relations to property and power. On the terrain of risk management, these professions recalibrated their descriptive practices with complex attitudes about probability and the importance of writing in its assessment.

These discursive contests also help us reframe the pervasive accidents of the novel as a genre. This chapter considers a novel trade in insurance in order to explore basic assumptions about realism and the trade of novelists. By locating the industrial novel within the discourse of risk management, I reframe its 'formal paradoxes' and even 'acute literary failure' in terms of its generic experiments with causality and Gaskell's professional status as a writer of loss.[6] Gaskell in *Mary Barton* recasts risk as something that novelists are uniquely suited to interpret. She asserts the novel's capacity

---

[5] *Specters of the Atlantic: Finance Capital, Slavery, and the Philosophy of History* (Durham, NC: Duke University Press, 2005), 16, 215.
[6] Catherine Gallagher, *The Industrial Reformation of English Fiction: Social Discourse and Narrative Form, 1832–1867* (Chicago, IL: University of Chicago Press, 1985), xv; Elaine Freedgood, *Victorian Writing About Risk: Imagining a Safe England in a Dangerous World* (Cambridge; New York: Cambridge University Press, 2000), 6.

to define the contested boundaries of this field by assessing risk and compensating for loss in a different currency. By exploring more affective dimensions of probability, Gaskell proposes that narrative itself might offer some readers as a compensatory experience for the disorientation and suffering of a modern, urban industrial condition. What results is a novel that takes accidents as thematic preoccupation as well as narrative opportunity. In direct contrast to what Henry James would deride as the Victorian novel's 'queer elements of the accidental and the arbitrary', *Mary Barton* instead reveals these elements as some of the most salient features of the cultural and aesthetic development of the genre.[7]

RISK WRITING IN CRISIS

Because of increased accidents, fraud, and arson often associated with labour disputes, factory and warehouse fires in the early nineteenth century were a prevalent and disturbing new problem to which few effective responses were possible.[8] Fire insurance emerged in England during the 1680s in consequence of the Great Fire of London, but it took on unprecedented importance for cities in the first half of the nineteenth century, particularly in the northern industrial belt.[9] Here, industrial construction far outpaced civic planning and oversight, factories suffered from haphazard operation and imperfect fire-prevention techniques, and political agitation brought unpredictable dangers. Touring the region in the 1840s, Engels claimed, 'it is precisely Manchester that has been built less according to a plan and less within the limitations of official regulations—and indeed more through accident—than any other town'.[10] The city seemed built by accident, accident prone, and beyond the regulatory reach of official oversight. Risk management was on uncertain ground. In an 1851 article for *The Assurance Magazine*, Samuel

---

[7] Henry James, 'Preface', in *The Tragic Muse*, VII, The Novels and Tales of Henry James (London: Macmillan, 1908).

[8] Robin Pearson, *Insuring the Industrial Revolution: Fire Insurance in Great Britain, 1700–1850* (London: Ashgate, 2004), 194.

[9] In the hyperbolic view of an 1839 article in the *London Saturday Journal*,

> *assurance* and *insurance* are two of the prime characteristics of the present age. They meet one everywhere—jostle us on the street, stare at us from the walls and the shop-windows, accost us on the Exchange and in the market-place, and twinkle on us in prospectuses, bills, and popular periodicals.
> (129)

[10] Friedrich Engels, *The Condition of the Working Class in England*, ed. Victor Kiernan (Harmondsworth, London; New York: Penguin, 1987), 86.

Brown complained that fire insurance especially lagged behind the business's curve.[11] Fire insurance firms, largely based in London, had little experience in the regions in which they hoped to expand and few dedicated employees to help adjust expectations and policies to compensate for risk in rapidly industrializing cities.[12] Many companies even doubted that fire followed regular patterns. Insurance companies accumulated data of past events in order to infer their future probability, but, with urban industrialization, they succumbed to a material version of Hume's epistemological quandary: 'Buildings and technologies changed too rapidly for past results to be generalized into the future'.[13] Not only were factory fires a new problem, but they also represented the problem of newness and the difficulty of imagining the future from the conditions of the present.

Gaskell's Manchester in *Mary Barton* is similarly an unprecedented amalgam of historical accretions and spasms of growth. The mill fire ignites on this threshold, a line that traces the political anxieties of the industrial city:

> Carsons' mill ran lengthways from east to west. Along it went one of the oldest thoroughfares in Manchester. Indeed, all that part of the town was comparatively old; it was there that the first cotton mills were built, and the crowded alleys and back streets of the neighbourhood made a fire there particularly to be dreaded.[14]

The mill offers another glimpse of Nead's Victorian Babylon in which the past continually interrupts the present: a dialectic of improvements and decay, light and darkness, order and anarchy. In Gaskell's Manchester, age and decrepitude are the combustible heartwood of the modernizing cityscape, and accident brings this paradox to light. Contemporary observers remarked how the factories at the heart of England's new industrial productivity and wealth were simultaneously the source of the nation's most conspicuous accidents and poverty.

As a business, insurance exploits and even exacerbates these very conditions of uneven property distribution. Writers like Gaskell on the

---

[11] Samuel Brown, 'On the Fires in London', in *The Assurance Magazine* (London: Charles & Edwin Layton, 1851), I, 31–62, <http://books.google.com/books?id=Fj0DAAAAYAAJ>.

[12] David Trevor Jenkins and Takau Yoneyama, eds., *The History of Insurance* (London: Pickering & Chatto, 2000), I, xxi.

[13] Theodore M. Porter, *Trust in Numbers: The Pursuit of Objectivity in Science and Public Life* (Princeton, NJ: Princeton University Press, 1995), 104. See also David Hume, *An Enquiry Concerning Human Understanding*, ed. Stephen Buckle (Cambridge: Cambridge University Press, 2007), 29–33.

[14] Elizabeth Cleghorn Gaskell, *Mary Barton: A Tale of Manchester Life*, ed. Jennifer Foster (Peterborough, ON; Orchard Park, NY: Broadview, 2000), 85–6. Subsequent references are to this edition and will be cited in line.

condition of England could find the 'two Englands' shadowed in insurance policies.[15] For instance, assurance companies (i.e. life insurance) discriminated heavily against workers in the selection and insurance of lives.[16] These companies instead focused on—and probably helped to define—an emerging professional class by 'selecting' as insurable lives less exposed to risk.[17] Discriminatory practices held true in fire insurance as well: since no provisions existed for *renters* in the 1840s, fire insurance imposed a de facto property qualification.[18] While fires on industrial properties may have resulted in claims for property owners, workers received no compensation and often lost their jobs. Injuries and loss of life were neither uncommon nor typically covered, save by ad hoc 'accident pools' or 'death pools' or by charities or Friendly Societies.[19] Additionally, liability claims for manufacturing accidents were much in dispute. Compensation for industrial injuries or accident victims ignored any damages that were not demonstrably physical, leaving sometimes debilitating emotional traumas unacknowledged and non-actionable.[20] While the asymmetries of insurance typically break along class lines, even the captains of industry with whom Gaskell was fascinated, such as Mr Thornton in *North and South* (1854–5), faced obstacles in the midst of the fire insurance crisis. Companies would refuse policies to factories, demand safety improvements, charge steep premiums, limit their coverage, or insure only parts of increasingly complex factories.[21] By some estimates, only half of the insurable property in Britain was covered by

---

[15] The word 'policy' extends an etymological root into the Middle French 'police', which, while denoting documents or written proof, also suggests the insurance industry's disciplinary and political functions. 'Policy' might readily substitute for its etymological kindred in scholarship on the politics of the industrial novel, or on the novel and the police.

[16] As Charles Babbage clarifies, 'The terms *insurance* and *assurance* have been used indiscriminately for contracts relative to life, fire, and shipping; [but] custom has rather more frequently employed the latter term for those relative to life'; see 'A Comparative View of the Various Institutions for the Assurance of Lives (1826)', in *The History of Insurance*, ed. Henry Jenkins and Takau Yoneyama (London: Pickering & Chatto, 2000), IV, 245.

[17] 'Lives' are described, in the insurance industry's own documentation, as its basic unit of trade. The term 'selection' reveals an implicit social Darwinism with profitability as the selection pressure on which 'lives' to insure: those with health, longevity, and non-dangerous work.

[18] My thanks to Tim Alborn for suggesting this and many other insights about types of insurances and their cultural functions.

[19] H. A. L. Cockerell and Edwin Green, *The British Insurance Business 1547–1970* (London: Heinemann, 1976), 39–40.

[20] Wolfgang Schivelbusch, *The Railway Journey: The Industrialization of Time and Space in the 19th Century* (Berkeley, CA: University of California Press, 1986), 135.

[21] Cockerell and Green, *The British Insurance Business 1547–1970*, 32; Pearson, *Insuring the Industrial Revolution*, 195.

1850 and policies frequently failed to the full extent of losses in cases like catastrophic fires.[22] Insurance companies themselves were losing money on fire insurance claims during the 1830s and 1840s.[23]

Much of this stemmed from the insufficiencies of their business practices, particularly on the part of fire insurers facing 'the increase in the size and complexity of risks, the rise of competition from new companies, and the growth of arson and fraud'.[24] In response, the insurance industry reviewed and refined its practices of assessing fire risk—practices in which writing and description, rather than quantification, took on perhaps unexpected roles. Fire insurers answered by employing agents and appointing committees to review properties, assess characters of potential clients, and interpret any fires in dispute. In the process, agents learned to observe closely, to record personal histories, and to describe with accuracy and vigour—making insurance archives a surprisingly rich resource of cultural data about economic relations, architectural spaces, and social identities.[25] As Baucom describes, the insurance industry developed 'thick descriptive protocols' and a 'historicizing operation' in its attention to particularity.[26] For example, the London-based Sun Fire Office blanketed their field agents with training documents about potential cases. These instructions stress the recording of all kinds of particulars as well as descriptions of objects, owners, and causal sequences. While this might not be surprising, an 1807 pamphlet emphasizes how such value depends on careful transcription: 'On delivering a new policy, read it over carefully, with the insured, when possible, and, if the buildings should be wrongly described, *which may vitiate the insurance*, or any other error be found therein, inform the office'.[27] Agents were responsible for transcribing persons and materials into a world of documentation organized by property values. These values were themselves insured by careful observation, writing, reading, and re-writing. The company warrants the otherwise problematic logic of fires through the representational fidelity of its contract.

The Sun Fire Office attempts to solve some of the unique problems of fires through its professional transactions in writing. Consider the Sun's instructions to their agents in the event of a fire:

---

[22] Trebilcock, *Development of British Insurance*, 1985, I, 11.
[23] Pearson, *Insuring the Industrial Revolution*, 194.
[24] P. G. M. Dickson, *The Sun Insurance Office, 1710–1960; The History of Two and a Half Centuries of British Insurance* (London: Oxford University Press, 1960), 140–1.
[25] Cockerell and Green, *The British Insurance Business 1547–1970*, 28, 32–3.
[26] Baucom, *Specters of the Atlantic*, 104.
[27] 'Instructions for the Agents of the Sun Fire Office', in *The History of Insurance* (London: Pickering & Chatto, 2000), I, 270. Original emphasis.

When a fire breaks out, you are, if possible, to repair to the place... It is particularly wished, that, at the instant you repair to a fire, you will endeavour to obtain every information from what cause the accident arose. You are immediately to acquaint the office of any loss, and procure for the sufferers, as soon as may be, as particular an account of the same as the nature of the case will admit.[28]

An agent covering a fire is compelled to rush to the scene, observe all of the particulars, make inquiries and interviews, and then transcribe the events. What seems especially striking is how the sufferers relate to their insurance agent who, at the instant of their trauma, procures for them no compensation but 'as particular an account of the same' as possible. He writes them not a check but a brief narrative, and then has the sufferers check his description. If he underwrites the value of their lost property, they underread (so to speak) its value as a contract, a guarantee of how property, life, and suffering signify in an emerging capital economy that depends on scribal practices. The protocols of the insurance industry demand the writing of particular accounts as well as the verification of the reading of those accounts by the insured.

In the immediate rush to the scene, the insurance agent would join a multitude already there. As suggested by the fire in *Mary Barton* (especially the crowd at Carsons' Mill and the scene's very conspicuousness in the novel), the description of risk was a crowded field. It included persons dissatisfied with how the professionalization of risk management was defining a whole range of cultural values and exclusions. In *Mary Barton* Gaskell contests these property-based values in favour of broader notions of mutual obligation. But she does so on risk management's very terrain. In his study of nineteenth-century American authors, Jason Puskar clarifies how novelists accepted the conceptual terms of a risk society in order to imagine 'new opportunities for fashioning systems of social and material independence'. Alongside the insurance industry, these authors helped produce a 'public consciousness of chance' by writing accidents into their narratives and imagining how they might afford new 'structures of mutual affiliation'.[29] Gaskell is similarly interested in how chance restructures social affiliations within the industrial city. Her own authorial practice parallels the insurance business in recalibrating description to new forms of industrial risk, displacing its uncertainties into the professional surety of writing and reading.

---

[28] 'Instructions for the Agents of the Sun Fire Office', 276–7.
[29] Jason Puskar, *Accident Society: Fiction, Collectivity, and the Production of Chance* (Palo Alto, CA: Stanford University Press, 2012), 3.

These overlaps are explicit in an 1869 letter that Gaskell wrote to her daughter Marianne. In giving encouragement and advice about how to become a proper novelist, Gaskell offers an analogy to reportage and street accidents:

> Then set to & imagine yourself a spectator & auditor of every scene & event! Work hard at this till it become a reality to you,—a thing you have to recollect & describe & report fully & accurately as it struck you ... If you but think eagerly of your story till *you see it in action*, words, good simple strong words, will come,—just as if you saw an accident in the street\that impressed you strongly/you would describe it forcibly.[30]

The successful writer channels a strong descriptive impulse—one that Gaskell can explain only by analogy to seeing 'an accident in the street'. Notably, the writer seems once removed: her task is not merely to imagine the story, but to imagine herself as its witness, to interpellate herself as a spectator, an auditor, a descriptive agent. Responding as if to an accident, this agent receives an imperative to 'work' and to 'describe & report fully & accurately'. To describe the accident is to reach for some form of representational integrity both in an agent's report free of vitiating errors and in a story comprised of 'good simple strong words'—the indisputable products of some 'action' just imaginatively witnessed.[31] Through close scrutiny and clear description, writing practices of insurance agents and novelists alike calibrate the event to its textual representations which then circulate in economies specific to each domain. Both economies depend on readers for the valuation of their representations, which are then offered as initial compensations for the traumatic events described. Beyond their shared attitude about the value of description, novelists and insurance writers employed a variety of similar strategies to make description 'become a reality'—or to persuade readers (and potential customers) to accept their representations of risk, loss, and compensation as such.

---

[30] J. A. V. Chapple and Arthur Pollard, eds, *The Letters of Mrs Gaskell* (Cambridge, MA: Harvard University Press, 1967), 542.

[31] Just as street accidents impress an observer to make forceful descriptions, these descriptions too—'good simple strong words'—are representational specie 'impressed' by the strong stamp of the accidental. The pose of author-as-bystander and the semiotic function of accident create what Jakobson has called 'the metonymical texture of realistic prose'. See 'Closing Statement: Linguistics and Poetics', in *Style in Language*, ed. Thomas A. Sebeok (Cambridge, MA: MIT Press, 1960), 375.

RISKY DESCRIPTIONS

The 'writing of loss', as Wertheimer has characterized this shared project, adds a different chapter to the history of description, especially in its reckoning with the accidental. With its English origins in the Restoration, the insurance business helps reconfigure 'the prose of things', as Cynthia Wall has argued of the eighteenth century's evolving attention to particularity, precision, and documentation. According to Wall, changing attitudes about description related to an epistemological shift: 'People—readers—were demanding to see the surfaces of their worlds and were prepared to read meaning rather than accident into idiosyncrasies and individualities'.[32] The 'writing of loss' takes this transformation even further. Its descriptions suture meaning and accident in new ways, as opposed to the either/or relation ('meaning rather than accident') that stretches from eighteenth-century neoclassical rhetoric and epistemology all the way back to Aristotle. That classical schema fails to meet the conceptual challenges of industrial catastrophes and fires in particular—the prose of uncertain things, as it were. At this moment, description must shift again with renewed emphasis upon its integrity, different attitudes about meaning and accident, and diverse textual practices including mixed modes and generic experiments by which the writers of loss—novelists and insurers alike—attempted to manage risk.

Reframing the description of risk in this way counters notions of insurance as dominated by Gradgrindian fact mongers and statisticians—the legacy of novelists who largely cleared the field in their own favour. The relation of insurance to quantification is more complex. Mapping the century's march toward an ideology of mechanical objectivity or 'trust in numbers', Theodore Porter suggests that, particularly with life insurance, agents and actuaries agreed on 'the importance of reliable statistical records. But they did not believe in the possibility of precise measurement, of reducing their work to calculational routines'.[33] Certainly insurers were deeply invested in quantifying phenomena and persons and accumulating statistics, but they also *resisted* quantification. The industry put up a fight when faced with Parliamentary pressure to standardize their measures, essentially to produce uniform actuarial tables for all persons and regions which could then be used to regulate insurance companies themselves. During hearings about the issue, actuaries argued that this was impossible:

---

[32] Cynthia Wall, *The Prose of Things: Transformation of Description in the Eighteenth Century* (Chicago, IL: University of Chicago Press, 2006), 6.
[33] Porter, *Trust in Numbers*, 102.

assessing risk required judgment and expertise. While Parliamentarian regulators wanted the transparency of numbers and facts, actuaries insisted on a 'subjective interpretation of probability'.[34] Interpreting risk depended on particulars, local contingencies, and myriad irreducible factors that demanded the reasoning mind.

In addition, while statistics and quantification had increased as a mode of social knowledge by the 1840s, they had yet to transform the business of assessing fire risk.[35] Fire insurers, while they collected vast amounts of data, did not take advantage of the statistical tools of probable inference which, as Samuel Brown pointed out, had invigorated the business of insuring lives, financial fidelities, and even railway accidents.[36] Robin Pearson states the matter more starkly: there remained in fire insurance 'a general lack of awareness, at times bordering on the stupefying, of the need for a systematic approach to data analysis'.[37] Unlike other insurances, no body of statistical or practical literature existed to help fire insurers assess risk. Their methods were less certain, established primarily through experience and imitation. Without standard practices, fire insurers had subjective leeway in assessing risk, though often to their cost.[38]

Responding to the problem, Brown urges fire insurers to pool data in the common interests of their threatened business. More interestingly, he suggests a way of processing the information that resembles non-statistical kinds of reading. Should the data and collected descriptions of fires be made available, 'a vast and novel field of observation would be open to the enquirer'.[39] Brown credits William Baddeley, an inventor and fire inspector, for attempting to create such an observable field in his annual reports of London fires in the *Mechanics' Magazine*. Brown praises Baddeley for offering 'a general narrative of the fires which have occurred in the year; and which have excited particular interest either from the magnitude of the losses, the destruction of human life attending them, or the unusual incidents which have made them notorious'.[40] If fires made for strong

---

[34] Porter, *Trust in Numbers*, 102.

[35] As a discourse, statistics had suffered some interestingly similar critiques, as Mary Poovey points out: 'Statistics...lacked a theoretical foundation, was thought to be governed by the values of its practitioners, and...was already embroiled in the political debate about the "condition of England".' See 'Figures of Arithmetic, Figures of Speech: The Discourse of Statistics in the 1830s', *Critical Inquiry* 19, no. 2 (1993): 256.

[36] Brown, 'On the Fires in London', 31–2.

[37] Robin Pearson, 'Moral Hazard and the Assessment of Insurance Risk in Eighteenth- and Early-Nineteenth-Century Britain', *Business History Review* 76, no. 1 (2002): 17.

[38] Pearson, 'Moral Hazard and the Assessment of Insurance Risk', 15.

[39] Brown, 'On the Fires in London', 32.

[40] Brown, 'On the Fires in London', 33.

impressions, then so did descriptions of fires that emphasized 'magnitude', 'destruction', and 'notorious' events which 'excited particular interest'. The prose descriptions, Brown implies, will give fire insurers insights into the statistical regularities which such events render so difficult to measure.

Brown and Baddeley try to resolve for fire insurance its curious incorporation of both anecdotal and statistical evidence, its attempts to negotiate between the singular, exceptional case described in prose and the general patterns of such events revealed in numerical tables.[41] As Poovey has argued, the discourse of statistics itself 'was (and remains) a mixed genre; it juxtaposed numerical, often tabular, formulations to discursive, sometimes historical or explanatory, narratives'.[42] In the 1830s and 40s, proponents of statistics worked hard to purify its quantitative integrity against 'figures of speech'.[43] By contrast, Brown and Baddeley invited such figures and narratives, as they already accepted that the object of their investigations—fires—escaped statistical certainties. Baddeley's annual reports employed both strategies at once. His 'general narrative' comprises short anecdotes and newspaper clippings of fires deserving 'special notice' punctuated by tables arranging the data in various ways.[44] While the tables suggest some regularities, they also reveal the persistent irregularities of fire risk which require other modes of interpretation: 'The causes of fires will be seen to be of the usual varied character, and a considerable number, notwithstanding the best intentions of all parties to elucidate them, remain enveloped in impenetrable mystery'.[45] With the array of contingencies and even personal motives in their ignition, fires seemed to demand more complex assessments of their causes and the extent of their liability. Fire insurers, in addition to sharing practices of description with novelists and journalists, also adopted narrative and even sensational techniques to enhance the assessment and marketing of risk.

Baddeley gathered his descriptions from newspaper accounts of fires, which tend to emphasize details about raging flames, howling mobs, narrow escapes, and brave rescues, as a sample of articles from the *Times*

---

[41] Elaine Hadley identifies this contest as central to debates about the Victorian marketplace, particularly regarding the New Poor Law. See *Melodramatic Tactics: Theatricalized Dissent in the English Marketplace, 1800–1885* (Palo Alto, CA: Stanford University Press, 1995), 88.

[42] Poovey, 'Figures of Arithmetic', 258.

[43] One could relate this to the simultaneous scepticism about the judicial integrity of a coroner's inquest verdict, as dataphiles like William Farr decried its almost total lack of statistical utility: 'It is using a phrase instead of giving a fact' (quoted in Ian A. Burney, *Bodies of Evidence: Medicine and the Politics of the English Inquest, 1830–1926* (Baltimore, MD: Johns Hopkins University Press, 2000), 68). See also Chapter 1.

[44] William Baddeley, 'London Fires in 1847', *Mechanics Magazine*, 29 July 1848, 102, <http://books.google.com/books?id=ihkFAAAAQAAJ>.

[45] Baddeley, 'London Fires in 1847', 108.

about major industrial fires in Manchester will suggest. Here is an 1836 description of a fire at a cotton-spinning factory in Manchester:

> some of the women and children were still in bed; they threw on a portion of their clothing and turned out of the building, whilst the other hands, after the immediate consternation into which they were thrown had subsided, took such measures as they could to impede the progress of the flames.
>
> ...
>
> Not only had Mr. Faulkner to bear up against disaster, but he had also to endure the insults and ribald screams of the brutal crowd.[46]

And here is an 1838 account of a fire at a Manchester factory that produced waterproof fabrics:

> A man was observed about this time forcing his way from one of the upper windows with his clothes all on fire, and although he was very much burnt, he happily effected his escape.[47]

Further details are provided the next day:

> the flames had burst forth with alarming fierceness, and although the engines immediately commenced playing on the building, in an incredibly short space of time the whole of the upper part was enveloped in one vast sheet of fire.[48]

Without gainsaying any damages or pain that these fires inflicted, there is a notable emphasis in these articles on such recurrent and eye-catching figures: vast sheets of fire, half-naked women and children, brutal injuries to bodies and reputations. Aled Jones claims that '[n]arrative, particularly in its melodramatic form, was... evolving as the newspaper journalist's favoured method of representing knowledge as news'.[49] The melodramatic conceits of these accident reports have specific commercial as well as narrative designs. They almost invariably transition to totals of property damage and the amounts for which the owners were insured—if at all. Consider this report of a fire at a Manchester card and machine factory in 1842: 'Since the flames have been subdued, however, the respective occupiers of the building have found themselves very serious sufferers beyond the amounts for which they are insured'.[50] (If only they had

---

[46] 'Alarming Fire in Manchester—Suspected Case of Incendiarism', *The Times*, 14 December 1836, 1.

[47] 'Dreadful Fire in Manchester, With Loss of Life', *The Times*, 28 August 1838, 5.

[48] 'Dreadful Fire at Manchester. Melancholy Loss of Several Lives', *The Times*, 29 August 1838, 5.

[49] Aled Jones, *Powers of the Press: Newspapers, Power and the Public in Nineteenth-Century England* (Aldershot, Hampshire: Ashgate, 1996), 82.

[50] 'Another Alarming Fire in Manchester. (From Our Own Correspondent.)', *The Times*, 8 January 1842, 6.

bought more coverage.) If the leading sensationalism 'excite[s]' particular interest', then the articles redirect this interest toward particulars, as if rolling over their readers' emotional attention to quantitative losses and the implied benefits of coverage. Their fairly consistent rhetorical pattern is less surprising considering that these stories, while sometimes deriving from newspapers' own correspondents, frequently digested reports from insurance companies themselves, as in this 1842 report: 'Yesterday morning the various fire insurance companies in the city received intelligence of disastrous fires having occurred'.[51] In extreme cases, some stories were anonymously planted by companies with ties to newspapers or by moonlighting editors.[52] Catastrophes could translate into big business for insurance companies and newspapers alike; they worked symbiotically through strategic publication of the 'alarming' and 'dreadful' and persistent ('*another* alarming fire') qualities of these events.

Big fires, incendiarism, and traumatic accidents had costs for insurers and hindered statistical models, but they also provided effective promotional tools, including 'frighten[ing] new clients into the market'.[53] Fire insurance transformed the very impediments to its operation into its best publicity. With their sensational and sympathetic storylines, fire reports doubled as advertisements for market-ready conceptions of loss and compensation.[54] Insurance marketers could promote their business's external consistency with moralizing interpretive frameworks—frameworks that writers like Dickens would use to critique insurance in general. Much as Timothy Alborn has described reactions to bank failures during the same era, catastrophic fires were a 'temporary text' whose interpretation was in dispute. Alborn argues that bankers, lacking an adequate discourse internal to their profession, had to 'import an interpretive framework from the novelists' in order to assure the public of the integrity of the financial system.[55] In a similar way, fire insurers, uncertain in their own methodology and lacking a predictive statistical approach, adapted anecdotes, narratives, and moralizing modes as part of their professional practice.

In playing up danger, loss, and the stark choices of being insured or risking catastrophic loss, insurance companies deployed several of the 'melodramatic tactics' that Elaine Hadley suggests were used instead to

---

[51] 'Yesterday Morning the Various Fire Insurance Companies', *The Times*, 28 January 1841, 3.
[52] Pearson, *Insuring the Industrial Revolution*, 183.
[53] Clive Trebilcock, *Phoenix Assurance and the Development of British Insurance* (Cambridge: Cambridge University Press, 1985), II, 238.
[54] Pearson, *Insuring the Industrial Revolution*, 283.
[55] Timothy Alborn, 'The Moral of the Failed Bank: Professional Plots in the Victorian Money Market', *Victorian Studies* 38, no. 2 (1995): 201.

resist commercialization.⁵⁶ A detail from an advertisement from 1847 (see Figure 2), although for a life insurance company, illustrates these tactics at work. The narrative follows its sight lines: an anxious child looks to her mother; mother the mortal sufferer looks imploringly up to heaven; a winged angel rides down beams of light bearing grace in one hand and in the other a 'POLICY' as she stares down the crowned skeleton of death whose tyranny has been denied. The slings and arrows of outrageous fortune are apparently only the concerns of the uninsured. The advertisement puts into high contrast the divisions of life and death, light and darkness, protection and danger by which melodrama made its moral types unmistakably clear to its audiences.⁵⁷ Those realms are divided by the policy document, at once the centre of pictorial attention and the boundary insurance invokes 'between property and loss, presence and absence, as no other nonreligious practice can do in the social world'.⁵⁸ Here, insurance practically claims to be a religious practice; the policy bridges the gap between material and ethereal realms depicted by the women's hands that almost but do not quite touch. No details about that policy are needed; indeed, they are hidden in the rolled document along with the implied signature of God as the underwriter, whose 'ascriptive power... promise[s] the ability to assign integrity without the connotation of marketable pleasure'.⁵⁹ The advertisement transfigures the choice to enter the insurance market as something beyond the market's sins. Purchasing a policy appears as a pious plea for divine mercy. Hadley identifies a trend in melodrama around mid-century that the advertisement's iconography seems to expressly perform: 'the curtain often fell on the solitary woman in a flood of light'.⁶⁰ Any lingering suspicions about the marketplace are further sublimated into a gendered maternal sphere.

Insurance's melodramatic tactics did not always impress the statisticians. William Cooke Taylor complained in 1835 that 'there are still people in the world, who prefer the figures of speech to the figures of arithmetic, and the rules of Longinus to those of Cocker. Pathetic tales, more than sufficient to supply a whole generation of novelists, prevailed over a dull, dry parade of stupid figures'.⁶¹ Taylor was describing debates about factory legislation in which the manufacturing industry's

---

⁵⁶ In this sense, the sensationalism of insurance complicates Hadley's claim about how 'melodramatic tactics' were used to confront commercialism. Straddling the very categories by which Hadley distinguishes commercialism and melodramatic resistance, insurance is at once individualist (protecting oneself) and communal (sharing risks and resources across policies), anecdotal and statistical.
⁵⁷ Hadley, *Melodramatic Tactics*, 68.   ⁵⁸ Wertheimer, *Underwriting*, 15.
⁵⁹ Wertheimer, *Underwriting*, 13.   ⁶⁰ Hadley, *Melodramatic Tactics*, 133.
⁶¹ Quoted in Poovey, 'Figures of Arithmetic', 260.

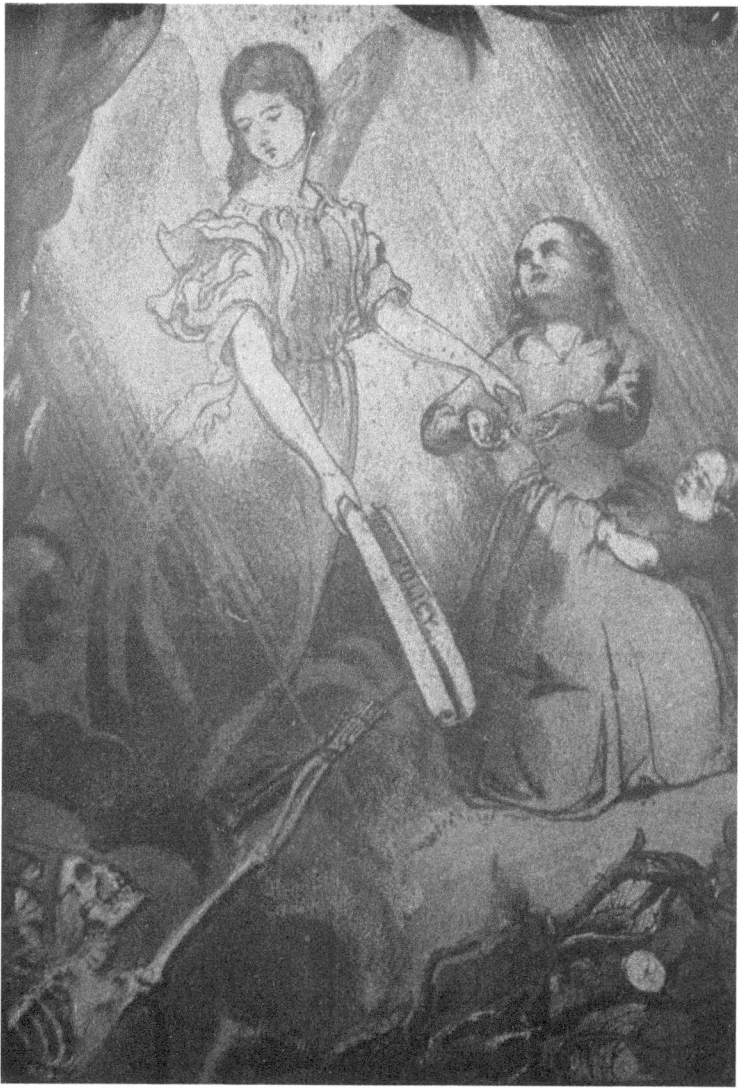

Fig. 2. Advertisement by the West of England Fire and Life Insurance Office, Exeter, April 1847

numbers-based defence lost out to the pathetic appeals of narrative. The insurance business played a different strategy, time and again deploying 'figures of speech' and sensation in lieu of arithmetic and transposing capital and political economy into domestic and gendered spaces—not dissimilar to how the cultural operations of the industrial novel, and *Mary*

Barton in particular, have been described.[62] Brown, seeking an answer to fire insurance's business failings, chose a suggestive phrase in crediting Baddeley's experiments with opening 'a vast and novel field'.

NOVEL FIELDS OF PROBABILITY

Accidents—and the mixed modes of describing them—opened 'a vast and novel field of observation' not only to fire insurers but also to novelists like Gaskell. Within such a 'novel field' these writers of loss could shape their professional credibility and their generic practice, including the 'field' of the novel itself. The discourse of risk management offers a different way to think about the generic inconsistencies and 'formal paradoxes' for which a novel like *Mary Barton* has received critical attention. According to Catherine Gallagher, the industrial novel develops its inconsistencies when it comes in contact with the so-called discourse of industrialism. Gallagher and others tend to judge based on standards of novelistic realism or formal integrity, but the industrial novel's inconsistencies may be solutions to different problems. Placing *Mary Barton* in the context of insurance reconsiders its 'formal eclecticism' as its greatest asset in the assessment of risk.[63] By experimenting with descriptive practices and attitudes toward probability, the novel proposes itself as a dedicated domain in which problems of risk can be considered. By her own descriptive heterogeneity, Gaskell asserts her novel's capacity to define the contested boundaries of this field and to compensate for loss in a different currency.[64]

---

[62] See Mary Poovey, *Making a Social Body: British Cultural Formation, 1830–1864* (Chicago, IL: University of Chicago Press, 1995), 145–7.

[63] Gallagher, *The Industrial Reformation of English Fiction*, 67.

[64] This argument runs parallel to the emotional compensation that Gaskell allegedly sought in writing the novel following the death of her son; see Jill L. Matus, *The Cambridge Companion to Elizabeth Gaskell* (Cambridge: Cambridge University Press, 2007), 28. In a similar context, Chapple and Wilson use the metaphor of insurance to characterize Gaskell's early diary, which 'served as a psychological insurance policy against the child's loss of her mother or the mother's loss of her child'. See J. A. V. Chapple and Anita C. Wilson, eds, *Private Voices: The Diaries of Elizabeth Gaskell and Sophia Holland* (Keele: Keele University Press, 1977), 77. Baucom distils the connection this way: 'insurance is the form that mourning takes when it equips itself for the market'; *Specters of the Atlantic*, 135.

Did Gaskell herself have insurance? This simple question is surprisingly difficult to answer. No direct mention is made in Gaskell's surviving correspondence. J. A. V. Chapple and Arthur Pollard note that there are significant gaps in which such information might have been documented: Gaskell's letters to her husband, as well as a cache of letters to the family's solicitor that—of course—perished in a fire. See *The Letters of Mrs Gaskell*, xiii. An 1850 letter to Eliza Fox, which now survives only in typescript, begins: '[. . .] is going to buy an annuity!!! think of that. May his shadow never be less!' (121). Unfortunately, the

Industrial Accidents and Novel Insurances 117

The raging factory fire in *Mary Barton* is part of Gaskell's exploration of the politics of risk management, particularly its implied divisions of propertied and working classes. She illuminates these questions with a catastrophe, or cata-strophe—classically the dramatic turn that produces the conclusion; the fire at Carsons' textile mill ignites early in the novel. For the Sun Fire Office, cotton mills were 'the most important class of industrial risk until well into the second half of the nineteenth century'.[65] Their field agent responding to such a fire must first and foremost 'obtain every information from what cause the accident arose'; based on his assessment, the agent would then narrate a particular account of the accident. Was the fire at Carsons' mill a crime of arson or fraud, a circumstance of a decaying and poorly managed factory, a chance spark from a careless worker, or could it have even been that disturbing Victorian phenomenon of spontaneous combustion?[66] Within the social cosmology that Gaskell imagines in her novel, there are clear motives for someone to have ignited the blaze. The mill owners might profit from insurance fraud; reports on prosecutions of false claims frequently appeared in newspapers as part of campaigns of insurance companies against such 'moral hazard'.[67] The workers are aggrieved enough to sabotage the master's factory, a suspicion reinforced by recent memories of the political incendiarism of the 1830s and 40s. Gaskell herself has a motive, using the mill fire as pretext to illuminate the depraved and dangerous conditions of factory work. So whodunit?

One of the only clues comes later in the novel and out of context, as John Barton lectures to a friend:

emended section refers to a page now lost, so the purchaser and beneficiary of that annuity remain unknown.

There is circumstantial evidence to suggest that Gaskell may have had some kind of insurance. In Manchester, the Gaskells' demographic was targeted by several emerging companies, such as *Clerical, Medical and General*. Gaskell's contemporary and sometime employer Charles Dickens—who loudly criticized speculative insurance in *Household Words*—had life insurance himself with two separate companies; Cockerell and Green, *The British Insurance Business 1547–1970*, 43. Along with references to insurance in *Mary Barton*, Gaskell's novel *Ruth* (1853) includes characters who converse about insurance products and correspondence with insurance companies (e.g. Chapter 30, 'The Forged Deed'). More certain answers might be located in archives of insurers in Manchester. The very lack of answers may be symptomatic of insurance's relatively low status in cultural history.

[65] Dickson, *The Sun Insurance Office*, 159.
[66] I refer, of course, to Dickens's canard in *Bleak House* (1852–3). While his detractors, including George Henry Lewes, lambasted the pseudo-scientific explanation of spontaneous combustion as a *cause* of Krook's death, this episode makes more sense in context of the broader cultural concern for the *uncaused* risks of combustion that are nonetheless a legitimate feature of industrial, urban, or narrative experience.
[67] Pearson, 'Moral Hazard', 29.

I've getten no head for numbers, but this I know, that by *far th' greater part o' th' accidents as comed in, happened in th' last two hours o' work*, when folk getten tired and careless. Th' surgeon said it were all true, and that he were going to bring that fact to light.

(126, original emphasis)

This passage connects with insurance's assessments of fire risk in two conspicuous ways. First, to explicate accident risk, John Barton offers anecdotal evidence from his own experience, having 'no head for numbers'. His observation gets confirmed as 'fact' by the professional surgeon, recalling how assessments of fire risk relied upon imitative professional practices in place of standardized numerical data. John Barton recognizes this as not his domain, but the surgeon's, who seems hardly more qualified as an actuary. Second, Gaskell includes otherwise unprompted italics on a phrase correlating accidents that 'comed in' with tired workers.[68] Within the novel's timeframe, Carsons' mill ignites just after sunset, so Gaskell retroactively implies that one of the workers may have accidentally caused the fire.[69] Not just any worker: the last to exit the building were Jem Wilson and his father. Jem Wilson is Mary's love interest who is later charged with the murder of the mill owner's rakish son, Harry Carson. Jem's trial hinges on the jury's interpretation of damning but not definitive circumstances which implicate him in the crime. The capital case against Jem dominates the second half of *Mary Barton*. As if foreshadowing that allegation, the fire suggests that Jem may have destroyed Carsons' mill as well as the son and heir.

Brown and Baddeley encourage a reading of fire risk inclusive of anecdote, memory, and factual correlation. Following theirs and John Barton's leads, we can form a strong suspicion about this fire's origins. But there the novel stops. After the blaze itself, it is not mentioned again—perhaps one of the novel's noted inconsistencies, or perhaps falling into the inquisitorial vacuum that so bothered William Payne. In a novel that becomes obsessed with the innocence or guilt of the alleged perpetrator of the story's defining murder, it seems strange that Gaskell has little interest in investigating the fire or determining its cause. Similarly, even when the novel does attend to the inquest on Harry Carson's murdered body, it notes the tension between seemingly abundant evidence and surprisingly cautious verdict. Old Mr Carson, seeking revenge, is seriously

---

[68] The italics present a kind of textual whodunit: the dialect is all John Barton, yet the italics must be the author's.

[69] Insurance companies and regional fire offices often pointed to worker carelessness as a cause of fires, publishing warnings and posting steep fines for any worker found responsible. See Cockerell and Green, *The British Insurance Business 1547–1970*, 32.

displeased, recalling prevailing legal complaints about the failure of inquests to make causal statements.[70] Those definitive statements must be made elsewhere. Though the novel requires a climactic trial and verdict to resolve its plot, Gaskell like the inquest also resists definitive interpretations of the narrative's signature events.

Departing from the interests of Brown, Baddeley, and Payne, Gaskell does not make the mill fire a mystery to solve: she does not care whodunit. Unlike coroners or the writers of loss in the insurance business, Gaskell has a different, even incurious, attitude. What Gallagher describes as a dominant impulse in *Mary Barton* 'to escape altogether from causality, to transcend causal explanation' may be better understood as Gaskell's concern with risk and how we interpret it.[71] Gaskell's novelistic assessment instead invokes a particular set of relations to accidents and risk. Two such relations are on display at the mill fire. Here is John Barton talking to his daughter on her way to the scene:

> Carsons' mill! Aye, there is a mill on fire somewhere, sure enough by the light, and it will be a rare blaze, for there's not a drop o' water to be got. And much Carsons will care, for they're well insured.
>
> (85)

The narrator suggests a much different relationship to risk with Jem's climactic escape from the burning building:

> The multitude did not even whisper while he crossed the perilous bridge, which quivered under him; but when he was across, safe comparatively in the factory, a cheer arose for an instant, checked, however, almost immediately, by the uncertainty of the result, and the desire not in any way to shake the nerves of the brave fellow who had cast his life on such a die.
>
> (89)

The industrial accident contrasts two economic relations to uncertainty or risk: the rich have insurance; the poor only gamble what little they have—their undervalued lives—'on such a die'. These two relations roughly characterize in *Mary Barton* the difference between what Benjamin Disraeli in *Sybil* called the 'two Englands' of the rich and poor. For each, happiness rises and falls with fortune, but at issue is the *mechanism* or rationale of fortune's movements: the insurance market versus the lottery. These concepts had only recently been disambiguated, as Lorraine Daston has argued.[72] Gaskell does not simply resurrect the lottery as a critique of

---

[70] Burney, *Bodies of Evidence*, 6.
[71] *The Industrial Reformation of English Fiction*, 67.
[72] As Daston suggests, insurance was frowned upon as a lottery or form of gambling, until the late-eighteenth century when new strategies of marketing and the increasing

insurance or financial speculation. Rather, she juxtaposes them in order to accentuate their difference, to characterize the gap between those with insurable property and those without. She uses the rising social acceptability of insurance to contrast the impoverished and exposed condition of England's working class.[73] For them the lottery is hardly a substitute for the predictive compensation for risk.

Gaskell uses accidents to characterize different positions within Victorian political economy. Standing for the insurance market is 'the employer; a being of another race, eternally placed in antagonistic attitude; going through the world glittering like gold, with a stony heart within, which knew no sorrow but through the accidents of Trade' (450). Gaskell in her Preface perceives that the poor 'were sore and irritable against the rich, the even tenor of whose seemingly happy lives appeared to increase the anguish caused by the lottery-like nature of their own' (29). Gaskell brings both perspectives into the frame of the spectacular mill fire, for which 'the accidents of Trade' furnishes an apt metaphor. The 'accidents of Trade'— whether market fluctuations or industrial accidents—are for mill owners bumps in a road that are smoothed out in the long run, or by the aggregate patterns of the self-regulating market, into an 'even tenor'. These same 'accidents of Trade' are insurmountable obstacles for workers, however, resulting in lost jobs, droughts of unemployment, and disfigured, sometimes fatally injured, bodies.[74] After their industrial accident, the Carsons suspend factory operations and, flush with insurance money, enjoy leisurely days while waiting out repairs and upgrades. Gaskell then splits the screen: 'There is another side to the picture. There were homes over which Carsons' fire threw a deep, terrible gloom' (95). The crisis for workers, then, is the irrationality of risk for an individual who cannot ride out the 'accidents of Trade', for whom circumstances do not aggregate, but happen one time only, usually with dire consequences.

influence of a capital economy on liberal subjectivity cast insurance as a responsible, defensive, and highly regulated choice; see 'The Domestication of Risk: Mathematical Probability and Insurance 1650–1830', in *The Probabilistic Revolution. Volume 1: Ideas in History*, ed. Lorenz Krüger, Lorraine J. Daston, and Michael Heidelberger (Cambridge, MA: MIT Press, 1987), 253. Geoffrey Clark concludes *Betting on Lives: The Culture of Life Insurance in England* (Manchester: Manchester University Press, 1999) with the Gambling Act of 1774, which banned speculative insurance practices and legislated that policy buyers must demonstrate a real and legitimate financial interest in the person or property at stake.

[73] A useful corrective to Gaskell's dichotomy can be found in Melanie Tebbutt's study of pawnbroking and working-class credit, wherein she explains how the poor used pawnbroking as a hedge against risk, among other reasons. See *Making Ends Meet: Pawnbroking and Working-Class Credit* (New York: St. Martin's Press, 1983).

[74] Gaskell gives an example with Jem's mother, the traumatized Jane Wilson, who was literally crushed by what seems an allegorical dead ringer for fortune's wheel in a factory where a large, uncovered gear caught and maimed her.

If *Mary Barton* makes industrial accidents an issue of class, it also invokes a contest between relations to probability. While the extent of historical interpretations of probability is vast, *Mary Barton* so emphasizes unprecedented, sudden, single-case phenomena as to invite scrutiny in this context.[75] In what patterns or predictable schema would such a catastrophe possibly fit? Porter suggests that actuarial thinking in insurance facilitates a transition from classical 'subjectivist' to modern 'frequentist' interpretations of probability.[76] The diverse and dissonant strategies of insurers to assess fire risk reveal both such interpretations operating at once. Frequentism, prominent in other insurances with better predictive statistical models, makes sense of probability in aggregates: cycles, cities, populations. Its laws are revealed in large numbers or after a series of quantifiable trials, such as flipping a coin. For any single flip, however, the theory tells you nothing.[77] Gaskell's novel confronts this threat of irrationality: the difficulty of interpreting the singular episode, or the strain upon individuals coming to terms with a probabilistic order which may or may not govern them. Gaskell in *Mary Barton* writes these conceptual challenges into the political landscape of England's industrial north. Further, she encodes concerns about probabilism into the novel's prominent accidents, where chance is still wild. Is the mill fire actually part of an aggregate order or a discernible plan? Is it a one-time-only, random, and traumatic catastrophe? The accident calls up each of these scenarios. The probability of a mill burning down, written into a mill-owner's insurance policy to insulate him from disaster, doubles as the odds of a game of chance, in which a worker gets one throw with everything at stake.

---

[75] Good overviews are also provided in Ian Hacking, *The Taming of Chance: A Philosophical Study of Early Ideas About Probability, Induction and Statistical Inference*, 2nd edn (Cambridge; New York: Cambridge University Press, 2006) and Douglas Lane Patey, *Probability and Literary Form: Philosophic Theory and Literary Practice in the Augustan Age* (Cambridge; New York: Cambridge University Press, 1984). Contemporary debates in statistics tend to emphasize two major approaches: frequentist and Bayesian; for example, see Henry Ely Kyburg and Mariam Thalos, *Probability Is the Very Guide of Life: The Philosophical Uses of Chance* (Chicago, IL: Open Court, 2003). By roughly sketching out those categories here, I do not mean to apply such a simplified schema retroactively; rather, I suggest that Gaskell identifies and dramatizes a version of this debate as a way of characterizing the 'two Englands' of the 1840s. Further, I hope to historicize such senses of probability in the early Victorian imagination of industrialism.

[76] Theodore M. Porter, *The Rise of Statistical Thinking, 1820–1900* (Princeton, NJ: Princeton University Press, 1986), 87.

[77] See Kavanagh for more on the paradoxes of Enlightenment probability theory: 'To the question, What *will* happen? it offers an exquisitely refined understanding of what *may* happen... Silent with regard to the one, it spoke endlessly of the many'; *Enlightenment and the Shadows of Chance: The Novel and the Culture of Gambling in Eighteenth-Century France* (Baltimore, MD: The Johns Hopkins University Press, 1993), 15–22.

Mary Barton hopes to resolve these contrasting relations to risk on its own terms; it does so by making contingency its prevailing narrative logic. On the one hand, mill owners must come to appreciate the 'lottery-like nature' of life on the job and in the streets. So, for example, the novel subjects Old Mr Carson to the murder of his son, Harry. This event is a catastrophic tragedy mediated through a chain of chance events. Harry Carson draws a comic sketch denigrating a delegation of workers, but when he throws the paper away, it accidentally falls short of the fireplace and gets recovered by the enraged men. These workers tear the same paper into pieces, mark one piece, and then hold a lottery to pick the man tasked with killing Harry. As opposed to the lucky payoffs that the term elsewhere suggests, this lottery can only be lost. On the other hand, workers must come to appreciate the 'accidents of Trade' and lottery-like circumstances of their lives as rational in the aggregate. Gaskell—perhaps not the Christian socialist that some critics have thought—resurrects through accidents what seems a kind of Christian laissez faire.[78] Although we cannot know, quantify, or predict the singular events and catastrophes of this fallen world, we can trust that the invisible hand of God's Providence directs and insures the greater order. Characters in *Mary Barton* must submit to and suffer through the accidents of trade as an article of faith.

This striking compromise is summed up within a few pages of the novel's conclusion by Job Legh, allegorically named as a resigned sufferer: 'It's true it was a sore time for the hand-loom weavers when power-looms came in: them new-fangled things make a man's life like a lottery; and yet I'll never misdoubt that power-looms, and railways, and all such-like inventions are the gifts of God' (472). Within this provocative claim, Job distinguishes the lottery from the assurance[79] of Providence, which, though he cannot know its workings, provides him a different and more secure relation to the risky business of life as a factory worker, one that pays off in the very long term. Eleanor Courtemanche points out that these characters have 'internalized a sacral version of the invisible hand metaphor' popularized in political economy by Adam Smith.[80] As

---

[78] This familiar conceptual elision of Adam Smith's 'invisible hand' as both God's Providence and the workings of capital has a long pedigree, including writers such as Defoe and Harriet Martineau in *Illustrations of Political Economy* (1832–4).

[79] The tension between theology and commerce in Job's resolution comes through in the etymology of 'assurance', in which Wertheimer finds 'a struggle between religious meaning, the long-sermonized "doctrine of assurance" which goes back to John Calvin, and its evolving commercial denotation of mutual insurance, which come to dominate its usage by the late eighteenth century'. See *Underwriting*, 25.

[80] *The 'Invisible Hand' and British Fiction, 1818–1860: Adam Smith, Political Economy, and the Genre of Realism*, Palgrave Studies in Nineteenth-Century Writing and Culture (Basingstoke, Hampshire; New York: Palgrave Macmillan, 2011), 180.

Courtemanche explains, Smith's invisible hand theory has a governing irony, seeming simultaneously to propose an autonomous 'emergent system' as well as 'the idea that God or possibly some devious elite is really pulling the levers'.[81] That tension between an emergent as opposed to a designed system is relieved by the 'the quasi-divine figure of *Providence*' with its power to rationalize the hidden benefits of catastrophe.[82]

Job seems like a mouthpiece for this conciliatory position, echoing industrial apologists like Andrew Ure in his *Philosophy of Manufactures* (1835) who claims that 'the new system of labour was destined by Providence' to be 'a benefaction, which, wisely administered, may become the best temporal gift of Providence to the poor'.[83] Such sentiments have annoyed readers of Gaskell's novel who have found its politics inconclusive and its genre overstrained. In the context of historical violence reacting to 'such-like inventions' that Job accepts as 'gifts of God', his passive testimony seems to complicate the reformist sentiments which *Mary Barton* sets out to express. But though the novel seems ambiguous from this perspective, muddling notions of Providence and political economy, it looks rather different in historically specific contexts of fire risk and loss.[84] In this sense, *Mary Barton* does not neatly fit the 'providential aesthetic' that had characterized so much of eighteenth and nineteenth-century fiction.[85] Rather, with its attention to accidents, the novel foregrounds the unresolved ironies within invisible hand theory and insurantial underwriting, including what Puskar calls 'the production of chance'.[86] Gaskell's goal is not to rationalize catastrophe, but to accentuate

---

[81] Courtemanche, *The 'Invisible Hand' and British Fiction*, 7.

[82] Courtemanche, *The 'Invisible Hand' and British Fiction*, 14. Original emphasis.

[83] Andrew Ure, *The Philosophy of Manufactures: Or, An Exposition of the Scientific, Moral, and Commercial Economy of the Factory System of Great Britain* (London: Charles Knight, 1835), 14, 17.

[84] That context also puts *Mary Barton* within a timeframe of effective reforms related to risk, coverage, and compensation. After mid-century, corporate and legislative changes to the insurance industry were significant: companies adapted business practices to new industrial cities; provided new products and coverage options for the poor; lobbied Parliament to legislate factory safety improvements, as with the Factory Reform Act of 1844; and began compensating for physical and non-physical trauma suffered on the job; see Cockerell and Green, *The British Insurance Business 1547–1970*, 39–40. Schivelbusch provides a good discussion of accidents, insurance, and liability with regards to the railroads, where laws requiring compensation were not instituted until 1864 in England; see *The Railway Journey*, 206. Mike Sanders offers a useful history of changes in compensation for factory incidents in 'Manufacturing Accident: Industrialism and the Worker's Body in Early Victorian Fiction', *Victorian Literature and Culture* 28, no. 2 (2000): 313–29.

[85] Thomas Vargish, *The Providential Aesthetic in Victorian Fiction* (Charlottesville, VA: University of Virginia Press, 1985).

[86] *Accident Society*, 62.

its heuristic complexities and displace its management into the domains of the novel and its readers.

NOVEL COMPENSATION OF ACCIDENTS

In *Mary Barton*, Gaskell engineers alternative notions of probability and compensation that respond to a contemporary discourse about risk management but that also significantly shape the generic parameters of the industrial novel and potentially the realist novel at large. At issue is the authorship of accidents, or how to settle the ironic agency that lies somewhere between autonomous and providential systems. Gaskell is writing at a time when liability claims for industrial suffering and manufacturing accidents were much in dispute. Who was responsible? Who would arrange compensation? Negligent employers, careless workers, faulty machines, a vengeful God? The writing of loss confronts these questions by imagining a spectrum of possibilities from blameless harm to more strict assessments of causality. In this context, *Mary Barton* extends MacPherson's argument about the eighteenth-century novel, shaped amid legal notions of 'strict liability' which made persons accountable for events they may not have intended, desired, or even been part of.[87] This 'tragic responsibility', she argues, runs counter to influential notions of *contract* within theories of the rise of the novel and the modern liberal subject. It requires instead 'a generalized social obligation' in which persons, things, and events are alike held equivalent.[88] In this context, the industrial novel's own 'formal and sociological interest in accidents' helps ask what social relations might better fit a technologizing world in which machines and humans mix, and in which responsibility has to be reconceived outside the contractual obligations that had defined nineteenth-century industrial labour.[89]

Accidents bring those social and obligatory relations into focus, providing the occasions to reinterpret liability.[90] Mike Sanders argues that by the mid-1850s the term 'accident' was finessed in the press and the law courts to mean that an event may have been caused but not intended. He contends that '"accident" made possible a compromise formula which

---

[87] Sandra MacPherson, *Harm's Way: Tragic Responsibility and the Novel Form* (Baltimore, MD: Johns Hopkins University Press, 2010), 4.
[88] MacPherson, *Harm's Way*, 38.   [89] MacPherson, *Harm's Way*, 190.
[90] N. N. Feltes was among the first to recommend liability as a keyword in broader thematic and formal analyses of the novel and the world it purports to represent. See 'Community and the Limits of Liability in Two Mid-Victorian Novels', *Victorian Studies* 17, no. 4 (1974): 355–69.

allowed industrial capitalism to accept responsibility for its casualties without having to admit its responsibility in producing those casualties'.[91] Mill owners took responsibility to pay compensation to injured workers, but refused the idea that any calamities or damages happened intentionally. Accidents were the endemic risks of industrial employment. Some deplored this view as splitting causation from conscience; Sanders' points to the sarcastic title that Dickens initially planned for *Little Dorrit* (1855–7): 'Nobody's Fault'. Gaskell too seems guilty of finessing the concept of accident, raising a troubling notion that industrial suffering may be uncaused and beyond critique. *Mary Barton* seems to displace accident into the resigned, even passive religion of Job, whose God is not liable for unprecedented acts.[92] But Job's Providential insurance, as it were, finds its compensation in a different currency: not in rewards for risk but in redefining its very assessment. In *Mary Barton*, Gaskell imagines a renovated relationship to probability: a third way that is neither the lottery-like Jobean hardship assured by God, nor the proleptic iteration of a modern property-based insurance underwritten by risk managers.

Gaskell reimagines the activity of risk assessment in novel terms. In a late conversation between Job and Mr Carson—a conspicuous meeting of the sufferer and the well-insured—Job tries to explain the problem. Like fire insurers sceptical about the regularity of risk, Job puts a rider on human nature; he declares: 'You can never work facts as you would fixed quantities, and say, given two facts, and the product is so and so. God has given men feelings and passions which cannot be worked into the problem, because they are for ever changing and uncertain' (473). As John Barton has 'no head for numbers', Job has little faith in what the novel elsewhere calls 'the science of consequences' (225). Compared to 'fixed quantities', God's accidental works or the eruptions of human 'feelings and passions which... are for ever changing and uncertain' cannot be predicted or reduced to equations of risk. Both John and Job remain active, however, in attempting to interpret extraordinary events. Confronted at one point with the seemingly insoluble problem of Jem's conviction and how he might help, Job 'went out into the street; and

---

[91] Sanders, 'Manufacturing Accident', 321.
[92] As the online dictionary law.com quips, 'acts of God' are the 'one time an insurance company gets religion'. 'Religion' is a moving target: 'acts of God' are defined by what an insurance company cannot pay, as when a catastrophe occurs across all of the company's assets. Larger companies that can distribute risk across more assets are more likely to cover these events, taking God out of the picture again.
  The position of underwriting vis-à-vis Victorian religion is not far from how the geological and biological sciences also deferred their uncertainties and speculations as God's domain. Looking at this another way, these disciplines were the colonizers advancing into religion's territory, and masking the materiality of their claims with the veneer of pious humility.

there he stood still, to ponder over probabilities and chances' (386). The faith that Job confesses is neither passive nor calculating, but based on evaluating 'probabilities and chances' in a more subjective and affective register. Accidents—whether industrial catastrophes, the vagaries of trade, or on-the-street collisions—are reimagined as moments of religious crisis which challenge the sufferer to forgive the acts of God.[93] In view of its working-class characters' plight—isolated, disenfranchised, and subject to the tragic lottery of their lives—the novel offers an industrial(-strength) Christianity that simultaneously works as a renovated probabilism.[94] To believe is to assess risk in a new way.

Job's probabilistic faith depends upon subjectively perceiving patterns in the accidents and randomness of experience. Keith Thomas has suggested that Protestantism urged its faithful to help themselves before calling for God's intervention, which results in a 'nascent statistical sense', or, as Pearson puts it, 'an awareness of patterns in apparently random behaviour'.[95] That nascent sense was rapidly maturing in Gaskell's own Unitarian community in Manchester. Among the influential members of the congregation of Cross Street Chapel where William Gaskell had presided as minister since 1828 was James Kay (later Kay-Shuttleworth), author of *The moral and physical condition of the working-class employed in the cotton manufacture in Manchester* (1832)—a source text for Engels and Gaskell alike. Cooperating with other leading Unitarians, Kay subsequently founded the Manchester Statistical Society, perhaps the first such established in Britain.[96] Though they promoted statistics to help document moral and physical hardships in Manchester, the Unitarians also subordinated numbers to their faith in human reasoning. Like Gaskell herself, they privileged outreach and sympathy in relating to the hardships of the poor. As Gallagher has shown, *Mary Barton* appears amid telling transitions within mid-Victorian Unitarianism,

[93] Consider the mid-street collision that strongly impresses Old Mr Carson, after which he decides to forgive John Barton for the murder of his son. Mr Carson happens to witness a brusque, working-class boy in full stride plough over an angelic girl. But, ventriloquizing the New Testament edict, she demands that her accidental assailant not be punished: '*He did not know what he was doing*' (453, original emphasis). In other words, it was an accident.

[94] As Courtemanche puts it, 'this book suggests it be read as an industrial-age supplement to the New Testament.' See *The 'Invisible Hand' and British Fiction*, 183.

[95] Keith Thomas, *Religion and the Decline of Magic* (New York: Scribners, 1971), 784; Pearson, *Insuring the Industrial Revolution*, 3. Gaskell's dissenting Protestantism brings her nearer to Thomas's claims about self-reliance and pattern-finding, as Unitarianism—just this side of Deism—deemphasizes the miraculous in favour of a more material understanding of Christ and his works.

[96] Monica Correa Fryckstedt, *Elizabeth Gaskell's Mary Barton and Ruth: A Challenge to Christian England*, Acta Universitatis Upsaliensis 43 (Uppsala, Sweden; Stockholm: [Uppsala universitet]; Almqvist & Wiksell International, 1982), 67.

moving from a strictly Necessarian 'Religion of Causality' to a 'Religion of Conscience'. While these debates focused on free will and voluntary righteousness, they underscore how 'competing theories of causality' were thoroughly diffused into Gaskell's cultural background at the time.[97]

In *Mary Barton*, Job has such a proto-statistical perspective (a head for patterns rather than numbers) in which industrial hardship does not call divine agency into doubt, but instead confirms its unpredictability. Accidents need other interpretive models than quantification and liability, so Gaskell emphasizes the affective and ethical dimensions of risk assessment. In so doing, she renovates Old Testament hardship, the lottery, and single-case probability into a new relationship to chance, whose probability cannot be measured except in terms of what persons and groups think about it.[98] Like Unitarianism, too, this faith-based probabilism is immediately available to the congregation, appealing to reasoned sympathy. Against the management of risk by a commercial clerisy, *Mary Barton* moves the ground of interpreting risk to collectives—including the novel's fictional jury weighing Jem's fate, the imagined community of Manchester agape at a factory fire, and even its own readership.

Gaskell's engagement with theological and actuarial debates about causation 'leads to a high degree of formal self-consciousness' in *Mary Barton*, recasting Gaskell's attempts to renovate probability in terms of description and narrative.[99] Aristotle long ago argued that narrative probability is determined by collectives, especially readerly collectives.[100] The relationship between novelistic practice and the conceptual evolution of

---

[97] *The Industrial Reformation of English Fiction*, 64.

[98] Gaskell follows the contours of conditional or Bayesian probability, which makes chance into an interpretive, rather than quantitative, event. In the Bayesian view, probability is not an objective property of the material world, but is conditional upon the subjective horizons against which it is measured; see Harri Valpola, 'Bayesian Ensemble Learning for Nonlinear Factor Analysis' (Ph.D. Dissertation, Finnish Academies of Technology, 2000), http://www.cis.hut.fi/harri/thesis/valpola_thesis/node12.html>. Bayes's theorem includes in its calculations how people's previous experiences or insights change the statistical probability of singular or hard-to-predict things; see Christopher D. Frith, *Making Up the Mind: How the Brain Creates Our Mental World* (Malden, MA: Blackwell, 2007), 121–2. For such catastrophic events like a mill fire or industrial trauma, Bayesian probability finds meaning in the collective reactions to that event, reactions that are themselves informed by prior experience, communal beliefs, and personal inspiration.

There are suggestive links between Gaskell, Bayes, and the cluster of actuarial concerns that I have identified in this chapter. Thomas Bayes was a nonconformist minister and mathematician. His work was publicized by another dissenting minister with interest in statistics, Richard Price, who also produced in 1780 tables on life expectancies used by insurance offices well into the nineteenth century. See Hacking, *The Emergence of Probability*, 114.

[99] Gallagher, *The Industrial Reformation of English Fiction*, 67.

[100] As part of their responsibilities, artists 'must necessarily in all instances represent things... as they are said or thought to be or to have been'. Aristotle, *Poetics*, in *The Basic*

probability has been widely acknowledged; drawing on Ian Hacking, Thomas Kavanagh sees almost 'a fundamental congruence, perhaps even a monadic harmony, between these two cultural phenomena: the rise of the novel and the elaboration of a science of probability'.[101] As probability moved into increasingly mathematical, quantitative, and frequentist domains, its relation to subjective and narrative domains had to be redefined. The writers of loss were elaborating such notions of probability through similar scribal practices and heterogeneous representational modes. Their eclectic writings manifest what historians of risk and insurance have noted: that probability judgments depend on descriptions, or on shared beliefs derived from those descriptions: 'The more vivid and accurate the account, the greater the propensity to assign a probability value to the event described'.[102] Insurance writers and novelists contained the uncertainties of risk by reframing them as a question of descriptive fidelity. And here the novel as a genre comes into its strength. *Mary Barton* garnered much praise for the vividness and accuracy of its portrayals. The *Athenæum* testified that Gaskell's forcible and fair 'pictures of life' were made with 'the fidelity of a Daguerreotype'.[103] The representative fidelity of these pictures notwithstanding, it is Gaskell's mimetic *credibility* that suggests the shared interests of insurance agents and novelists both to transcribe the improbable into particular accounts and to claim that function as their unique professional or generic province.

Gaskell offers the novel itself—if not as a substitute for probability thinking, then as a laboratory for the study of its contingencies, limitations, irrationalities, and human quanta. To interpret them, *Mary Barton* foregrounds the logic of accidents in terms of sentiment, political economy, and God's Providence. The deconstructive—indeed, destructive—potential of accidents, however, reveals contradictions in the novel's ideologies. Ironically, to recover the ethical and affective dimensions of chance, the industrial novel must *produce* accidents and uncertainties and

---

Works of Aristotle, ed. Richard McKeon (New York: Random House, 1941), 1483. See also Chapter 9 of *Poetics*.

[101] Kavanagh, *Enlightenment and the Shadows of Chance*, 107. Patey identifies the Augustan novel as the preeminent form demonstrating the effects of probability on literary practice, and argues that it manifests, through didactic narratives, 'the conditions of knowledge and learning, the need for the methods of cultivating probable inference'. See *Probability and Literary Form: Philosophic Theory and Literary Practice in the Augustan Age* (Cambridge; New York: Cambridge University Press, 1984), 176.

[102] Pearson, *Insuring the Industrial Revolution*, 3. See also Peter Bernstein, *Against the Gods: The Remarkable Story of Risk* (New York: Wiley, 1996), 279.

[103] Henry Fothergill Chorley, 'Review of Mary Barton', *Athenæum* 1095 (21 October 1848): 1050.

refuse to make absolute sense of them. Gaskell displaces much of this work onto the instability of markets, the modernizing cityscape, and the threats of industrial injury, but her fascination with accidents potentially implicates the novel in celebrating the suffering that it seeks to alleviate.[104] Factories burn; children collide in the streets; workers' bodies are traumatized in the production of sensational, descriptive, and narrative forms that depend on the uncertainties of risk as much as they attempt to manage them. Like insurance, the industrial novel visits destruction proleptically upon its subjects to guarantee their value.[105] In this sense, it was *Gaskell* who torched Carsons' cotton mill; the motive was not simply reform, but an authorial pyromania,[106] the production of spectacles that necessarily border on the inexplicable.[107]

Gaskell is more than a writer of loss: she is an author of accidents, which she refashions as the novelist's profession. If, as Wertheimer claims, 'accidents and destruction can be made providential by pointing us toward the commons', then Gaskell uses them to make common the valuation of risk, at the time so strongly linked to the writing and reading of loss.[108] She claims the iteration of accidents as the domain of the novelist and the generic privilege of the novel. Not everyone accepted this as an innovation. Consider Henry James's famous denigration of the Victorian novel: 'what do such large loose baggy monsters, with their queer elements of the

---

[104] Bruce Robbins offers a related perspective on Dickens, who, in venturing into the terrain of statistics and political economy in *Bleak House*, exhibits 'complicity in the inhumanity he attacks'. See 'Telescopic Philanthropy: Professionalism and Responsibility in *Bleak House*', in *Nation and Narration*, ed. Homi Bhabha (London; New York: Routledge, 1990), 225.

[105] Baucom, *Specters of the Atlantic*, 105.

[106] Consider that in writing *North and South*, Gaskell toyed with the idea of using a factory fire to precipitate that novel's great reconciliation. In 1854, she wrote to Catherine Winkworth: 'What do you think of a fire burning down Mr Thornton's mills *and house* as a *help* to failure? Then Margaret would rebuild them larger & better & need not go & live there when she's married.' Chapple and Pollard, *The Letters of Mrs Gaskell*, 310, original emphasis.

[107] At the mill fire, Mary passes out: 'the heated air, the roaring flames, the dizzy light, and the agitated and murmuring crowd, had bewildered her thoughts' (87). In its sublimity, accident reveals itself as potentially illegible, entirely beyond description or economies of compensation. In this sense, accidents are the most obvious instances of Jean Baudrillard's sense of catastrophe as the radical play of surfaces which other critics, such as Julian Wolfreys, have extrapolated as the metropolitan condition itself. See David F. Bell, *Circumstances: Chance in the Literary Text* (Lincoln, NB: University of Nebraska Press, 1993), 90–1; Julian Wolfreys, *Writing London: The Trace of the Urban Text from Blake to Dickens* (Basingstoke, Hampshire: Macmillan, 1998).

[108] Wertheimer, *Underwriting*, 32. Jill Matus makes a similar point about 'the commonality of suffering' in *Mary Barton*: a community of Gaskell-as-author, her aggrieved characters, and her readership. See Matus, *The Cambridge Companion to Elizabeth Gaskell*, 29. Thus, Gaskell makes suffering an emotional property in common, a literary analogue to how Friendly Societies or mutual companies also shared risk and loss.

accidental and the arbitrary, artistically *mean*?'[109] James's 'baggy monsters' sound bite is better remembered than what immediately follows about the novel's 'queer elements of the accidental and the arbitrary'. Gallagher and others have extended this aspect of James's critique, noting how, to take the case of *Mary Barton*, the novel's paradoxes, arbitrary coincidences, and accidents call increased attention to the unsettled issue of genre.[110] James cannot answer his question about artistic meaning without implied reference to his own aesthetic; similarly, Gallagher understands the 'generic eclecticism' of Gaskell's novel in terms of 'later British realism'.[111] But realism is not the only game in town. Regarding the arbitrariness and accidents of the Victorian novel, the history of description offers just as promising an interpretive framework, and one that illuminates broader contexts for how novelists like Gaskell developed literary realism. Further, to denigrate accidents or arbitrary elements or dismiss them as 'reality effects' is to overlook their cultural dynamics and to miss the opportunity to elaborate more nuanced histories of novelistic realism in interdisciplinary terms.

Situating *Mary Barton* this way suggests how the novel's generic parameters—particularly its eclecticism and accidents—develop as part of Gaskell's writing of loss, itself part of a discursive field about probability and risk in the industrializing city. Following professional and moral imperatives to distinguish the 'subjective probability' and writing practices that she shares with insurers, Gaskell reimagines risk in a form that the novelist and her readers are uniquely suited to interpret. Further, Gaskell accentuates accident and its contradictions in order to develop a reading practice that is willing to be expansive and inconclusive. Rather than merely manage accidents, *Mary Barton* accentuates their generative paradoxes in order to give prominence to subjective and collective measurements of risk in narrative form. Thus, the logic of accidents becomes one and the same with the novel's own contrivances, improbabilities, and seemingly uncaused happenings. It makes sense that the Providence of *Mary Barton* should echo the era's juridical shift to limit employer liability. Gaskell elides her own novelistic enterprise with an act of God: both enjoy

---

[109] James, 'Preface'.
[110] Gallagher, *The Industrial Reformation of English Fiction*, 68.
[111] Gallagher, *The Industrial Reformation of English Fiction*, 87. George Levine, though he takes issue with James, also situates the accidental and the arbitrary within realism's framework: '[t]he nonstructural detail, apparently thematically irrelevant, provides the primary evidence of the antiliterary thrust of realism, and ironically, the case for its trustworthiness.' See *The Realistic Imagination: English Fiction from Frankenstein to Lady Chatterley* (Chicago, IL: University of Chicago Press, 1981), 151. For Levine's specific response to the James quotation, see *The Realistic Imagination*, 141–2.

a creator's license to cover the totally unexpected, to authorize the random catastrophe, to plot the impossible narrative coincidence, to plunk down spectacular and even arbitrary episodes within the novel. As Courtemanche says, 'though we cannot really read novels themselves as evolving without design, they often grapple with the tension between emergent orders, random accident, and the human desire to read experience as orderly'.[112] Indeed, it is nonsense to claim that Victorian novels were written by accident. However, many were written *through* accident and a keener sense of such generic engagements helps to reveal their multiform structures and cultural concerns. Gaskell risks the coherence of her own work on the order we infer from its accidents. If *Mary Barton* bears family resemblance to the kind of 'large loose' Victorian novel that James critiques, then its 'queer elements of the accidental and the arbitrary' are among the most significant features in its narrative and cultural designs.

[112] *The 'Invisible Hand' and British Fiction*, 155.

4
Street Literature and the Remediation of Accident

> And Mary turned out of the house, which had been *his* home, where *he* was loved, and mourned for, into the busy, desolate, crowded street, where they were crying halfpenny broadsides, giving an account of the bloody murder, the coroner's inquest, and a rawhead-and-bloody-bones picture of the suspected murderer, James Wilson.
>
> Gaskell, Mary Barton

It would not take long for the printers of broadsides and street ballads to transform such sensational news into printed sheets to circulate amid the busiest streets. Mary Barton has barely recovered from hearing the news herself when she encounters a crying vendor in the crowds, hawking a cheap single-page report of the coroner's inquest, perhaps in verse and likely illustrated with a reusable 'murderer' woodcut kept in stock. This broadside capitalizes on the suspicion of Jem Wilson as the jealous criminal—the topic itself a generic stock-in-trade for such publishers. The scene is a one-off in *Mary Barton*, but it starts to suggest the ubiquity of broadsides and ballads in the cases with which this book is concerned. It also sets the terms by which street literature—and cheap or popular literature in general—was coming to be conceived and denigrated. Gaskell's novel implicitly competes with other texts responsive to urban happenings: specifically, the newspaper and the halfpenny broadside, with their abiding interest in reporting trials, coroners' inquests, accidents, temptations, suicides, and crimes. Such half-penny broadsides proliferate in the same elbowing scrum which inspired Gaskell to write *Mary Barton* in the first place: 'I bethought me how deep might be the romance in the lives of some of those who elbowed me daily in the busy streets' (29). But Gaskell has no sense that street literature possesses any such interesting depth. In this distaste for the opportunistic broadsides, we can read Gaskell's contempt for their immediate, unabashed commerce of cheap urban bathos sold to any (and every) passer-by on the street.

Broadsides and ballads were a conspicuous element within an even-more conspicuous flood of cheap, ephemeral texts in the mid-nineteenth century. The ways in which Victorian writers like Gaskell responded are suggestive of a broader struggle for literary and cultural authority in which notions of ephemerality, randomness, and authorial design were pivotal concepts. A surge of cheap texts printed for street-level and popular consumption occasioned debates not necessarily about *what* people were reading, but *how* and *why*.[1] As a number of novelists and periodical writers protested, the incredible proliferation of printed things seemed only to allow for discovering texts by accident and reading in casual, desultory, rapid, and random ways. Indeed, the accidental became a preferred descriptive term within debates about the diffusion of knowledge and even the status of literature, particularly applied to those metropolitan productions which characterized the explosion of cheap print. Accidents or accident news supplied content for these texts, particularly broadsides, but more significantly they offered heuristics for understanding the sea changes in Victorian print media at mid-century.

Near the beginning of his three-part survey on the new proliferations of print, E. S. Dallas outlines what he believes to be the essential question of the age:

> What is to be the destiny of all this popular literature which is now produced in almost incredible quantities, and of which the so-called 'press' is but a single branch? In the whole range of political thought, there is not a subject that at the present moment is half so suggestive.[2]

Much was at stake, including, as Mary Poovey argues, the modern form of the literary field: 'This issue, made more urgent by the dramatic increase in the number and kinds of printed materials..., involved the evaluation and, ultimately, the definition of "literature"'.[3] Mapping her own ideas of the field in 1858, Margaret Oliphant declares much of popular literature out of bounds in 'The Byways of Literature: Reading for the Million'.[4] She recognizes the enormous readership for such productions while displacing them from literature's main street into the back alleys. Oliphant's ghetto-izing metaphor seems more hopeful than accurate: these ephemeral

---

[1] Kelly J. Mays, 'The Disease of Reading and Victorian Periodicals', in *Literature in the Marketplace: Nineteenth-Century British Publishing and Reading Practices*, ed. John O. Jordan and Robert L. Patten (Cambridge; New York: Cambridge University Press, 1995), 166.

[2] E. S. Dallas, 'Popular Literature—The Periodical Press. [Part 1]', *Blackwood's*, January 1859, 99.

[3] Mary Poovey, 'Forgotten Writers, Neglected Histories: Charles Reade and the Nineteenth-Century Transformation of the British Literary Field', *English Literary History* 71, no. 2 (Summer 2004): 433.

[4] Margaret Oliphant, 'The Byways of Literature: Reading for the Million', *Blackwood's* 84 (August 1858): 200–16.

publications could not be overlooked; according to a writer in the *Bookseller*, they proliferated to cover the walls and shop windows of England's 'great centres of population'.[5] One need not even peek into 'by-streets or small shops', suggests Thomas Wright, but visit 'the largest booksellers or newsagents of leading thoroughfares' to witness the dynamics of an emerging mass media.[6] Mary Barton encounters the spectacle of printed ephemera by just wandering out into the crowded street.

This chapter analyses how mid-century literary commentators responded to the proliferation of popular print in forms of penny journals, broadside ballads, magazines, tracts, ephemera, and periodicals at large. We can and should discriminate between them, noting how each category is conditioned by its own particular historical and material circumstances. That said, Victorian commentators frequently did not discriminate in their surveys of the field, reacting to (or imagining) such collective entities as apparently embraced all forms: 'cheap literature', 'popular literature', 'reading for the million', and 'the unknown public'. Furthermore, these writers characterized such a literature as itself undiscriminating, and—as we shall see—used indiscriminate selection as a method to sample this vaguely defined ocean of print. In many cases, 'print' is hardly even the point. The problem was the non-discriminating public whom 'popular' literature seemed to index.

This conspicuous, bustling publishing market was synonymous with the complicated and often worrying concept of the popular. To many Victorians, the condition of England expressed the condition of England's readership, whose influence and dimensions were expanding and uncertain.[7] Oliphant's title presumes a million readers. Imagining this body as 'the unknown public' in an eponymous article in *Household Words*, Wilkie Collins raises the number to three million.[8] Just who were these readers, 'the mysterious, the unfathomable, the universal public of the

---

[5] 'Illustrated Periodical Literature', *Bookseller*, 30 November 1861, 681.

[6] Thomas Wright, 'Concerning the Unknown Public', *Nineteenth Century* 13 (February 1883): 283.

[7] Scholarship has complicated Victorian assumptions about the existence, composition, extent, and cultural ramifications of such a public. For a brief overview of the complexities of the cultural and educational developments of the working class and the reactions they inspired, see Brian Maidment, '"Penny" Wise, "Penny" Foolish?: Popular Periodicals and the "March of Intellect" in the 1820s and 1830s', in *Nineteenth-Century Media and the Construction of Identities*, ed. Laurel Brake, Bill Bell, and David Finkelstein (Basingstoke, Hampshire: Palgrave, 2000), 104. See also the useful survey of perspectives on the popular in Andrew King and John Plunkett, eds, *Victorian Print Media: A Reader* (Oxford; New York: Oxford University Press, 2005), 165–9.

[8] Thomas Wright put the number even higher. Though impossible to accurately answer, questions about the nineteenth-century reading public have enjoyed the attention of bibliography-minded scholars from Richard Altick to William St. Clair, Jonathan Rose,

penny-novel Journals'?[9] What were they getting from the floods of broadsides and 'pennorths' of serial fiction and sensational stories? What was to be the destiny of printed literature and even of print itself? Many Victorian critics were paternalistically concerned with sensationalism and its deleterious influence, although by mid-century observers were suggesting that education had changed popular taste for the better, away from, for example, the salacious stories of Edward Lloyd and G. W. M. Reynolds; many conceded that cheap literature posed few threats to morality.[10] Their concerns are also frequently understood as anxiety 'about the unpredictability of reading and its effects' on a new mass public.[11] But reading is only half the story; rather, the entire production–reception complex of popular literature seemed unprecedented, unpredictable, and immense. As summed up by a writer in the *British Quarterly Review*:

> More astonishing than Gas, or Steam, or the Telegraph, which are capable of explanation on scientific grounds, is that flood of Cheap Literature which, like the modern Babylon itself, no living man has ever been able completely to traverse, which has sprung up, and continues to spring up, with the mysterious fecundity of certain fungi, and which cannot be accounted for in its volume, variety, and universality by any ordinary laws of production.[12]

No scientific explanation could account for the explosion of cheap literature, whose expanse and profusion seemed analogous only to the growth of the modern metropolis. This writer offers a development hypothesis of spontaneous generation, identifying in the efflorescence of cheap literature 'the mysterious fecundity of certain fungi'.[13] Oliphant, denying that the

---

and Franco Moretti, all of whom crunch numbers to reshape our understanding of the English reading nation.

[9] Wilkie Collins, 'The Unknown Public', *Household Words*, 21 August 1858, 217.

[10] Patrick Brantlinger thinks that Collins was in the critical minority for taking this view; see *The Reading Lesson: The Threat of Mass Literacy in Nineteenth Century British Fiction* (Bloomington, IN: Indiana University Press, 1998), 17–18. But it was widely present in reviews of popular literature, as a few examples might suggest. Oliphant finds very little objectionable content in her purchased miscellany, and 'no one who is minded to repeat the experiment need fear a contrary result'; see 'The Byways of Literature', 212. As the *Bookseller* suggests, 'in the majority of our present periodicals there is nothing to shock and but little to alarm the most moral and fastidious'; 'Illustrated Periodical Literature', 682. Charles Manby Smith concludes that even the presses of Seven Dials publish materials which 'are neither so rancorously seditious, nor so grossly indecent as we can recollect them to have been in times past'. See 'The Press of the Seven Dials', in *The Little World of London; Or, Pictures in Little of London Life* (London: A. Hall, Virtue & Co., 1857), 266.

[11] Brantlinger, *The Reading Lesson*, 17.

[12] 'Cheap Literature', *British Quarterly Review*, April 1859, 316.

[13] Biological metaphors to explain the ephemerality and boundary problems of Victorian periodicals have descended without much modification into even recent scholarship. Margaret Beetham calls them 'amoeba-like' in 'Towards a Theory of the Periodical as a

diffusion of popular literature results from rational recreation, offers a similar metaphor of extraordinary fungal metamorphosis:

> So the [edifying] penny cyclopædias dropped one by one into oblivion, and nobody missed them; and lo, rushing into the empty space, the mushroom growth of a sudden impulse, rapid and multitudinous to meet the occasion, came springing up a host of penny magazines—spontaneous and natural publications, which professed no artificial mission, and aimed at no class-improvement, but were the simple supply of an existing demand.[14]

Oliphant reimagines change in early nineteenth-century literary products as the competition and replacement of species.[15] So doing, she makes a tidy metaphor from the rhetoric of natural history and Victorian political economy, whose ideologies could be seamlessly stitched by reference to the spontaneous, the sudden, and the self-directed. While Oliphant certainly scorns the 'cash nexus', she and others are more preoccupied with large numbers, chance processes, and the '[*extra*]ordinary laws of production' of new literary phenomena. As the *British Quarterly Review* writer suggests, cheap literature 'cannot be accounted for' by (as Oliphant tries to claim) 'the simple supply of an existing demand' or other conventional economic models. '[T]he usual distributive agency' does not apply, Charles Manby Smith suggests of the notorious presses of Seven Dials; instead, cheap literature 'creates its own market wherever it goes'.[16] Its logic, not only *un*usual, seems adaptable to circumstances entirely local and contingent. Oliphant's very diction—'million', 'multitudinous', 'mysterious', 'natural', 'spontaneous'—suggests a profound concern about stochastic processes, about the mysteries of sudden, random development as they seem to structure the publishing market, popular texts, and the metropolis in which they concentrated.

Confronted with the spectacle of popular literature, a cohort of Victorian commentators set out to explore its urban byways. Their curiosity about its mushroom-like profusion and spontaneity manifests in their very approach to this material: each takes random samples to investigate and classify. They grab handfuls of ballads or pick any new miscellany to read

---

Publishing Genre', in *Investigating Victorian Journalism*, ed. Laurel Brake and Aled Jones (New York: St. Martin's Press, 1990), 24. Joel Wiener cites A. P. Wadsworth in comparing newspapers to butterflies and mushrooms; see 'Sources for the Study of Newspapers', in *Investigating Victorian Journalism*, ed. Laurel Brake and Aled Jones (New York: St. Martin's Press, 1990), 156.

[14] Oliphant, 'The Byways of Literature', 203.

[15] Studies of 'new' media are often drawn to the development paradigms of natural history, 'applying the evolution paradigm to media generation'; see Lev Manovich, *The Language of New Media* (Cambridge, MA: The MIT Press, 2002), 68.

[16] Smith, 'The Press of the Seven Dials', 264.

through, reporting their findings in essays that adopt the classificatory rhetoric of natural history. The profusion of print media required a mode of knowing beyond a reader's capabilities of perusal; statistics came in handy, but for some they glossed over the textual particularities that made all the difference for judging the popular mind. As Dallas says of his lengthy survey, 'It would be easy to heap up statistics, but, unfortunately, statistics are signs rather than ideas'.[17] If reading provided more robust ideas, that task was stymied by the sheer variety, inconsistency, and ephemerality of the textual objects to be somehow generalized and exemplified. The most fundamental problems were where to begin and what to select. Many commentators concurred with Dallas: 'It is impossible to pick and choose. Selection can only proceed on arbitrary principles'.[18]

Such indiscriminate selection looks like the right, impartial strategy to deal with the directionless profusion of popular literature. So frequently repeated, the strategy reveals its motive pattern: to confront the potentially random generation of media forms, markets, and a reading populace. Oliphant, Collins, and others register popular literature as a kind of accidental media, antithetical to the structured literary market in which they are deeply invested. This chapter tracks their surprisingly consistent responses to it, and then turns to examples of urban broadside ballads which take randomness as their very subjects. Using examples of texts about accidents—including the tragic Regent's Park ice accident of 1867—I suggest how these ephemeral texts come to 'remediate' accidents. In other words, the new 'mass media' of Victorian popular print can be characterized by the accidentalness it absorbs into its material and commercial designs. Broadsides and penny periodicals reveal the enfranchisement of randomness in print culture, which Oliphant and other commentators so assiduously denigrate. Furthermore, their surveys of this mass media borrow the same discourse of disorientation, accidental discovery, and spontaneous growth which popularly characterized the Victorian metropolis. Not only does cheap literature emerge from the city, it shares the emergent properties by which both were coming to be understood.

Randomness also has a contemporary saliency to which the end of this chapter will return. For we today, witnessing a similar profusion of

---

[17] Dallas, 'Popular Literature—The Periodical Press. [Part 1]', 101.
[18] Dallas, 'Popular Literature—The Periodical Press. [Part 1]', 96. Random sampling had contemporaneous parallels in the mathematics of probability. For Laplace and Gauss, random observations were the means to discover order within apparent chaos and large data sets; according to the 'bell curve' or Central Limit Theorem, 'the sum or mean of a great number of *independent random observations* is approximately normally distributed.' See Deborah J. Bennett, *Randomness* (Cambridge, MA: Harvard University Press, 1998), 99.

materials in electronic archives and on the web, are better placed than our scholarly predecessors to appreciate what fascinated the Victorians. In their responses to the expanse and seeming randomness of metropolitan print media, we can realize an analogue to the nascent critical insights of the digital humanities. Reflecting on archives now—including the dynamics of remediation, random access, the serendipity of the database, the problems of classificatory encoding—we see in contemporaneous reactions to Victorian popular literature a compelling attention to such contingencies. These writings offer critical analogues for the study of Victorian new media in the new media of our own.

PROFUSION AND CLASSIFICATION

> The critic is fairly distracted by the infinite variety that besets and captivates him. The only way, therefore, in such a garden of roses, is to begin boldly, pluck the first flower that comes to hand, and arrange the bouquet as best we may.
>
> Bennett G. Johns, 'The Poetry of the Seven Dials'

In his survey of popular broadsides and ballads published in the *Quarterly Review*, Bennett Johns sets out to catalogue 'The Poetry of Seven Dials': the anonymous, cheap, one-page one-offs that celebrated accidents, catastrophes, scandals, executions, dastardly crimes and murders, and other such lurid or timely events. While Johns remarks on the sensational elements of these texts, he also notes—explicitly in his descriptions and implicitly through his investigative approach—the randomness permeating their production and circulation. His taxonomy is nearly thwarted as 'the modes of treatment are so curious, the metres employed so lawless, the beauties and the blots so many and so unexpected, that the difficulty is where to begin and what to select'.[19] The investigator is stymied at the level of his fundamental abstraction: an organizational framework in which to assimilate the data. Judging their contents and material production to be ungoverned by any organizing principles, Johns undertakes a random sample—an approach better suited to the phenomenon of efflorescent texts.

The arbitrary or indiscriminate selection of cheap literature became standard practice for journalists writing on its phenomenal success and mysterious, 'lawless' character. Justifications for this approach varied. For writers like Johns, the unprincipled selection of texts seemed the

---

[19] Johns, 'The Poetry of Seven Dials', 385.

method—or the explicit anti-method—most appropriate to these 'lawless' objects of study. Others including Collins had no guidance or recourse except to buy 'hap-hazard'; randomness seemed endemic to the popular literary market. Like Dallas, many claimed that arbitrary selection was the only expedient for surveying a vast amount of material. It was commonplace to remark upon its scope. Oliphant describes the abundance as 'wastes of print' and 'wildernesses of words'.[20] According to the *British Quarterly Review*, 'the subject [of cheap literature] is too vast to be dealt with as a whole, or to be treated fully'; the best the author can do is to bring before the reader 'incomplete and fragmentary' materials.[21] For this writer, perceptions of vastness of 'that flood of Cheap Literature' are homologous to an awestruck sense of the city's expanse: 'like the modern Babylon itself, [which] no living man has ever been able completely to traverse'.[22] The familiar metaphors of the city as labyrinth, a hell of endless documents, an uninterpretable Babylon, are easily transferred to the cheap literature plastering its walls and windows.[23] According to the *British and Foreign Review*, the 'signs in the present literary times' are not hard to find: 'they stand plainly evident in the highways' and add cacophonous voice to 'all that Babel of mingled discord and harmony' that echoes through England and its great centres of population.[24] To discover or read the signs, one needed to take to the streets and take in, inter alia, *street signs*; as Dallas suggests: 'The most vivid idea of the enormous diffusion of periodical literature will be obtained by a visit to any flourishing newsvender' in the metropolis.[25]

---

[20] Oliphant, 'The Byways of Literature', 202.
[21] 'Cheap Literature', 316, 345.   [22] 'Cheap Literature', 316.
[23] See Lynda Nead's introduction to *Victorian Babylon*. J. Hillis Miller sees the trope of documents as fundamental to London as revealed in *Bleak House*: 'a document about the interpretation of documents... an imitation in words of the culture of a city'. See J. Hillis Miller, *Victorian Subjects* (Durham, NC: Duke University Press, 1991), 179.
[24] 'Popular Literature of the Day', *British and Foreign Review; Or, European Quarterly Journal* 10 (January 1840): 435. The allusion is to scripture as well as Carlyle's 1829 *Edinburgh Review* essay 'Signs of the Times'. His sweeping invective against a materialist, mechanized age includes an observation about 'mysterious' change that resonates with other observations about the press: 'The casual deliration of a few becomes, by this mysterious reverberation, the frenzy of many'. 'Signs of the Times', in *The Spirit of the Age: Victorian Essays*, ed. Gertrude Himmelfarb (New Haven, CT: Yale University Press, 2007), 32.
[25] Dallas, 'Popular Literature—The Periodical Press. [Part 1]', 101. Thackeray's survey of cheap knowledge opens with such an excursion and an ironically 'judicious' purchase: 'A walk into Paternoster Row, and the judicious expenditure of half-a-crown, put us in possession of the strange collection of periodical works... We know not how many more there may be of the same sort; but, at least, these fifteen samples will afford us very fair opportunity for judging of this whole class of literature'. See William M. Thackeray, 'Half a Crown's Worth of Cheap Knowledge', *Fraser's Magazine*, March 1838, 279.

The metropolis—most often its seedier localities—and its print media were assumed to share qualities of chaos and randomness. J. Hepworth Dixon turns the perusal of cheap literature into a stroll through the slums: 'Their virtues and their vices... are in no way referable to the same standard. The ethics which flourish in the inferior hemisphere of thought, sufficiently differ from those which are recognised in the upper, to startle the accidental intruder into the unaccustomed domain'.[26] Somewhere beyond standards, customs, or ordinary laws lay darkest London and its mysterious, popular texts. Johns and Dixon deploy figures of ungoverned chaos and the labyrinth that characterized descriptions of the neighbourhood: 'what involutions can compare with those of Seven Dials?' asks Boz, who takes the perspective of '[t]he stranger who finds himself in "The Dials" for the first time', just as Dixon goes slumming as an intruder into its literature.[27] Dickens helped to make that neighbourhood infamous for the strange and surprising encounters that Johns and Dixon adapt as a bibliographic procedure, an accidental approach to the collection and evaluation of metropolitan media.[28] From the 'infinite variety' Johns will 'pluck the first flower that comes to hand': a metaphor that ironically prettifies the encounter with these texts for sale on London streets, outgrowths of the dingy urban labyrinth of Seven Dials. As if tidying up the mess, Johns arranges his 'bouquet' according to the loose style of social taxonomy that Dickens so comically deploys in *Sketches by Boz*.

Johns's floral collection has its roots in early modern *florilegia*—written compilations or commonplace miscellanies of quoted texts.[29] But it has a different valence amid the early Victorian popularity of classificatory social theories when 'the heroic age of scientific classification' was in full bloom.[30] Commentators on popular literature joined a wave of scientific

[26] J. Hepworth Dixon, 'Literature of the Lower Orders (Batch the First)', *Daily News*, 26 October 1847, 3.
[27] Charles Dickens, *Sketches by Boz: Illustrative of Every-Day Life and Every-Day People* (London; New York: Oxford University Press, 1966), 69.
[28] So too does it transfer certain class anxieties about working and non-working urban poor into their seemingly disordered spaces and 'lawless' literature. Consider where, for instance, Collins 'discovers' the unknown public: 'I made my first approaches to [this discovery], in walking about London, more especially in the second and third rate neighbourhoods'. 'The Unknown Public', 217.
[29] Ann Blair, *Too Much to Know: Managing Scholarly Information Before the Modern Age* (New Haven: Yale University Press, 2010), 124–5.
[30] Harriet Ritvo, *The Platypus and the Mermaid, and Other Figments of the Classifying Imagination* (Cambridge, MA: Harvard University Press, 1997), 15. Foucault in *The Order of Things* claims that the eighteenth century was the heroic age of classification and the nineteenth century turned to historicism. As Merrill points out, the vogue for classification in the nineteenth century was based on identifying *species*, rather than articulating a vast classical taxonomy. See Lynn L. Merrill, *The Romance of Victorian Natural History* (New York: Oxford University Press, 1989). It may be this attention to singularity, to the

investigators whose primary resource for understanding was the taxonomy. In this context, natural history offers a useful background discourse for these investigations into the unknown regions of popular print. With the profusion of specimens from Britain's military and commercial expeditions into previously unexplored territories, 'the discovery, naming, and classification of new species was a routine feature—indeed the staple employment—of natural history'.[31] Lynn Merrill points out additional reasons for its popularity: almost anyone could set out to identify species and doing so could generate celebrity.[32] New species were celebrated in the shows of London as well as in the press; the first issue of *The Penny Magazine* includes an article on a few remarkable specimens from the Zoological Gardens.[33] Like journalists writing on popular media, Victorian naturalists were fascinated with how particular specimens fit into a teeming mass. Further, classification engendered an 'awareness of the tenuousness, the impermanence' of each singular example.[34] Naturalists and commentators on cheap literature were fascinated with how ephemeral specimens, profuse and seemingly chaotic, were also elements of a structured ecology.

In his *Dictionary of Natural History*, William Martyn describes the challenge of classifying 'the sublime disorder of Nature herself, too prolific to enumerate or arrange'—terms familiar to contemporaneous investigations of other teeming, tangled banks: the metropolis and its print media.[35] The rhetoric of classification was deployed in the urban jungle, as in naturalists' field studies, to subordinate chaos to its principled order of things. If the advertised goal was to sort and understand, a taxonomic approach also segmented and striated an otherwise undifferentiated 'mass' of the populace whose potential for collective insurgency was yet unmeasured. Partly as a result, classification flowered in early Victorian urban sociology; its application to popular literature was a logical offshoot. Henry Mayhew does both at once, a kind of literary sociology of the urban underclass. In such chapters as 'Of the Publishers and Authors of

---

ephemeral individual within the class, which suggests how nineteenth-century classification fits into Foucault's framework.

[31] Ritvo, *The Platypus and the Mermaid*, 10.

[32] Merrill, *The Romance of Victorian Natural History*, 87. Such accessibility was one of several reasons for the emerging split between descriptive natural history and the 'hard' biological sciences during this period, as Merrill points out. In terms of celebrity, Boz made his name in part by 'identifying' social species like the 'shabby-genteel'.

[33] Paul Lawrence Farber, *Finding Order in Nature: The Naturalist Tradition from Linnaeus to E. O. Wilson* (Baltimore, MD: Johns Hopkins University Press, 2000), 30.

[34] Merrill, *The Romance of Victorian Natural History*, 52.

[35] William Frederic Martyn, *A Dictionary of Natural History* (London: Longman et al., 1806), iii.

Street Literature' in *London Labour and the London Poor*, Mayhew uses the same rhetorical framework for the professionals and their wares alike: 'Specimens [of street literature] will be found adduced, as I describe the several classes [of salesmen]'.[36] Mayhew makes the equivalence through his orthodox faith in an influence model of reading. He argues for 'the history and character of our street and public-house literature' as important political phenomena: 'I say, *important;* because the street-ballad and the street-narrative like all popular things, have their influence on masses of the people'.[37] Many writers went beyond an influence model to argue for cheap literature as a veritable index to the popular mind. Oliphant reads it as symptomatic of a mass psychology: the 'multitudinous public... opens its own mind to us, all unawares and unconsciously, by means of those penny papers'.[38] Perusing the reading for the million, she claims to read as many minds. Charles MacKay agrees that the masses testify through their popular poetry: 'What a faithful index to the national mind may be found in the songs which delight the people!'[39] This presumed indexical relationship allows the classification of reading materials to apply to readers. Further, the thorough subdivisions of popular literature seemed to overlay the stratigraphy of specialized professional classes and a diversifying reading public. Dallas was struck with the extent of specialization in the popular press: 'the great point to be kept in view is that periodical literature is essentially a classified literature. No matter on what principle the classification proceeds, the result is still the same—to divide and subdivide this kind of literature more and more'.[40] Tracing the dividing branches becomes an exercise—as Mayhew attempts it—in understanding the working and non-working populace.

The naturalists' imperative to identify and sort new species appears frequently in journalistic investigations of popular literature. In 'The Unknown Public', Collins plays with the taxonomic approach as he seeks, collects, and sorts 'these all-pervading specimens of what was to me a new species of literary production...: this locust-flight of small publications'.[41] Such classification is at once an exercise in genre theory and a mode of knowledge that flattens its objects into types: 'small publications' for display in a cabinet of journalistic prose. Thackeray collects 'a dozen specimens' by walking into a shop in Paternoster

---

[36] Henry Mayhew, *London Labour and the London Poor* (London: G. Woodfall, 1851), 220.
[37] Mayhew, *London Labour and the London Poor*.
[38] Oliphant, 'The Byways of Literature', 204.
[39] Charles MacKay, 'On Popular and National Poetry', *Bentley's Miscellany*, March 1838, 251.
[40] Dallas, 'Popular Literature—The Periodical Press. [Part 1]', 102.
[41] Collins, 'The Unknown Public', 217.

Row.[42] In 'Popular Serial Literature', Coventry Patmore selects 'specimens of an immense and increasing body of publications, in many respects peculiar to our own times'.[43] Oliphant constrains her investigation to a mere fraction of 'that reading for the million which has become so multitudinous. We have not even attempted to notice the *countless swarms* of serial stories'.[44] Collins explains the peculiarity of these 'new specimens' of literary production as a 'locust-flight' with the capacity to become 'all-pervading specimens'. Like Oliphant among the mushrooms, Collins expresses some concern for the demolition of other literary harvests. The locust metaphor clarifies the potential insurgency of popular literature (and by extension the reading populace) which these taxonomies attempt to discipline: exponential growth, swarming behaviour, voracious consumption. By metonymy, these specimens suggest huge numbers of absent readers about whom Collins cannot find any 'positive information'.[45] The language of specimens—mushrooms, locusts, flora—allows these authors to transpose the 'immense and increasing body' of the unknown public and its literature onto knowable objects, subordinated to a hierarchical taxonomy; and also allows their removal to a position of critical authority beyond the popular swarm.

RANDOM SELECTION AND DIFFUSION

Collins plays many roles in 'The Unknown Public', including the amateur natural historian out to discover new species.[46] He also traces the idling path of the urban *flâneur* 'who goes botanizing on the asphalt', as Benjamin says—and thereby performs a particularly masculine, bourgeois urban fantasy.[47] Collins's interest in an 'unknown public' derives not from encountering the public as persons, but from passing shop windows with the latest penny journals on display. He adopts the role of Dixon's 'accidental intruder' into the 'unaccustomed domain' of the literature of the lower orders. Collins intrudes into the domain of what Lorna Huett

---

[42] Thackeray, 'Half a Crown's Worth of Cheap Knowledge', 280.
[43] Coventry Patmore, 'Popular Serial Literature', *North British Review* 7 (May 1847): 111–12.
[44] Oliphant, 'The Byways of Literature', 214. My emphasis.
[45] Collins declares that 'it is only possible to pursue the investigation which occupies these pages by accepting such negative evidence as may help us'. 'The Unknown Public', 210.
[46] Merrill, *The Romance of Victorian Natural History*, 37.
[47] Walter Benjamin, *Charles Baudelaire: A Lyric Poet in the Era of High Capitalism*, trans. Harry Zohn (New York: Verso, 1997), 36.

calls the 'literary Other' for his own particular purposes.[48] As Andrew King argues, Collins imports a colonial paradigm to the metropolitan centre, seeking 'exotic artifact[s] from a dark continent ready for cultural colonization and exploitation'.[49] He is also window-shopping: an urban performance independent of purposeful purchasing or utility, such as Rachel Bowlby has described.[50] As such, the chance encounters and accidents of a city stroll allow Collins to defend his experiment as impartial. In collecting penny journals to read, Collins claims to sample randomly: he buys 'five specimen copies, at five different shops' and insists that each sample copy was 'bought hap-hazard':[51]

> I have not maliciously hunted them up out of many numbers; I have merely looked into my five sample copies of five separate journals,—all, I repeat, bought accidentally, just as they happened to catch my attention in the shop windows. I have not waited for bad specimens, or anxiously watched for good: I have impartially taken my chance.[52]

Accident works both as a method of discovery and a characterization of popular literature's own haphazardness to which Collins will bring orderly knowledge. Collins's whole approach to the penny journals (and by extension the unknown public) depends on the accidental opportunities of *flâneurism* and the market for these texts. He describes the principles of

---

[48] Lorna Huett, 'Among the Unknown Public: *Household Words, All the Year Round* and the Mass-Market Weekly Periodical in the Mid-Nineteenth Century', *Victorian Periodicals Review* 38, no. 1 (2005): 63.

[49] Andrew King, 'A Paradigm of Reading the Victorian Penny Weekly: Education of the Gaze and *The London Journal*', in *Nineteenth-Century Media and the Construction of Identities*, ed. Laurel Brake, Bill Bell, and David Finkelstein (Basingstoke, Hampshire: Palgrave, 2000), 80. King and Plunkett suggest Collins's essay 'must be read with enormous suspicion', explaining how Collins strategically wrote 'The Unknown Public' to defend his friend Mark Lemon after his firing from the *London Journal*; *Victorian Print Media: A Reader*, 13. Huett finds 'an inherent ambivalence' in 'The Unknown Public'; she argues that Collins, while seemingly focused on a lower-class readership, is 'employed in simultaneously addressing and creating a middle-class audience for [*Household Words*]'; 'Among the Unknown Public', 61. As Collins investigates the 'unknown public', so the narrator in Poe's story tries to identify 'The Man of the Crowd', who ultimately represents his own alienated self; in the same way, Collins identifies only his own preconceptions.

[50] Bowlby argues that window shopping or 'just looking' becomes possible by mid-century because of the intertwined transformations of display architecture and conceptions of commodities that shift from use value to exchange value. To this she traces 'the episodic structure of naturalist novels' and—suggestive of the random method Collins employs—the coincidences of their plots: 'a necessity implicit in the irreconcilable doubleness of what Lukács identifies as the modern alternation of monotony and novelty, whereby events and changes cannot but seem random'. See Rachel Bowlby, *Just Looking: Consumer Culture in Dreiser, Gissing, and Zola* (New York: Methuen, 1985), 13, 15.

[51] Collins, 'The Unknown Public', 217.

[52] Collins, 'The Unknown Public', 219.

popular literature attuned to the city's consumerist rhythms not of supply and demand, but glance and opportunity.

In each shop, Collins impersonates a member of the mysterious unknown public (dubbing himself 'Number Three Million and One') and approaches the shopkeepers for advice on what to buy, hoping 'to hear a little popular criticism, and to get at what the conditions of success might be' in mapping the unfamiliar genre of the penny journal.[53] Thus disguised and seeking knowledge, Collins plays a disciplinary role as an undercover detective, carrying out Dixon's imperative that 'the springs of that literature should be well watched'.[54] But, as the *British Quarterly Review* points out, 'the sources, nature, [and] extent' of cheap literature are beyond the scope of any single investigation.[55] To his frustration, Collins fails to discover the wellsprings of popular literature, finding himself instead upon a floodplain without a compass. His interviews are of no apparent help. He provides a sample conversation with a salesman, a dialog between buyer and seller:

> *Number Three Million and One.*—'I want to take in one of the penny journals. Which do you recommend?'
>
> *Enterprising Publisher.*—'Well, you see, some likes one, and some likes another.... Take 'em all the year round, and there ain't a pin, as I knows of, to choose between 'em. There's just about as much in one as there is in another. All good pennorths'.[56]

Try as he may, Collins cannot extract any other opinion concerning these journals save that one is as good as another; he might as well choose haphazardly. Just as Johns struggles with 'where to begin and what to select', 'there ain't a pin' of distinction by which Collins can disaggregate the mass. Venturing into another shop, he notes of its keeper: 'He had a perfect snow-drift of penny journals all over his counter—he snatched them up by handfulls, and gesticulated with them cheerfully; he smacked and patted them, and brushed them all up in a heap, to express to me that "the whole lot would be worked off by the evening"'.[57] Rather than a careful, page-by-page handling of a book, the shopkeeper shovels and piles texts as a kind of maniacal manual labour, turning not leaves but

---

[53] Collins, 'The Unknown Public', 210.
[54] Dixon, 'Literature of the Lower Orders (Batch the First)', 3. Brantlinger characterizes 'The Unknown Public' in similar generic terms to Collins's fictional work: 'a mystery story, with Collins as literary detective'. The detective exposes his author for anxieties about his own authority: 'The emergence of the detective seems to be linked to a weakening or defaillancy of narrative authority'. See *The Reading Lesson*, 17, 146.
[55] 'Cheap Literature', 316.   [56] Collins, 'The Unknown Public', 218–19.
[57] Collins, 'The Unknown Public', 219.

indistinguishable commodities.[58] Piling up like snowdrifts and flying out the door in careless commerce, these journals circulate according to the indiscriminate logic of the cheap print market.

Oliphant mocks these same instabilities of the popular literary market in 'The Byways of Literature'. She writes of a family holiday trip to a cathedral town (Canterbury), an occasion for which they 'invested a sixpence in a most miscellaneous and varied collection of literature'.[59] Contrasting with the 'decorum and dignity' of the great, grey cathedral in the background, the miscellany represents to Oliphant all the sins of the commercial world: vanity, inconstancy, ignorance.[60] Cheap literature's ephemerality contrasts with the gradualist aesthetics and political conservatism embodied by the cathedral: 'It is so many hundred years since, chapel by chapel, and pile on pile, that fair old minster rose into the poetic perfection of its present moment'.[61] In its shadow, popular literature seems as alacritous and ephemeral as daisies in the grass. Reclining upon the lawn, Oliphant notes: 'scattered over the daisies, with the wind among their leaves, lay the unauthoritative, undignified, unlearned broadsheets'.[62] In the easy pun on leaves/pages—'the wind among their leaves'—Oliphant whispers her contempt for the modishness, transience, and fatuity of the broadsheets. The texts are 'scattered' on the grass in haphazard array. Chance carries no literary authority for Oliphant; in her follow-up article 'New Books', she derides a popular travelogue by William Hepworth Dixon whose 'little accidental information' is gleaned

[58] Reminiscent of the rag-and-bottle shop in *Bleak House*; its shopkeeper, the illiterate Mr Krook, similarly cannot discriminate among the textual contents of his mercantile chaos. Smith has a similar experience to Collins while visiting a Seven Dials press, 'turning over a massive bundle' of the 'five thousand different samples [kept] constantly on hand'; Smith, 'The Press of the Seven Dials', 253. The Victorian depiction of hands and 'manual' labour is a surprisingly consistent index to social distinctions, as Peter Capuano explores in 'Novel Hands: Manual Activity and Victorian Fiction' (Ph.D. Dissertation, University of Virginia, 2009).

[59] Oliphant, 'The Byways of Literature', 200.

[60] The implied contest between the cathedral and the periodical press shows up in Trollope's *The Warden* (1855) as the aged warden Mr Harding is attacked by the newspaper *The Jupiter*, which disturbs his sanctuary and ruins his reputation.

[61] Oliphant, 'The Byways of Literature', 201. Such sentiments line up with the traditional Tory defence of the English constitution, whose own contingency is ameliorated by its longevity. In *The English Constitution* (1867), Bagehot makes the connection explicit: '[the constitution] contains likewise historical, complex, august, theatrical parts, which it has inherited from a long past... Its essence is strong with the strength of modern simplicity; its exterior is august with the Gothic grandeur of a more imposing age'; *The English Constitution*, ed. Miles Taylor (Oxford; New York: Oxford University Press, 2001), 10–11. Other examples include Edmund Burke in *Reflections on the Revolution in France* (1790) and Coleridge in *On the Constitution of Church and State* (1829) who affirms the constitution as an idea gradually realized through history.

[62] Oliphant, 'The Byways of Literature', 201.

only 'here and there by chance'. Of its author Oliphant says, 'Perhaps he tossed up [a coin] before he set out on his journey to decide which country it should be'.[63] Oliphant's day trip to the cathedral was no such accident. Taken together, her articles imply that the market for popular literature is chaotic and incoherent; if self-organizing, it does not organize itself toward quality.

'The Byways of Literature' suggests that rational recreation no longer structures (if it ever did) the reading habits of the lower classes.[64] Oliphant challenges assumptions, popularized by the Society for the Diffusion of Useful Knowledge, about the value of reading for its own sake and faith in individual tendencies of self-improvement.[65] For Oliphant, 'diffusion' of reading and knowledge operates according to other, abstract laws, first revealed to her through statistics: 'the horrid numerals of a statistical account disclosed to us the fatal certainty that the multitude, like ourselves, loved amusement better than instruction'. The charitable phrase 'like ourselves' belies the contempt Oliphant has for the multitude of readers who 'share with the children and the savages' a desire for facts before philosophy and have a simple love of stories.

More interesting than Oliphant's derisive claim is how she gets there: she argues that the social and material conditions of working-class lives structure their receptiveness as readers. The working class are constrained to an identity dictated by circumstance alone; they lack leisure for thinking; have no conceptual horizon for sustained narrative or intellectual inquiry; live lives not of contemplation but of activity: 'all these accidents of their condition give colour to the character of the masses, and are faithfully reflected in the literature they patronize'.[66] They must want active, engaging literature, and 'the qualities of mind concerned in its production are quite a secondary consideration'.[67] The *primary* circumstances

---

[63] Margaret Oliphant, 'New Books', *Blackwood's Edinburgh Magazine* 108 (August 1870): 172, 168.

[64] Michael Hancher points out that the 'march of the intellect' was already being satirized in the 1820s before the Society for the Diffusion of Useful Knowledge got underway. See 'From Street Ballad to *Penny Magazine*: "March of Intellect in the Butchering Line"', in *Nineteenth-Century Media and the Construction of Identities*, ed. Laurel Brake, Bill Bell, and David Finkelstein (Basingstoke, Hampshire: Palgrave, 2000), 93.

[65] Newman provides another perspective, attacking the triumvirate of Sir Robert Peel, Bentham, and the Brougham Society for the secularist assumption that increased knowledge of the physical sciences necessarily leads to moral improvement: 'the veriest of pretences which sophist or mountebank ever professed to a gaping auditory. If virtue be a mastery over the mind, if its end be action, if its perfection be inward order, harmony, and peace, we must seek it in graver and holier places than in Libraries and Reading-rooms'; see 'The Tamworth Reading Room' (1841), 268.

[66] Oliphant, 'The Byways of Literature', 215.

[67] Oliphant, 'The Byways of Literature', 205.

of its production, like its reception, must also be 'brief and rapid' and outside of the essentials of philosophical contemplation. Oliphant understands the logic of such readers and literature as one and the same: each structured by the 'accidents of their condition'. The accidental characterizes both text and reader as if, as Kelly Mays puts it, 'the individual reader, having no principle of organization, no self-coherence, came to mirror the indiscriminate, unorganized chaos of texts he read'.[68]

Like so many of her peers, Oliphant is less concerned with the contents than with the production and reception of popular literature, especially as it seems structured (or scattered) by the changeable, uncertain logic of the mass. In other words, she reacts to its potentially *random* diffusion. That same apprehension of randomness, figured within the accident, characterized representations of the metropolitan environment for these textual species. It also figured in industrial and transport contexts which this book investigates in other chapters—and to which popular literature was frequently compared. 'Omnivorous' reading practices seemed to turn people into machines; the rapid and desultory reading it required was said to discompose the mind as when 'whirled through a country in a railway-carriage' as if 'hurrying at lightning speed from one part of chaos to another'.[69] Now including mass print media, such urban-industrial phenomena seemed barely controlled at scale and speed, haunted by the accidental possibilities which would throw them into disarray.

This growing sense of the potential randomness of mass literature was what came to bother Victorian authors more invested in the ideologies of literary design. As James Mussell suggests, the profuse circulation of nineteenth-century ephemera sets up a 'hermeneutic struggle' to reestablish the grounds of textual meaning.[70] Oliphant attempts to contain the logic of cheap literature to simple and simplistic formulae—supply and demand; the baseline childish/savage love of stories—but these fail to address the complexities she herself recognizes in the 'varied and fluctuating mass, ... uncertain and changeable', of popular literature.[71] Some strange catastrophism is reshaping the literary landscape; some unscrupulous species is overpopulating the terrain. Oliphant finds, scattered across the daisies, texts whose ephemerality and miscellaneity reflect the seemingly lawless processes of mass phenomena.

[68] Mays, 'Disease of Reading', 176.
[69] 'Reading as a Means of Culture', *Sharpe's London Magazine*, December 1867, 317; C. H. Butterworth, 'Overfeeding', *Victoria Magazine*, November 1869, 503; quoted in Mays, 'Disease of Reading', 171–2.
[70] 'The Passing of Print: Digitising Ephemera and the Ephemerality of the Digital', *Media History* 18, no. 1 (February 2012): 83.
[71] Oliphant, 'The Byways of Literature', 214.

THE REMEDIATION OF ACCIDENT

> If he would learn the secret of the immense successes that have been achieved by modern publishers, he must go even further, and examine for himself the nature and particularities of the best-known works patronized by the poor, the half-educated, and the uneducated; he must carefully study the broad sheets issued in weekly and monthly portions at the cheapest possible rates.
>
> *Bookseller*, 'Illustrated Periodical Literature', 1861

The *Bookseller*'s author encourages the literary historian to 'examine for himself' the source documents that conspicuously bedeck the walls and windows of the city. With the advent of electronic archives making some of these documents widely accessible, we can adopt the investigator's pose and sample this 'reading for the million'. From the swarms or snowdrifts of possible materials, I will select some halfpenny sheets of street ballads which are explicitly about accidents. In contrast to texts of more intelligent design, Oliphant characterizes popular print as a spontaneous media, reflecting the 'accidents' of its readers' condition. This section takes Oliphant at her word to investigate how accidents might actually condition these texts. Because, as this book suggests, accidents owe their absorbing interest not simply to sensation but to an interpretive contest between design and chance, street literature about accidents focuses this dynamic as a feature of metropolitan print media. Documents like street ballads not only report or versify upon metropolitan accidents; they also come to remediate them in the very conditions of their textual production and reception. They are accidental texts through and through.

The term 'remediation' has taken on a generalized definition as translation of something from one medium into another. But it was initially used by new media theorists Jay Bolter and Richard Grusin to explain how media transform at moments of significant technological change. Remediation, in their stricter definition, comprises a dynamic between immediacy and hypermediacy, or between transparency and the proliferation of opaque interfaces, which is a primary characteristic of the digital age.[72] Interestingly, Victorian commentators consistently explained the advent of cheap literature in terms recognizable in almost any discussion of 'new media', digital or otherwise. Cheap literature for the Victorians manifested analogous changes to traditional print production and access. In the next

---

[72] Jay David Bolter and Richard Grusin, *Remediation: Understanding New Media* (Cambridge, MA: MIT Press, 1999).

section, I draw out more clearly the rhetorical parallels between reactions to digital and print media. Here, I want to argue that the dynamics of remediation are present within street ballads as they characterize Victorian popular media as something strikingly new. The dynamics of immediacy and hypermediacy in street literature spawned all sorts of speculation about the characteristics of an emerging mass media in print. Though certainly not limited to broadsides and ballads, those documents help bring its dynamics into focus.

Charles Manby Smith boldly (and anecdotally) claims that these 'productions surpass in number and popularity those of any other press in the kingdom'.[73] Though the aforementioned critics have been mainly concerned with penny journals and periodical fiction—'the great hebdomadal vortex', as the *British Quarterly Review* describes the gaping periodical maw—street ballads held a similar interest for Victorians as a mass medium and window on the masses.[74] Bennett Johns says of street ballads that, 'though they teach little or no history, they show, at least, what kind of Poetry finds the most favourable reception and the readiest sale among our lowest classes'.[75] Johns is one of numerous critics who paraphrase or (variously) cite a quote about how balladry might represent or even legislate the true character of a nation, irrespective of its laws: 'if a man were permitted to make all the Ballads of a nation, he need not care who should make the laws'.[76] In his article 'On National and Popular Poetry', Charles MacKay offers another version: 'Give me the writing of songs for a people: let who will make their laws'.[77] Dixon is also a believer: 'The man who declared that any one might make the laws of a country—so that he was permitted to write its popular ballads—probably did not exaggerate the power of the people's literature in producing and determining the national character'.[78] But Johns, wary of granting too great an influence to popular literature and more sensitive to the fragmentation of the reading public, pointed out what in 1867 was obvious: 'the Nation no longer speaks as a whole'.[79] To Johns, street ballads were not national poetry but

---

[73] Smith, 'The Press of the Seven Dials', 252.   [74] 'Cheap Literature', 321.
[75] Johns, 'The Poetry of Seven Dials', 404.
[76] Johns, 'The Poetry of Seven Dials', 382. The range of attribution is surprising. Johns credits the Scottish patriot Andrew Fletcher. It also gets attributed to Francis Bacon, Robert Burns, and William Cobbett. (See MacKay, 'On Popular and National Poetry', 251.) It has also been traced back to pre-Confucian Chinese scholars by James Legge, *The Sacred Books of China: The Texts of Confucianism* (New York: Scribners, 1899), 290.
[77] MacKay, 'On Popular and National Poetry', 251.
[78] Dixon, 'Literature of the Lower Orders (Batch the First)', 3.
[79] Johns, 'The Poetry of Seven Dials', 383. King and Plunkett suggest that the second Reform Bill renewed interest and anxiety about the politics of popular culture. See King and Plunkett, *Victorian Print Media: A Reader*, 127.

specimens of a particular enterprise. Nor did he credit them with any political franchise; instead, they seemed 'lawless', fixed only by whatever news or circumstances might drive a successful print run. In fact, what street ballads so colourfully demonstrate are the laws of lawlessness, or the enfranchisement of randomness in popular print media.

Broadsides and broadsheets were 'the first medium of mass communication', according to Michael Hughes.[80] Though they appeared throughout the country, they were metropolitan products and as a literary institution they reflected the 'teeming, gregarious, convivial life, affluent or penurious' of the inner London streets.[81] Broadsides originated in the early sixteenth century and much about them remained unchanged over their long career, but they enjoyed a renaissance in the developing urban culture of the nineteenth century, providing a de facto (because inexpensive) source of entertainment and news for an expanding and increasingly literate working class. Facing competition from penny newspapers after the 1855 abolition of the newspaper stamp tax (among related reasons), the broadside presses would finally halt.[82] As a working-class cultural form, broadsides were widely ignored in the mainstream press though '[o]n the few occasions when they were seriously noticed in contemporary journals their popularity was generally a cause for amazement'.[83] Echoing Oliphant's interpretation of periodical miscellanies, Hughes suggests of broadsides that 'their main concern was to tell a story'. Commentators left quite a record about *what* stories broadsides told, but at the time they were more amazed with *how* these stories were told: how formed, and how—in extraordinary fashion—produced and circulated. Broadsides seemed to take ephemerality to an extreme.

In classifying the poetry of Seven Dials, Johns includes a pseudo-journalistic category of 'Modern Events': any versified report on extraordinary events or accidents which succeeds 'not by the wit, beauty, or

---

[80] In Charles Hindley, ed., *Curiosities of Street Literature* (New York: Augustus M. Kelley, 1970), 5. Hughes provides some useful distinctions: broadsides were 'single, unfolded sheets of paper printed on one side only' while broadsheets were printed on both sides. They were first printed in 'black letter' or Gothic font, though by the nineteenth century most appeared in 'white letter' or Roman font. Beginning with the late-eighteenth century fascination with folk culture, 'black letter' ballads became collectible while their 'white letter' street-ballad counterparts were usually and strategically ignored.

[81] John Holloway and Joan Black, eds., *Later English Broadside Ballads* (London: Routledge & Kegan Paul, 1979), II, 1.

[82] Hughes gives a summary: 'Popular taste had become more sophisticated and demanding for detailed, accurate news; Victorian street life and activity altered, assisted by the laws against hawking and signing in the streets; the abolition of public executions in 1868, and the spirit which brought this about, worked against the broadsides.' In Hindley, *Curiosities of Street Literature*, 10.

[83] Hindley, *Curiosities of Street Literature*, 9.

aptness of the verse, but by the absorbing interest of the calamity which it describes'.[84] According to Mayhew, these are known in the trade as 'Ballads on a Subject' and their interest derives not only from the topicality of an 'exciting public event' but also their just-in-time production, a temporality of print with a full head of steam: 'the celerity with which one of them is written, and then sung in the streets is in the spirit of "these railroad times"'. The time interval from event to ballad varied, but Mayhew suggests that they were 'often enough written, printed, and sung in the street, in little more than an hour'.[85] Mayhew reports that 'the patterers laugh at telegraphs and express trains for rapidity of communication, boasting that the [mainstream] press strives in vain to rival *theirs*'.[86] Street ballads claimed contemporaneity as a mass medium practically *because* they bypassed the mainstream press, including by means of plagiarism, forgery, and repurposing 'stock' content. As is well known, execution ballads were sometimes executed before the prisoner was, printed in advance to be sold on site. For many critics, these circumstances were partly to blame for the raggedy composition and poor production value of the broadsides. From another perspective, their rickety forms and break-neck pace contribute to broadsides' distinction as a cultural phenomenon. In his anthology of street ballads, John Ashton claims that '[t]hey owe a great deal of their charm to the fact that they were absolutely contemporary with the events they describe, and, though sometimes rather faulty in their history, owing to the pressure under which they were composed and issued, yet those very inaccuracies prove their freshness'.[87]

Ballads seemed shaped by the pressures of absolute contemporaneity, but their 'freshness' should be qualified: Smith and Mayhew report that they gathered much of their content from newspapers.[88] Further, when news cycles were slow, some unscrupulous publishers produced 'cocks'—the trade slang for fake stories or wondrous accounts. These broadsides sometimes rehashed calamities or sensational murders that had occurred

---

[84] Johns, 'The Poetry of Seven Dials', 221.
[85] Mayhew, *London Labour and the London Poor*, 275.
[86] Mayhew, *London Labour and the London Poor*, 229. Original emphasis.
[87] John Ashton, *Modern Street Ballads* (London: Chatto & Windus, 1888), vii.
[88] Smith, 'The Press of the Seven Dials', 258; Mayhew, *London Labour and the London Poor*, 220. Hepburn raises serious doubts about the integrity of previous ballad collectors and investigators; see *A Book of Scattered Leaves: Poetry of Poverty in Broadside Ballads of Nineteenth-Century England* (Lewisburg, PA: Bucknell University Press, 2000), I, 18; *A Book of Scattered Leaves: Poetry of Poverty in Broadside Ballads of Nineteenth-Century England* (Lewisburg, PA: Bucknell University Press, 2000), II, 536. But this chapter is interested in how such presumptions, however mistaken they look to Hepburn, help to reveal a prevailing sense of contingency in the ballads.

elsewhere or long ago.[89] 'Cocks' exploited the public credulity that such events were constantly occurring, especially in London: 'Now it is an earthquake, now a conflagration, now a horrible thunder-storm and shipwreck. In London, this species of illustrated cock is everlastingly on the alert'.[90] The particulars were almost beside the point. Though not exactly fakes, ballads on the 1834 burning of the Houses of Parliament successfully sold varying versions of the same story: 'It was the work of incendiaries,—of ministers, to get rid of perplexing papers,—of government officers with troublesome accounts to balance,—of a sporting lord, for a heavy wager,—of a conspiracy of builders,—and of "a [sic] unsuspected party"'.[91] The alternating currents of accident and rumour made metropolitan broadsides changeable and charged. 'Freshness' did not always mean historical contemporaneity, either; many broadsides recycled old materials into fresh stories through a perspectival immediacy. *Curiosities of Street Literature* collected by Charles Hindley includes the 'Full Particulars of the Horrible & Dreadful Great Fire in London'—the Great Fire of 1666, that is, whose ashes are stirred again by this nineteenth-century broadside. As the document explains in a head note:

> Of this dire catastrophe, all our histories give a general, and some of them a detailed, account; but no relation hitherto published is so minutely descriptive as that written at the time, and as it were on the smoking embers of the city, by the ingenious John Evelyn; from whose memoirs we have therefore extracted the whole narration.[92]

What follows are selected diary entries in which Evelyn, in the present tense, tracks the fire's progress. The broadside adopts Evelyn as its eye-witness, its on-the-spot reporter; it claims the absolute timeliness of his descriptions, written 'as it were on the smoking embers of the city'. The phrase also superimposes Evelyn's text on the smoking embers; his words are literally written upon them. The Victorian broadside, hot off the presses so to speak, likewise offers itself as a still-smouldering artefact of the historical calamity. Whether 'cocks', rekindled news, or earnest reportage, urban broadsides were expected to be up-to-date with a vengeance.

Accidents triggered quick reactions from all sorts of publishers. Shortly after 4:00 p.m. on Tuesday, 15 January 1867, a thinning sheet of skating ice in Regent's Park broke up under the weight of 150–200 people, mostly

---

[89] This practice was hardly unique to ballad writers. Penny-a-liners writing in the mainstream press were frequently guilty of the same thing. See 'Penny-a-Liners', *Chambers's Edinburgh Journal* NS 57 (1 February 1845): 68.
[90] Smith, 'The Press of the Seven Dials', 260.
[91] Mayhew, *London Labour and the London Poor*, 230.
[92] Hindley, *Curiosities of Street Literature*, 7.

men and boys, who were skating, sliding, and promenading across it.[93] Many were precipitated into the freezing water and panicked rescue attempts ensued. By that evening, the bodies of eight men had been recovered and taken to a nearby workhouse for identification. By the next afternoon, rescuers had recovered the bodies of thirty more. An official inquest into their deaths began, and although various theories about the accident were proposed, no answer emerged as to why the ice disintegrated. In the wake of the accident, the *Times* published long articles every day for two weeks along with assorted letters to the editor, eye-witness accounts, and reports on the inquest. Other newspapers followed suit. Public and press reactions were furious, in large part because the victims were mostly well-to-do or professional males between 10–40 years of age. As Wendy Neal demonstrates, the uproar was not so loud for that same winter's deep freeze of the indigent: 'attitudes towards calamity reflected in the press varied according to the class of those involved'.[94] For the Regent's Park accident, everyone seemed to blame the government, overlooking the efforts of the Royal Humane Society which employed 'Icemen' as lifeguards, ready to rescue and revive anyone who might fall through such frozen lakes. On that day, the Icemen had even warned people and posted signs about dangerous ice conditions—to no avail. Nonetheless, the *Illustrated London News* proposed a Minister for London whose business would be exactly to know whether people should be on the ice or not.[95] The *ILN*'s sincere recommendation of an ice czar nearly amounts to a bureaucratic parody. But it suggests how management and accident, governance and unruly crowds came to structure the interpretations of the Regent's Park catastrophe, echoing similar debates about the metropolis itself.[96]

Responses to the Regent's Park accident also came from other, less authoritative quarters, including the broadside presses of Seven Dials.

---

[93] See Wendy Neal, *With Disastrous Consequences: London Disasters 1830–1917* (Enfield Lock, Middlesex: Hisarlik, 1992), 107–18 for a thorough account of the accident as well as insightful background on how 'ice' provided recreation and excitement for the well-to-do and profound stresses upon livelihood and survival for those on the edge. In collapsing those extremes, the accident caused an uproar.

[94] Neal, *With Disastrous Consequences*, 117.

[95] Neal, *With Disastrous Consequences*, 115. The *ILN*'s comments are from the issue of 19 January 1867.

[96] The official report of the inquest into the Regent's Park accident suggests the political lessons that Matthew Arnold would extrapolate from the Hyde Park disturbance. In fact, the first instalments of *Culture and Anarchy* began later that same year. The ice accident happened because (officially speaking) of 'a large body of persons on the ice at the same time' and the 'rottenness and partial thaw' of the ice. The inquest finally recommended that the Legislature 'consider the propriety of investing the police or other authority with the power to prevent the public venturing on the ice'. 'The Catastrophe in Regent's-Park. The Inquest and Verdict of the Jury', *The Times*, 29 January 1867, 5. Perhaps they should have put up railings.

Presenting a ready and cheap alternative to newspapers, their broadsides reported such events but also remediated them in contrasting ways. The most famous of the Seven Dials presses, the Catnach Press, almost immediately produced a ballad titled 'Awful Accident On the Ice In the Regent's Park' which circulated its own sentimental version of the event on a broadsheet for sale in the street:[97]

> You feeling Christians, both high and low,
> O listen to this sad tale of woe:
> On that fatal Tuesday, boys and men so brave
> In the Regent's Park they met a watery grave
> Their cries were dreadful—see the parents wild,
> O God of Heaven, in mercy, save my child!
> For the ice gave way, the people lined the shore,
> Upwards of fifty sank to rise no more.
>
> (ll. 1–8)

The first stanza sets the tone for the ballad's 'sad tale of woe', not a narrative but a short and mixed catalogue of sentimental scenes ('see the parents wild') and facts of the matter ('fifty sank to rise no more'). It gets some facts wrong, though so did initial reports from the *Times*, which also ratcheted up a dolorous sensationalism in its subsequent articles. But the ballad's sentimental imperatives ('O listen', 'O see') and inconsistent detail are features unique to the species of street literature. In its hasty reproduction and short lifespan, the ice accident ballad reveals the interesting contingencies of its genesis.

For Johns, Catnach's ice accident ballad is a signature example of the form. He uses it to roughly sketch how the balladeers and presses of Seven Dials transform such 'Modern Events' into print:

> Thus, say, an appalling accident happens in London; the news spreads like wildfire throughout the city, and gives rise to rumours, even more dreadful than the reality. Before night it is embalmed in verse by one out of five or six well-known bards who get their living by writing for Seven Dials, and then chanting their own strains to the people. The inspiration of the poet is swift, the execution of the work rapid, but the pay is small.... A thousand or two copies are struck off instantly, and the 'Orfle Calamity' is soon flying all over London from the mouths of a dozen or twenty minstrels.[98]

---

[97] Hindley collected another ballad on the subject printed by H. Disley in St. Giles: 'Terrible Accident on the Ice in Regent's Park, and Loss of Forty Lives'. See Hindley, *Curiosities of Street Literature*, 125.
[98] Johns, 'The Poetry of Seven Dials', 392.

Notable in Johns's report are the uncertainties invited by rumour and oral transmission which amplify and distort the news so much as to become objects of fascination in their own right. News of such calamities 'spreads like wildfire' by the very haphazard logic of the accidents they describe. A printed version is likewise 'soon flying all over London' from minstrels' mouths, a remediation of the rumour now in print. Pens and presses, too, are set flying: the work of versifying is executed in great haste and a flight of copies are 'struck off instantly'. For Johns and other commentators, ballad composition has neither time nor interest in typographical, factual, and metrical accuracy.[99] Describing victims of an appalling accident, the ballad becomes the event 'embalmed in verse', itself a morbid body for a fascinated public to gaze at in the street. The encounter with the 'embalmed' broadside replicates the 'view' of inquest jurors tasked with interpreting death by accident or design. Here, the body in question is not a corpse, but a text.

Johns imagines that its opening lines produce a 'dismal horror' that grows as rapidly as the public audience: 'The dismal horror attending on a dozen such verses shouted out *con spirito* in the midst of a busy thoroughfare, spreads rapidly, and the crowd thickens as they stand aghast, all intently listening, and all eager to buy'.[100] The ballad works to appal, to recreate the potential threat of just such an accident by juxtaposing its unwitting victims with the ballad's chance auditors: 'They little thought as they went on their way / They'd never live to see another day' (ll. 11–12). Listeners/buyers encounter the performance/text by whatever chances bring them to that busy urban intersection. Like onlookers at the scene of the accident, a crowd gathers to witness the horrific event which has been remediated—according to how Johns traces it—through wildfire-like news, dreadful rumour, poetic inspiration, hasty execution, immediate printing, couriers/minstrels flying all over London with texts, public performance of the ballad, its subsequent display on walls and windows,

---

[99] While Johns and other commentators deride such stylistic carelessness, these ballads may find an unlikely defender in Thomas Carlyle, who suggests that such speed and fracture are characteristic of the age. In a letter to John Sterling defending the scattered style of *Sartor Resartus*, Carlyle cites a revolution in language that has made a pure style impossible:

> But finally do you reckon this really a time for Purism of Style; or that Style (mere dictionary style) has much to do with the worth or unworth of a Book? I do not: with whole ragged battalions of Scott's-Novel Scotch, with Irish, German, French and even Newspaper Cockney (when 'Literature' is little other than a Newspaper) storming in on us, and the whole structure of our Johnsonian English breaking up from its foundations,—revolution *there* as visible as anywhere else!

Thomas Carlyle, 'Letter to John Sterling', 4 June 1835, The Carlyle Letters Online, <http://carlyleletters.dukejournals.org>.

[100] Johns, 'The Poetry of Seven Dials', 393.

and its happenstance reception or eventual purchase. The ice accident becomes and is superseded by the 'Orfle Calamity'.

With great success for the publisher. Johns suggests that industrious chanters could sell 250–350 copies per day; the printed edition would eventually run from 5,000 to 10,000 copies. The poets were paid poorly and, to supplement their income, often sung and sold the ballads themselves. For them as for the publishers, financial success required producing these songs any time a ballad-worthy 'modern event' came to public notice and getting them to the streets as fast as possible. In their heightened attention to accidents, the balladeers were not unlike 'penny-a-liners' who were 'perpetually going about in watch for what the chapter of accidents may throw in their way'.[101] As Johns suggests of street ballads, 'A murder always sells well, so does a fire, or a fearful railway accident'.[102] The calamities market is unpredictable at best. As the *British Quarterly Review* reports, the larger market patterns of cheap literature are practically unknown even to its writers: 'The actual sale seems to depend upon fortuitous circumstances, and it would appear that the fluctuations are so great and unmanageable that the conductors are at a loss to arrive at an average by which to regulate their calculations'.[103] The logic of cheap literature's reception, in short, seems to share all the uncertainties of its production, keyed to accidents. Like the freelancing penny-a-liners, the broadside presses pursue accidents as topical materials and as context for the happenstance marketing of their printed work. The street balladeer not only takes from the chapter of accidents, he prints a page of it to throw in the way of passers-by.

In the final part of his survey of periodical literature, E. S. Dallas gathers such fugitive publications under the heading of 'Tracts'. This is a broad category for Dallas, including religious pamphlets, solicitations, and almost any chance prose from the street. Like much of the popular literature Dallas reviews, these texts are omnipresent and extensive: '[this] species of literature... is of infinite variety'. But Dallas argues for a special characteristic of their production: 'They are written with a purpose sometimes very absurd, often very mischievous, but almost always calculated for instant effect... to give a sudden shock, to catch us unawares, *to hit us at random*'.[104] What Dallas implies, a broadsheet ballad like 'Ice Accident' makes clear: the relationship between the unexpected shocks of city living and the popular print media whose production and reception tap the same

---

[101] 'Penny-a-Liners', 65.   [102] Johns, 'The Poetry of Seven Dials', 404–5.
[103] 'Cheap Literature', 345.
[104] E. S. Dallas, 'Popular Literature—Tracts', *Blackwood's*, May 1859, 516, 517. My emphasis.

insurgent logic of chance. The Regent's Park ballad remediates the ice accident into a textual object whose generation and street-level audition have accident-like properties in their own right. Quickly on the scene and on the streets, the broadside claims immediacy which is dynamically related to the hypermediacy of its peculiar textual condition and the proliferation of competing texts. Like the 'modern event' that precipitates the broadside, such a text hits its readers at random. By making accidents their business, street balladeers transform the business of writing into a practice more accidental than designed. And this is precisely the problem.

The anonymous balladeer seems not to discriminate in his address to 'You feeling Christians, both high and low'. But responses from journalistic elites to such textual productions reveal a snobbery which lines up with the politics of chance. Oliphant and Collins applaud things designed over things random, especially as regards literature in the marketplace; Johns credits his own orderly, bouquet-like taxonomy over the contingent publications of Seven Dials; as I have argued, Gaskell in *Mary Barton* uses chance to distinguish between the insured wealthy and the lottery-dependent poor. These writers frequently locate lower social orders in an epistemological category of uncertainty; in Oliphant's words, 'this large portion of the community... is a varied and fluctuating mass,... uncertain and changeable... acted upon by peculiar and not very favourable circumstances'.[105] We can quickly identify the political imperatives here. But insofar as these terms are problematic, they are also appropriate: popular literature seems *delighted* to be chaotic and cheap and lawless, finding therein opportunities for comedy, community, public performance, and profits, all exploiting the possibilities of contingency in textual production.

Consider another example, this one connecting the streets to another contested cultural domain, the music hall.[106] Publishers frequently sold the lyrics of popular songs on halfpenny sheets and broadsides. A particularly interesting example, published by J. Pitts of Seven Dials some time between 1819 and 1844, appears as one of four ballads on a sheet titled 'Braham's Delight'.[107] The first song, 'Chapter of Accidents', is the life story of a luckless man who would now be identified as 'accident prone':

---

[105] Oliphant, 'The Byways of Literature', 214.
[106] Barry J. Faulk, *Music Hall & Modernity: The Late-Victorian Discovery of Popular Culture* (Athens, OH: Ohio University Press, 2004) offers the most sustained work on the music hall's contested status and its significance in formalizing a cultural modernity.
[107] 'Braham's Delight' (J. Pitts, 1844 1819), Harding B 11(436), Bodleian Library Broadside Ballads, <http://bodley24.bodley.ox.ac.uk/cgi-bin/acwwweng/ballads/image.pl?ref=Harding+B+11(436)&id=01324.gif&seq=1&size=1>. The lyrics might be memorized or lifted from sheets like 'Chapter of Accidents, Popular Comic Song' (London: H. White

Street Literature and the Remediation of Accident 159

> I'll tell you of sad accidents a long & dismal chapter
> For if had [sic] luck ever had a form they to my back have strapped her
> I never once a wooing went in all my woeful life sir
> Or ten to one but I had got Miss Fortune for my wife sir,
>
> (ll. 1–4)

Virtually married to misfortune, the singer knows that the odds are against him ('ten to one') in this woeful life. The gambling metaphor, his bad luck, and the comic/weak rhymes quickly establish a social context for the singer. The broadside prominently advertises these lyrics as currently 'Sung at the Various Places of Public Amusement' where we will probably not find Margaret Oliphant. Like other popular and inexpensive prints displayed for quick sale, 'Chapter of Accidents' is pitched to the less economically fortunate. In appealing to this populace, the ballad depends on its readers/auditors to self-identify with fractured biographical narratives. The song seems appropriate for working-class life conceived by Oliphant wherein individual character is not self-directed, but governed by circumstances and misfortune. Oliphant would judge 'Chapter of Accidents' a song for its own sake, a fragmentary testimonial composed for amusement in 'brief and rapid' moments of leisure. Seen a different way, the ballad echoes what Regenia Gagnier argues about lower-class autobiography as it problematizes the literary devices and publishing models more common to producing middle-class literary subjectivities.[108]

The singer offers the chapters of his 'woeful life' as a gleeful catalogue of misadventures, material misfortunes, and injuries.[109] Across nine stanzas, slapstick accidents plague the singer and the unfortunate others who fall—quite literally—in his path:

> One day at play my teacher cried mind what you're with that ball about
> So taking care to strike it low I knock'd my master's eyeball out
> And being frightened tried to find myway [sic] out by a shorter cut
> But running down a flight of steps I fell into a water butt
> . . . .
> Beneath a scaffold walking once with Fribble and his daughter
> In looking up plump on my head came down a hod of mortar
> A voice above cried Mind below, to run I tried to tell her
> But flurried pushed in the mud her father down a cellar

& Son, [n.d.]), which include both music and lyrics of 'A Celebrated Comic Song Sung with universal Applause by Mr Wilkinson, in his Entertainment of Trifles Light as Air: Arranged for the Piano Forte, by Mr Wm West'.

[108] Regenia Gagnier, *Subjectivities: A History of Self-Representation in Britain, 1832–1920* (New York: Oxford University Press, 1991), 125.

[109] By which, as Mayhew reports throughout various interviews in *London Labour and the London Poor*, the working or non-working class frequently account for their status.

....
Some thieves one night the parlor robbed but they could get no higher,
Watch'd next night fell fast asleep and set the house on fire
(ll. 9–12, 17–20, 33–34)

For the singer, 'accidents' include a wide range of circumstances: personal injury and disability, happenstance encounters and coincidences, falling objects, and fires. The comedy of sensational misfortunes drives the sales of 'Chapter of Accidents' and also generates fellow feeling during its performance, vocalized in every ensemble refrain of 'Oh oh oh!'—whether signifying exaggerated alarm, sympathetic groans, or group laughter. Accidents fill the chapters of his 'woeful life', but—unlike the folio sheet music version—they also come to represent the slapdash condition of the ballad itself, bearing no resemblance to a 'chapter', sprinkled with typographical errors[110] and metrical irregularities, and ending almost arbitrarily. The length of his 'chapter' depends on what audiences might tolerate in the duration of a song; approaching that limit, the story abruptly ends. In the last stanza quoted above, he sets a house on fire and then—almost a *non sequitur* if logical sequence were even the point—declares that he has lost the rest of the story: 'More accidents I would recount in hopes that you would note them / But by mistake I've thrown away the book in which I wrote them' (35–6). He breaks faith with narrative to keep faith with accidents, having literally 'thrown away the book' and frustrated his intent to have his auditors 'note' his troubles sympathetically or as a didactic warning. The lyrics suggest a chain of mediation: he experienced accidents, transcribed them into a book, and then shared them in/as song which itself ends by mistake. The ballad then circulates as an ephemeral object in the market for popular literature.

Accidents reveal the contingencies of popular print media on multiple levels. 'Chapter of Accidents' draws its contents from assorted incidents and then remediates them as an ephemeral experience of song/print. As with the Regent's Park ballad, accident structures the internal narrative as well as the context of the ballad's publication and reception. As representatives of curious species or a class of texts for journalistic investigators, these accidental texts are demoted largely because of their class affiliations. When Oliphant writes about how working-class readers prefer a literature which reflects the 'accidents of their condition', she suggests how the condition of the accidental is itself a classed phenomenon. Its impingement on Victorian print culture spurred authors like Oliphant to

---

[110] Errors by the compositor that twentieth-century bibliographers W. W. Greg and Fredson Bowers would come to call 'accidents'.

denigrate chance. Collins has similar misgivings about this change—which he does not well understand, or wilfully misunderstands—in the modes of literary production, access, and reading. For instance, after the 'unknown public' becomes a commonplace phrase, Thomas Wright in 1883 reveals it to be a complete fabrication. Collins could never discover this public, Wright argues, because it never existed. Presuming a reading populace coextensive with penny journals, Collins misunderstands the relation of cheap literature to potential readers whose 'appetite... though not discriminative—perhaps *because* not discriminative—is omnivorous'.[111] Nor can Collins (or Oliphant) decipher the logic of miscellaneity, which, as Dallas points out, is the textual condition of omnivorous reading: 'it is a necessity of [a periodical's] popularity that it should also be to a very large extent miscellaneous'.[112]

What is 'unknown' about the reading (or listening) public, about the 'destiny of all this popular literature' is not necessarily a mystery. Instead, the 'unknown' represents a condition of unknowing, a contingent, even insubordinate approach to reading and cultural literacy. The 'unknown' is a variable in an equation beyond solution, describing the random diffusion between texts and readers. Wright outs himself as a member of the so-called unknown public, explaining that he read light literature as well as shelves of classic and contemporary texts.[113] There is no clear demarcation between domains; readers and texts intermingle in ways that do not presume distinction or design. As Jonathan Rose describes the 'promiscuous mix of high and low' in the intellectual lives of the British working class, '[t]heir approach to literature was a random walk'.[114] Collins himself takes random walks to sample the miscellany of popular literature, but he and others disdain randomness as a means of accessing and understanding the immense print resources of Victorian culture. Richard Altick finds a 'deep-seated prejudice against random reading', against 'a random flitting from one subject to another' to which he traces 'much of the opposition to free libraries and cheap periodicals in the second half of the century'.[115]

---

[111] Wright, 'Concerning the Unknown Public', 281. Original emphasis.
[112] Dallas, 'Popular Literature—The Periodical Press. [Part 1]', 101.
[113] Richard Altick notes that cheap imprints of classics and masterpieces became increasingly available after 1847. See *The English Common Reader: A Social History of the Mass Reading Public, 1800–1900*, 2nd edn (Columbus, OH: Ohio State University Press, 1998), 308.
[114] Jonathan Rose, *The Intellectual Life of the British Working Classes* (New Haven, CT: Yale University Press, 2001), 371. A 'random walk' refers to a mathematical model of movement through a temporal sequence of random steps. The concept has been used across many disciplines to describe stochastic processes, including diffusion models and Brownian motion.
[115] Altick, *The English Common Reader*, 133.

Interestingly, that trajectory has recently taken a different turn. Victorian critics associated randomness with an unfamiliar mass media in ways that anticipate how the internet and 'new media' proper have been discussed. Their questions about scale, classification, access, and remediation have been revived by the proliferation of electronic texts requiring new modes of access.

VICTORIAN NEW MEDIA; OR, PRINT 2.0

Like their Victorian predecessors, scholars of the Victorian periodical press have been no less intimidated by the methodological challenges of understanding its contours and characteristics as a whole. Joanne Shattock and Michael Wolff concede this while introducing their pioneering collection of essays:

> for the press as a whole, we appear to have little choice except to be satisfied with a casual or glancing knowledge, believing that anything broader or deeper or more systematic is beyond the bounds of reasonable humanistic ambition. The sheer bulk and range of the Victorian press seem to make it so unwieldy as to defy systematic and general study.[116]

The subtitle of their collection is *Samplings and Soundings*, announcing a method entirely consistent with the seemingly unsystematic approaches of their Victorian forebears. However, in the decades since Shattock and Wolff's 1982 volume, the digitization of print materials and research methods has allowed scholars to reconsider these problems less apologetically. Many scholars have even come to celebrate the potentials of spontaneity and randomness in how we encounter cultural materials in new media. The rhetoric of serendipity and random results permeates the web, particularly those sites built for managing its proliferation whether in general search or in specific databases.[117] Randomness has returned as a keyword in current critical conversations about the remediation, collec-

---

[116] Joanne Shattock and Michael Wolff, eds, *The Victorian Periodical Press: Samplings and Soundings* (Leicester: Leicester University Press, 1982), x.

[117] To name only a few examples: the 'I'm Feeling Lucky' button on Google's home page (<http://google.com>); the social media plug-in StumbleUpon (<http://www.stumbleupon.com>); the Oxford English Dictionary's 'Lost for Words? Get a random entry' below its primary search box (<http://www.oed.com>); the British Library's 'random selection' of images from its Evanion Catalogue of nineteenth-century ephemera (<http://www.bl.uk/catalogues/evanion/GalleryDisplay.aspx>). For further discussion and examples, see Paul Fyfe, 'Technologies of Serendipity', *Victorian Periodicals Review* (forthcoming, 2015).

tion, and accessibility of cultural materials in electronic archives and databases. For Jerome McGann, the digitization of humanities materials and methods invites a 'stochastic critical process', a self-critical reflection of the contingencies of the cultural past: 'This is a place where we glimpse the intellectual authority of chance and randomness, those swerves from orderliness that order itself demands—as Lucretius argued so long ago'.[118] In her groundbreaking book on remapping genre, Wai Chee Dimock hopes for 'an archive that is as broad-based as possible, as fine-grained as possible, an archive that errs on the side of randomness rather than on the side of undue coherence'.[119] James Mussell and Suzanne Paylor, among the editors with Laurel Brake of the *Nineteenth-Century Serials Edition*, are challenged and encouraged by the 'unexpected cross references, echoes, and subjects that occur across the edition, coupled with the potentially endless ways in which readers can navigate' their electronic archive.[120] These sentiments are echoed by Ed Folsom, one of the co-editors of the online *Walt Whitman Archive*, in his keynote essay for a *PMLA* forum on 'Database as Genre: The Epic Transformation of Archives'.[121] Folsom is delighted by the serendipitous discoveries and accidental insights that electronic collections make possible, a kind of 'random access' of cultural memory aided by machine. He cites Lev Manovich's *The Language of New Media* to suggest how narrative knowledge is ceding to database, scrambling our inherited equations for coherence. Manovich imagines the two terms as antagonists: 'As a cultural form, the database represents the world as a list of items, and it refuses to order this list. In contrast, a narrative creates a cause-and-effect trajectory of seemingly unordered items (events)'.[122] Manovich severely simplifies the definitions and relationship of database and narrative, and several of Folsom's respondents attempt corrections.[123] However, this simplification may

---

[118] Jerome J. McGann, 'The Rationale of Hypertext', in *Radiant Textuality: Literature After the World Wide Web* (New York: Palgrave, 2001), 19, 83.
[119] Wai Chee Dimock, *Through Other Continents: American Literature Across Deep Time* (Princeton, NJ: Princeton University Press, 2006), 79.
[120] James Mussell and Suzanne Paylor, 'Mapping the "Mighty Maze": Nineteenth-Century Serials Edition', *19: Interdisciplinary Studies in the Long Nineteenth Century* 1 (2005): 2–3, <http://19.bbk.ac.uk/index.php/19/article/view/437>.
[121] Ed Folsom, 'Database as Genre: The Epic Transformation of Archives', *PMLA* 122, no. 2 (October 2007): 1572–9.
[122] Manovich, *The Language of New Media*, 225.
[123] See Jonathan Freedman et al., 'Responses to Ed Folsom's "Database as Genre: The Epic Transformation of Archives"', *PMLA* 122, no. 5 (October 2007): 1580–612. Meredith McGill suggests that Folsom describes 'not a transformation but a "remediation" of archives' (1593). Manovich does offer examples back to the Renaissance and suggesting that database and narrative are 'two competing imaginations, two basic creative impulses, two

illuminate Oliphant's and others' concerns for the Victorian 'new media' of popular literature and its uncertain readership.

I do not mean to confirm Manovich's binary or his progressivist story. Instead, I mean to suggest how such a simplified opposition between database and narrative informed responses to new media since the 1820s as well as before.[124] Cheap literature in its indiscriminate abundance represented to commentators like Oliphant and Collins something of 'the first stirrings of the attack of database on narrative'.[125] They wilfully misunderstood popular literature as a kind of database, an index to the popular mind, whose abundant component objects could be flattened into indiscriminate equivalence. Collins derides the weekly papers for their scrappy variety, replete with '[p]ickings from *Punch* and Plato', noting sarcastically that 'all appear in the most orderly manner, arranged under separate heads, and cut up neatly'.[126] The text becomes a tabular index of arbitrary pickings from which he can pick arbitrarily—a process that parallels his haphazard sampling of publications on a grander scale. The 'random access' credited to databases and digital media became a robust feature of cheap literature with the unprecedented magnitude, distribution, and affordability of periodical and other print forms. It recasts the disorderly revolution in the production and distribution of Victorian media as what might be called 'Print 2.0'.

Victorian commentators as well as contemporary scholars describe nineteenth-century print media as a revolution in information technology in terms that uncannily prefigure (and probably structure) discourse about the Internet, networked information culture, and Web 2.0+.[127] In crediting 'Gas, Steam, and the Electric Telegraph' as signal innovations of the

---

essential responses to the world'; see *The Language of New Media*, 233. Still, McGann identifies this as an 'easy binary' that 'install[s] the progressivist story that underpins *The Language of New Media*' (1589).

[124] For a thorough and fascinating discussion of the prehistory of information overload, see Blair, *Too Much to Know*. In particular, Blair points out several contexts in which 'haphazard order' became the privileged mode of access, as in some Renaissance reference books: 'This clear embrace of the miscellaneous order inspired humanist imitators who hailed the virtues of the *ordo fortuitous*, or random order'; see Blair, *Too Much to Know*, 127. Random access also has a prehistory as a mode of reading reaching back to the *Sortes Virgilianae*, *Sortes Homericae*, and *Sortes Sanctorum*—forms of bibliomancy in which one opens a book (the *Aeneid*, *Odyssey*, and Bible, respectively) to a random page and accepts its contents as divination. Charles O. Hartman, *Virtual Muse: Experiments in Computer Poetry* (Hanover, NH: University Press of New England, 1996), 89–90.

[125] Folsom, 'Database as Genre: The Epic Transformation of Archives', 1574.

[126] Collins, 'The Unknown Public', 221.

[127] For an accessible introduction to the distinguishing features of Web 2.0 and its potential applications to humanities studies, see Cathy N. Davidson, 'Humanities 2.0: Promise, Perils, Predictions', *PMLA* 123, no. 3 (May 2008): 707–17.

nineteenth century, the *British Quarterly Review* includes 'the Art of Printing amongst modern acquisitions, since, although moveable types were invented in a former age, the discovery of their full capability belongs to our own.... it is a hundredfold more astonishing than the original discovery, or invention of types'.[128] It is notable that these are prefatory remarks to a survey of 'Cheap Literature'. On the proliferation of 'literary rubbish' and ephemera, Dallas argues that 'by the mere fact of that increase, it has introduced new processes and habits, and it inaugurates a new era'.[129] 'Literature', for Dallas, can no longer be defended as an exclusive category but includes every cultural atom; nor can 'authorship' be reserved for a select few: 'Everybody is reading, every class is writing'.[130] Prefiguring overheated claims about the Internet's potential for radical democracy and free culture, the *Penny Magazine* celebrates how 'ready and cheap communication breaks down the obstacles of time and space' and 'greatly reduces the inequalities of fortune and situation'.[131] Victorian celebrants of 'our literary democracy' squared off with more conservative critics citing a version of what Yokai Benkler in *The Wealth of Networks* explains as the Babel objection to networked information culture: profusion tends to chaos.[132] In countering that argument, Benkler points to the regional and local clusters, rather than undifferentiated mass, that can be shown to structure the Internet and its topology of cultural influence. This response too has its Victorian anticipation, when Dallas insists 'that periodical literature is essentially a classified literature' whose dividing and subdividing branches roughly map the topology of Victorian professions and leisure interests. Dallas also elucidates the necessary connection between the robustness of popular media and miscellaneity.[133] Victorian popular media have their own versions of niche markets, long tails, and the characteristics of superabundance and miscellaneity that David Weinberger credits to Web 2.0 in his book *Everything is Miscellaneous: The Power of*

[128] 'Cheap Literature', 315.
[129] Dallas, 'Popular Literature—The Periodical Press. [Part 1]', 97.
[130] Dallas, 'Popular Literature—The Periodical Press. [Part 1]', 96; E. S. Dallas, 'Popular Literature—The Periodical Press. [Part 2]', *Blackwood's*, February 1859, 188.
[131] 'Preface', *Penny Magazine*, December 1832, iv. By comparison, see the libertarian manifesto by John Perry Barlow, 'A Declaration of the Independence of Cyberspace', *Electronic Frontier Foundation*, 8 February 1996, <https://projects.eff.org/~barlow/Declaration-Final.html>. Manovich among others points out that such a 'California ideology' ignores the potential totalitarianism of networked surveillance, and overlooks the subjective interpellation into a network that we misrecognize as our own creation; *The Language of New Media*, 61.
[132] Christian Johnstone, 'On Periodical Literature', *Tait's Edinburgh Magazine*, 1 July 1833, 491; Yochai Benkler, *The Wealth of Networks: How Social Production Transforms Markets and Freedom* (New Haven, CT: Yale University Press, 2006), 10, 237.
[133] Dallas, 'Popular Literature—The Periodical Press. [Part 1]', 101–2.

the New Digital Disorder.[134] The disorderly alleys of cheap Victorian literature were tantamount to an information superbyway.

As King and Plunkett suggest, '[w]ays we discuss media influence today are often developments of nineteenth-century models'.[135] Mussell and Paylor extrapolate this when they observe the 'similar problems of plenitude' in navigating the 'mighty maze' of Victorian periodicals for readers then and scholarly editors and researchers now.[136] As Benkler and others characterize networked information culture, Mussell and Paylor note that nineteenth-century print forms are 'exceptionally malleable and fragmentary'.[137] They also realize, as does virtually everyone who has worked on the digital markup of texts, the almost hapless enterprise of 'classifying' objects (whether phrases, physical features, genres) through encoded description and metadata.[138] The attempt to impose on texts a schema of tags, elements, and attributes—necessarily rigorous so that the encoded text will jibe with the informational structures of its host archive, related encoding projects, and search engines—reveals instead radiant textuality and the already rhizomic features of genre. Analogous classification problems bothered Victorian natural historians, as 'the profusion and variety of the world' continually challenged their basic classificatory schema and elements. The painstaking work of description (taxonomic markup) paradoxically impeded the efforts to recognize new species as they proliferated.[139] Remarkable family resemblances to these problems appear in Victorian efforts to classify textual media which can even be seen as a precursor to hypermedia. Mussell and Paylor offer the example of W. T. Snead, finding metaphors for linked hypermedia in his cataloguing of the 'the vast and multifarious world of periodical literature' in *Index to the Periodicals of the World* (1893): users would need help navigating the informational maze; librarians would provide 'living fingerposts to the literature of the world'.

---

[134] David Weinberger, *Everything Is Miscellaneous: The Power of the New Digital Disorder* (New York: Times Books, 2007).

[135] King and Plunkett, *Victorian Print Media: A Reader*, 36.

[136] Mussell and Paylor, 'Mapping the "Mighty Maze"', 3. The phrase 'mighty maze' comes from W. T. Snead's introduction to his *Review of Reviews* (January 1890). It resonates not only with print media but with the perennial metaphor of the labyrinthine metropolis. Though Mussell and Paylor do not mention it, the labyrinth was one of several tropes used to characterize both mass media and the cityscape.

[137] Mussell and Paylor, 'Mapping the "Mighty Maze"', 18.

[138] The fullest articulation of these issues can be found in McGann, 'The Rationale of Hypertext'. See also Folsom, 'Database as Genre: The Epic Transformation of Archives', 1576.

[139] Ritvo, *The Platypus and the Mermaid*, 87–8.

There are compelling homologies in contemporary new media and the media that seemed to Victorians radically new. We perceive them better because, as McGann suggests, digital access to cultural materials helps us realize the extent to which such processes were active in the past. Dimock reminds us that genres have always been as fluid and interconnected as celebrants of 'database' have recently suggested. The digital era only exposes this insight:

> The links and pathways that open up suggest that knowledge is generative rather than singular, with many outlets, ripples, and cascades, randomized by cross-references rather than locked into any one-to-one correspondence.... The input network here is vast, washing up a largely unregulated mass of material, blurring the line between intention and accident.[140]

Dimock's phrases echo many of the responses to Victorian popular media, that 'largely unregulated mass of material' whose model of knowledge diffusion did not correspond to directed, rational recreation but rather emerged in the course of a reader's 'random walk' through its superabundant, variously classified materials. The seemingly spontaneous, random generation of popular literature undermined its status as a stable object of knowledge, blurring 'the line between intention and accident' in the logic of its production and reception.

If there are correspondences between approaches to new media then and now, there are also risks in following them too closely. As if updating Shattock and Wolff's apprehensions, Dallas Liddle argues that

> One of the few bodies of text comparable to the Victorian periodical press in size, heterogeneity, variety of contributors, and resistance to categorization is the modern World Wide Web. We can surely understand why the most common methodological observation made by scholars of the Victorian press is that no existing methodology can describe or explain it.[141]

This chapter has endeavoured to show the appropriateness as well as the shortcomings of such a claim. Similarly frustrated that 'no existing methodology' will suit their investigations, Oliphant, Collins, Johns, and others, faced with cheap literature's seeming madness, abandon method—or so it seems. They deploy (or displace onto these publications) a rhetoric of randomness which masks their own particular modes of navigating and arranging their materials. The problem recurs in Manovich's metaphor of the database because the seeming equivalence of its data renders invisible

---

[140] Wai Chee Dimock, 'Introduction: Genres as Fields of Knowledge', *PMLA* 122, no. 5 (October 2007): 1378.
[141] Dallas Liddle, *The Dynamics of Genre: Journalism and the Practice of Literature in Mid-Victorian Britain* (Charlottesville, VA: University of Virginia Press, 2009), 149.

the structured ways of accessing data, modes which are fundamentally programmatic.[142] In each case, the 'accidentalness' of discovery erases some important cultural and technical designs. In thinking about the potential of electronic scholarship, we must not fail to recognize, though it is less easily seen or conceptualized, the 'computer imagination' as our own critical prosthesis: 'Because our computer tools are models of what we imagine we know—they're built to our specifications—when they show us what they know they are reporting ourselves back to us'.[143] In other words, digital Victorian studies disclose Victorian culture and the digital culture of Victorianists alike. Mussell and Paylor are particularly sensitive to the 'bibliographic intervention' of their electronic edition: '[i]t is incumbent upon researchers to recognise that the digitisation process enforces a reconfiguration of material and that the process of marking up texts is simultaneously one of re-making them'.[144] Fortunately, re-making—digital remediation—offers some extraordinary opportunities that may help, in Andrew King's phrase, to '[return] the reading of periodicals at least partially to the dispersion, disruption and seriality' which characterized their Victorian encounters.[145]

Electronic archives link us to Victorian culture not only through *what* we can read but also *how* we encounter the materials in 'the endless reaches of the Library of Babel'.[146] With the advent of projects like the *ncse*, databases of British newspapers, periodicals collections, digital libraries, and electronic archives of cultural objects, Victorian print materials are accessible now as at no time since their original publication. They have been remediated electronically, but the dynamics of remediation were already present in the production and reception of popular literature. The Babylon of the English metropolis saw a profusion of materials whose cataloguing seemed utterly beyond reach and instead invited other modes of access. Victorian readers took random walks. Commentators made random samples, amazed at the stochastic potential of the popular literary marketplace. Popular texts seemed imprinted with the miscellaneity and accidentalness of metropolitan experience. Increasingly preoccupied with potentials of haphazardness, the Victorians found in 'popular literature' and its metropolitan environs some perplexing cultural contexts in which to articulate notions of random or stochastic

---

[142] For a thoughtful discussion on the invisibility of codes of composition, transmission, and access, see Alan Liu, 'Transcendental Data: Toward a Cultural History and Aesthetics of the New Encoded Discourse', *Critical Inquiry* 31, no. 1 (Autumn 2004): 49–84.
[143] McGann, 'The Rationale of Hypertext', 143.
[144] Mussell and Paylor, 'Mapping the "Mighty Maze"', 2, 18.
[145] King, 'A Paradigm of Reading the Victorian Penny Weekly', 81.
[146] McGann, 'The Rationale of Hypertext', 181.

development. They were mapping the development of what Castells calls the 'informational city', a 'space of flows' described by evolving media forms and the emerging networks of their production and circulation.[147] And they were articulating the patterns and politics of accident in new media, then and now.

[147] Manuel Castells, *The Informational City: Information Technology, Economic Restructuring, and the Urban-Regional Process* (Oxford; Cambridge, MA: Blackwell, 1989).

5

Chaos and Connections on the Victorian Railway

> I'm going by the Rail, my dears, where the engines puff and hiss;
> And ten to one the chances are that something goes amiss;
> And in an instant, quick as thought—before you could cry 'Ah!'
> An accident occurs, and—say good-bye to poor Papa!
>
> *Punch*, 'The Railway Traveller's Farewell to His Family', 1851

Between the 1840s and 1870s, perhaps nothing symbolized accident as strongly as the railway. A devoted reader of *Punch* at the time might conclude that no train journey was taken without one. For the pessimistic Papa about to board his train in 'The Railway Traveller's Farewell' (1851), 'going' by the rail suggests an untimely demise as much as a journey. The chances, he figures, are 'ten to one' in favour of a catastrophic event. This probability might be disputable; the following year, F. S. Williams calculated a passenger's odds of being killed in a railway accident as 1 in 420,437.[1] Nonetheless, *Punch*'s Papa marks the comic extreme of a broad association of the railway with disaster. Accidents, particularly those involving passengers or spectacular aftermaths, were inextricably coupled to the railroad as it spread through the British landscape and Victorian consciousness.[2] This association came early in the railroad's

---

[1] Frederick Smeeton Williams, *Our Iron Roads: Their History, Construction and Social Influences* (London: Ingram, Cooke, and Co., 1852), 369, <http://books.google.com/books?id=cycOAAAAQAAJ>. The *Times* offered even better odds: 'As to the safety of this mode of travelling, it must now be surely beyond question even in the minds of the most timid... the odds of more than 6,000,000 to 1 in favour of the traveller's safety'. See 'The Present State of the Railway Interest', *The Times*, 12 January 1850, 4.

[2] Compare the drastically higher probability of accidents for railway workers: according to government data, between July and December of 1855 there was 'one serious accident for every 190 workers'. Jamie L. Bronstein, *Caught in the Machinery: Workplace Accidents and Injured Workers in Nineteenth-Century Britain* (Palo Alto, CA: Stanford University Press, 2008), 9–10. Bronstein points out that more quotidian accidents in the day-to-day workings of the railway garnered far less press coverage, one of several factors that accidents to railway workers were largely absent from public view. This essay, while acknowledging the complex and discrete histories of 'railway accident', takes up the umbrella term to examine certain patterns in its production in the popular press.

career. The triumphal opening of the Liverpool and Manchester line in 1830—a gala celebrating the world's first proper passenger railway—was infamously marred by a fatal injury to MP William Huskisson. Huskisson was an enthusiastic supporter of the railway who ended up thrown to the tracks as a train came on, and his story is well known.[3] But as reported by Edward Stanley in *Blackwood's*, Huskisson's injury was one of *several* accidents occurring to the multiple trains participating in what was supposed to be a highly orchestrated event. Earlier that day, a wheel fell off the engine pulling Stanley's train: 'a trifling accident', he says, as the carriages just slowed to a stop. But then the following train failed to stop in time and the passengers experienced 'a crash upon our rear, sufficiently loud and forcible to give an idea of what would happen, if by any strange chance it had charged us with the unrestrained impetuosity of its powers'.[4] Here, Stanley isolates two elements whose combination could ignite the Victorian imagination as much as it wrecked trains: 'strange chance' and its 'unrestrained impetuosity', or the opportunity for accident and the raw, chaotic force of its consequences.

For many travellers, 'strange chance' seemed ever-present on the lines, producing anxieties about 'lives being at the mercy of a tin pipe, or a copper boiler, or the accidental dropping of a pebble on the line of way'.[5] For railway managers, sympathizers such as Williams, and later engineers like L. T. C. Rolt, trains were highly engineered and regulated for safety. Accidents did not disclose 'strange chance' but human error. Blame was frequently shifted onto workers or onto passengers, who, as Williams and others were at pains to point out, were at no one's mercy but their own: sometimes leaping from cars, riding on the roof, and wandering on the tracks.[6] According to Williams, *Punch*'s paranoid Papa should climb aboard for his own safety: 'In view, however, of the accidents on railways to passengers, from causes beyond their own control, we make bold to utter... that, after all, as things now are, *it is safer to travel by railway than to stop at home*'.[7] Williams cites numbers of physical injuries reported in

---

[3] Simon Garfield, *The Last Journey of William Huskisson* (London: Faber, 2002); Paul Fyfe, 'On the Opening of the Liverpool and Manchester Railway, 1830', *BRANCH: Britain, Representation and Nineteenth-Century History* (Romanticism and Victorianism on the Net, 2012), <http://www.branchcollective.org/?ps_articles=paul-fyfe-on-the-opening-of-the-liverpool-and-manchester-railway-1830>.
[4] Rev. Edward Stanley, 'Opening of the Liverpool and Manchester Railroad', *Blackwood's Edinburgh Magazine* 28 (November 1830): 825.
[5] Edwin A. Pratt, *A History of Inland Transport and Communication in England* (London: K. Paul, Trench, Trübner & Co., 1912), 245.
[6] Bronstein, *Caught in the Machinery*, 32.
[7] Frederick Smeeton Williams, *Our Iron Roads: Their History, Construction and Administration*, 2nd edn (London: Cass, 1968), 437. Emphasis original.

London to prove how railway injuries are few when compared to the myriad quotidian risks to which everyone is exposed. But the provision Williams strains to make about accidents 'from causes beyond [passengers'] control' was precisely the driving wheel of railway anxieties in the nineteenth century. Accidents—if only the anticipation of them—brought into focus the tension between engineered design and uncontrolled chance that came to characterize the Victorian railway.

As Wolfgang Schivelbusch has argued, the railway categorically shifted the experience of travel toward a passive vulnerability. Passengers relinquished control to the machines whose profound momentum could result in accidents that, when they did happen, were catastrophic on an unprecedented scale. The 'unrestrained impetuosity' that Stanley identifies as a train's destructive potential is precisely a product of technological restraint. This is Schivelbusch's 'technological accident', arriving in full force with steam power: 'the more civilized the schedule and the more efficient the technology, the more catastrophic the destruction when it collapses. There is an exact ratio between the level of the technology with which nature is controlled, and the degree of severity of its accidents'.[8] An essentially impetuous molecule, steam, wreaks havoc upon the system which presses it into service. But accidents were not simply a product of the railway's development: they offered Victorian observers discursive opportunities to arrest and examine this development in mid-career. The accident concentrates the problem not only of technological control, but of apprehending the degree to which human design and regulation could function in a system increasingly large, fast, and interconnected. The railway accelerated the conceptual distortions of the Victorian metropolis it seemed to radi(c)ally extend.

The railroad's connections to the metropolis were geographical as well as metaphorical. As trunk and feeder lines connected distant regions and swelled English cities, the railway was frequently characterized as transforming the nation into one giant city. Paralleling the difficulties of finding a discourse appropriate to the emerging metropolis, railway travel brought its own set of representational challenges, particularly in terms of spatio-temporal disorientation—the so-called annihilation of space and time. How such profound warping was accommodated has been the subject of diverse critical studies. This chapter takes a different track to consider how accidents paradoxically became a solution to the

---

[8] Wolfgang Schivelbusch, *The Railway Journey: The Industrialization of Time and Space in the 19th Century* (Berkeley: University of California Press, 1986), 133. Paul Virilio makes a similar argument about twentieth-century technologies in *Unknown Quantity* (London; New York: Thames & Hudson; Fondation Cartier pour l'art contemporain, 2003).

representational dilemmas the railroad seemed to introduce, dilemmas that register in the abundance of visual metaphors, language of disorientation, and subjective alienation in much writing about railway travel at the time. Accidents arrested the dialectics of urban-industrial development which either confounded or escaped apprehension. If, as Williams and Rolt tried to claim, accidents were overrepresented compared to their actual occurrence, this may testify to their useful descriptive function in urban-industrial discourse, or to their forensic capacity to interrogate what Schivelbusch calls the 'machine ensemble', 'consisting of wheel and rail, railroad and carriage, expanded into a unified railway system, which appeared as one great machine covering the land'.[9] From this perspective, scenes of accidents might actually compensate for what so many Victorians—especially Victorian novelists—complained the railway erased: knowledge of intermediary places, particulars, and the contingency of their relations.

This chapter follows the railway's growing association with randomness to arrive at a different perspective on accidents. Their prevalence in representing the Victorian railway is neither *prima facie* evidence of so many historical catastrophes nor an overwhelming critique of the physical and cultural deformations the railway heralds, as literary critics tend to suggest. Rather than accepting them as merely evidence of suspicion about the powers of metropolitan improvement or industrial modernity, I argue that accidents became imaginative sites for Victorian writers to arrest the dynamics of massive and contingent change. If the railway's growth seemed random, accident offered moments to reckon with the agencies shaping or deforming its development. Furthermore, if railway travel seemed to annihilate the richly particular experiences of the local, as novelists like George Eliot and others claimed, railway accidents provided a paradoxical solution: they returned close attention to local particularity, the contingencies shaping the everyday, and the dynamic connections within the sprawling network they outwardly tracked. Seen especially in Dickens's and Trollope's changing thoughts about the railway over its most tumultuous decades, accidents compel the reconstruction of the chronotopes the railway seemingly destroyed. These writers' changing representations of railway accident also suggest an emerging apprehension of cosmos within chaos, an attitude about growth and change more accepting of complex, potentially unknowable causalities. Ultimately, accident is not a destructive force opposed to engineered design, but a lens through which to see more contingent models of growth and

---

[9] Schivelbusch, *The Railway Journey*, 37.

form, whether as a feature of a transport network or the literary genres they facilitated.

'THIS LATERAL BABYLON'

> For instance, supposing that railroads, even at our present simmering rate of travelling, were to be suddenly established all over England, the whole population of the country would, speaking metaphorically, at once advance en masse, and place their chairs nearer to the fireside of their metropolis... As distances were thus annihilated, the surface of our country would, as it were, shrivel in size until it became not much bigger than one immense city.
>
> Sir Francis Bond Head, 'Railroads in Ireland', *Quarterly Review*, 1839

The 'annihilation of space and time' was a phrase widely circulated in early discussions about the railway. Michael Freeman traces its first usage to an article in 1833 and suggests the phrase was soon common to both celebrations and critiques of the railway.[10] For some, the roaring, shrieking monster gobbled up time and space as a kind of destruction: 'On—on—the mighty monster pursues its headlong course, mindless and merciless, destroying alike time and space'.[11] For others, such annihilation worked in service of economy, nation, and empire. Sir Francis Bond Head's *Quarterly Review* article is nominally titled 'Railroads in Ireland', but dilates to an omnivorous survey of railway travel, its dangers, and its economic opportunities for Britain at large. In these terms, the 'mighty monster' of empire is hardly a train engine but the metropolitan geography which railway tracks circumscribed. As Williams argued in his popular railway history *Our Iron Roads*: 'the extremities of the island are now, to all intents and purposes, as near the metropolis as Sussex or Buckinghamshire were two centuries ago. The Midland counties are a mere suburb. With the space and resources of an empire, we enjoy the compactness of a city'.[12] Quoted above, Head also describes the railway's annihilation of space in terms of an imperial metropolis, as the country transforms into 'one immense city'. Head strains to give a domestic

---

[10] Michael J. Freeman, *Railways and the Victorian Imagination* (New Haven, CT: Yale University Press, 1999), 21. Schivelbusch suggests that the phrase had lost its currency by the 1860s as passengers accommodated the experience of visual disorientation and annihilated time.

[11] Julia Pardoe, *Reginald Lyle* (New York: Burgess & Day, 1854), 104, <http://books.google.com/books?id=CwQnAAAAMAAJ>.

[12] Williams, *Our Iron Roads*, 1968, 284.

character to this sprawling city in his political hopes that rails might allow all of England's disparate populations to pull up a chair, united, at the metropolitan hearth. From fire-breathing monsters to fireside chats, the railway created and likewise connected antipodal reactions to its impact, annihilating and augmenting at once.

With its connection of distant points and erasure of much of the intervening experiences of travel, the railroad seemed to rupture the 'traditional space–time continuum' of old transport technologies and the social geography they engendered.[13] As Nicholas Daly argues, 'for the Victorians [the railway] stood as both agent and icon of the acceleration of the pace of everyday life; it annihilated an older experience of time and space, and made new demands on the sensorium of the traveler'.[14] Daly follows Benjamin by including the railway in a modern urban-industrial context which produces a hyperstimulated subject. For Benjamin, the defining experience of modern life is shock: in the jolts felt by the factory worker, the pedestrian jostled on the city streets, and—Daly adds—the jarring, anxious experience of railway travel. As Daly shows, the railway produced in travellers a new set of nervous preoccupations: heightened attention to temporality and its disruptions, the consciousness of sudden death, and the uncanny experience of distant points brought into immediate proximity—or the 'collision' of distant points, as Schivelbusch provocatively suggests. Though he does not, Daly could easily have drawn upon the conspicuous references to the metropolis in Victorian writing about the railway, connecting to mainline theories of urban modernity from Simmel onwards.

For the Victorians, a metropolitan frame of reference could partially accommodate the disorientation, unmeasurable expanse, and uncertain social forces that the railway seemed to herald. With its own ready associations with disorder, the city was a touchstone in debates about the railway's social and geographical effects. Resistance to the railway

---

[13] Schivelbusch, *The Railway Journey*, 43. Other theorists and cultural historians have used the concept of space–time compression to describe the very conditions of an emerging modernity; see David Harvey, *The Condition of Postmodernity: An Enquiry into the Origins of Cultural Change* (Oxford; Cambridge, MA: Blackwell, 1989); Stephen Kern, *The Culture of Time and Space 1880–1918* (Cambridge, MA: Harvard University Press, 1983). Whitman had long since famously called railways 'the type of the modern' in 'To a Locomotive in Winter', in *Leaves of Grass* (Boston, MA: James Osgood and Co., 1881), 359, <http://www.whitmanarchive.org/published/LG/1881/poems/269>. Such claims are still prevalent in criticism which accepts the railway as 'the central symbol for nineteenth-century modernity'; see Ian Carter, *Railways and Culture in Britain: The Epitome of Modernity* (Manchester; New York: Manchester University Press, 2001), 4.

[14] Nicholas Daly, 'Railway Novels: Sensation Fiction and the Modernization of the Senses', *English Literary History* 66, no. 2 (1999): 463.

sometimes became a histrionic defence of an idealized town/country divide, particularly by the gentry whose land might be appropriated by eminent domain.

> Mountains were to be cut through; valleys were to be lifted, the skies were to be scaled; the earth was to be tunnelled; parks, gardens and ornamental grounds were to be broken into; the shrieking engine was to carry the riot of the town into the sylvan retreat of pastoral life.

The anonymous member of Parliament quoted here complains about the invasion of the working class across geographically encoded social boundaries.[15] The 'levelling' of Arcadian landscape and the 'riot of the town' each suggest the political upheavals made possible by the railway's remapping of population, capital, and power. Even railway sympathizers were concerned about the effects of railway redistribution: would it empty the countryside of every able-bodied person? Would it evacuate the city centres of their productive workforce? Arguments went back and forth, but ultimately so did the railway's demographic influence, allowing people out of as well as into cities: 'Their action, in this respect, was centripetal as well as centrifugal'.[16] The railway perforated the already osmotic boundaries of the metropolis, permanently changing its complicated structure and demography.

As the railroad reconfigured the social geography of the Victorian city, it contributed to a changing notion of cities themselves. The railway circumscribed diverse persons and distant things within the horizon of an imperial metropolis. In other words, it decentralized the metropolis into a national or even imperial phenomenon. Jack Simmons points out that, in the 1830s and 1840s, the railway 'seemed to offer almost unlimited possibilities for the future development of the city'.[17] Although the first significant railway lines connected Stockton to Darlington and Liverpool to Manchester, railway companies chose London for their terminal stations. That London became a railway hub was collectively unplanned and

---

[15] Quoted in C. Hamilton Ellis and Susan Hyman, *Railway Art* (Boston, MA: New York Graphic Society, 1977), 27. For a useful overview of contemporary debates, see 'The Railway's Vandalism' in Jack Simmons, *The Victorian Railway* (New York: Thames and Hudson, 1991), 155–73.

[16] Samuel Smiles, *The Life of George Stephenson, Railway Engineer* (London: John Murray, 1857), 335, <http://books.google.com/books?id=yjkBAAAAQAAJ>. For details and historical perspectives on this shift, see John R. Kellett, *Railways and Victorian Cities* (London: Routledge & Kegan Paul, 1979); Jack Simmons, *The Railway in Town and Country, 1830–1914* (Newton Abbot, Devon; North Pomfret, VT: David & Charles, 1986); Jeffrey Richards and John M. MacKenzie, *The Railway Station: A Social History* (Oxford: Oxford University Press, 1986), especially Chapter 2 'London' and Chapter 3 'The Expansion of London'.

[17] Simmons, *The Railway in Town and Country, 1830–1914*, 96.

perhaps unwise. As Simmons suggests, railway companies overlooked the incredible expense, difficulty, and disruption this decision entailed. But 'they assumed at once that London must continue to play the part laid down for it by the old main roads, so that it became first the railways' great point of convergence' and then a great junction by the 1860s.[18] The railways cemented London's metropolitan centrality and expanded its capacity for geographical and imperial projection. London's status as a transport hub would reinforce perceptions of the railway as a metropolitan phenomenon, radiating into the country.[19] Conversely, railways accelerated the on-going physical and metaphorical transformation of London into its characteristic form of a Victorian Babylon. As London was made into a great junction, 'it also became a great tangle'.[20]

In his 1858 novel *The Three Clerks*, Anthony Trollope voices some of the geographical ambiguities the railway had created:[21]

> it is very difficult nowadays to say where the suburbs of London come to an end, and where the country begins. The railways, instead of enabling Londoners to live in the country, have turned the country into a city. London will soon assume the shape of a great starfish. The old town... will be the nucleus, and the various railway lines will be the projecting rays.[22]

As Trollope suggests, sprawling suburbs have erased the boundary of the rural. The phrase 'turned the country into a city' literally implies the metropolitan transformation of England. At the same time, the city becomes more amoebic, a strange suburban species. The railway subjects London to an ambiguous transformation into a shape with flexible boundaries and radiating arms. The 'great starfish' expands the biomorphic logic of 'the Great Wen', London as tumour, already in place by the 1820s. For Trollope, it is London which 'assume[s] the shape'; the railway

---

[18] Simmons, *The Railway in Town and Country, 1830–1914*, 96.
[19] As Dickens describes the chaotic transformation radiating from 'Staggs's Gardens'— the community radically transformed by the railway in *Dombey and Son*: 'The carcasses of houses, and beginnings of new thoroughfares, had started off upon the line at steam's own speed, and shot away into the country in a monster train'. *Dombey and Son*, ed. Andrew Sanders (London; New York: Penguin, 2002), 245.
[20] Simmons, *The Railway in Town and Country, 1830–1914*, 96.
[21] Simmons sees Trollope as the only Victorian writer besides Dickens who seriously engaged the railway. He offers a fascinating detail: in 1857–8, *Barchester Towers* and *The Three Clerks* were both written 'largely in trains, with the aid of a simple device [Trollope] fashioned for the purpose'. Simmons, *The Victorian Railway*, 202. See also Anthony Trollope, *An Autobiography* (New York: Harper, 1883), 93, <http://books.google.com/books?id=u4YIAAAAQAAJ>. Thus, beyond what the text describes, *The Three Clerks* is imbued with the material traces of the urban ambiguity that Trollope experienced with pencil in hand.
[22] Anthony Trollope, *The Three Clerks* (New York: Harper, 1860), 25, <http://books.google.com/books?id=GBoGAAAAQAAJ>.

seems to subordinate physical London, its dimensions already difficult if not impossible to perceive, to a node on a map of radiating lines. An 1845 issue of *Punch* includes an imaginary 'Railway Map of England' (see Figure 3) in which the dense connections of railway lines cover the country from coast to coast, a tangle of roads concentrated in the cities

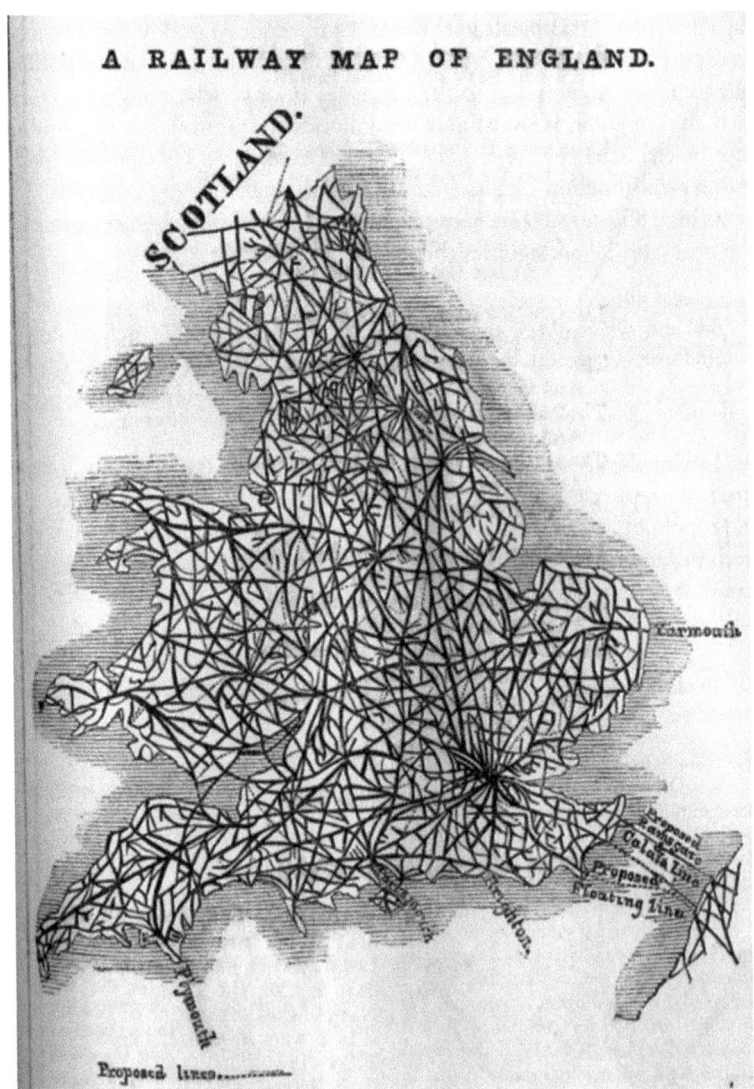

Fig. 3. 'A Railway Map of England'
Punch, 27 September 1845, 163.

they extend, London most conspicuously.[23] The comic map visualizes the centrifugal and centripetal forces which blurred the thresholds of metropolitan and national space: 'The nation's contraction into a metropolis... conversely appeared as an expansion of the metropolis: by establishing transport lines to ever more outlying areas, the metropolis tended to incorporate the entire nation'.[24] The *Punch* map frames only the island landmass, but the geographical coverage of the railway web would extend beyond its shores. Because the railway could accommodate contradictory notions of a cohesive metropolis and its impossible extent, it facilitated the imagination of a nation unbounded by geography and spatio-temporal constraints.[25] It created the material networks and imaginative interconnection to subordinate distant places, persons, and property to empire.

The radiating, lateral expansiveness of the metro-railway complex appears to striking effect in Edward Churton's *The Railroad Book of England* (1851). Curiously, Churton begins with almost no mention of the railway at all, providing instead a lengthy prose tour of 'the wonders of the metropolis':

> In a work especially intended as a guide to the Railroads of Great Britain, ... it will naturally be expected that we should say something of the capital from whence issue the main lines: we therefore offer the following brief account of the wonders of the metropolis... [And it] defies the calculation of man as to the ultimate boundaries of this lateral Babylon.[26]

The bulk of Churton's weighty book describes locations along England's major railway lines. Many of these lines have no direct connection to London, but Churton puts London front and centre in his guidebook anyway. London 'will naturally be expected' as the railway's centre, anchoring the otherwise amorphous network with its formidable status as metropolis and becoming a newly accessible travel destination. In 1850, the *Times* ranked such tourism among the railway's most notable

---

[23] 'A Railway Map of England', *Punch*, 1845, 163. Richard Altick surveys the tropes of the railway in fiction and suggests that 'fully one-quarter of all brief topical allusions in metaphorical form were inspired by the railway's presence and the proliferation of its lines'. See *The Presence of the Present: Topics of the Day in the Victorian Novel* (Columbus, OH: Ohio State University Press, 1991), 783.

[24] Schivelbusch, *The Railway Journey*, 35.

[25] Matthew Beaumont and Michael J. Freeman, eds, *The Railway and Modernity: Time, Space, and the Machine Ensemble* (Oxford; New York: Oxford University Press, 2007), 19.

[26] Edward Churton, *The Railroad Book of England: Historical, Topographical and Picturesque; Descriptive of the Cities, Towns, Country Seats, and Other Subjects of Local Interest, With a Brief Sketch of the Lines in Scotland and Wales* (London: Sidgwick and Jackson, 1973), 1.

consequences: 'Thirty years ago not one countryman in 100 had seen the metropolis. There is now scarcely one in the same number who has not spent the day there'.²⁷ As if furnishing his visiting countrymen with a guidebook, Churton offers lists of London's notable bridges, parks, places of recreation, and such like, but only before elaborating on the city's extraordinary size. His geographical interest is once preeminent and impossible to satisfy, for London 'defies the calculation of man as to the ultimate boundaries of this lateral Babylon'. *The Railroad Book of England* soon departs for increasingly distant destinations, following the radial tracks to their 'ultimate boundaries' whose tenuous connections to London suggest the extent of the metropolis's imagined community. Churton's apt metaphor of 'this lateral Babylon' suggests how the railway elaborates the tropes by which London was characterized: central, massive, ambiguous, and resistant to representation.

In an 1847 issue, *Punch* takes the railway's lateral reconfiguration of the metropolis even further, reversing the image of nation and railway network:

> It is quite evident that the old Geographies and Road-Books must be getting useless.... The geographical questions which will shortly be in use have reference to nothing but railways. Instead of saying, 'What is the capital of England?'—the instructor of youth will inquire, 'What is the capital of the London and Birmingham railway?'²⁸

According to Churton's geographical road-book, the answers are one and the same: London. However, *Punch* implies that the capital city is no longer anchored to the Thames banks, but floats outward on the rails which have redefined national geography. The joke also plays upon the transfer of economic and political capital to the railway: the seat of national power is not in London, but in a railway company's boardroom. Taking the conceit to an extreme, *Punch* suggests that the railway may evacuate signifiers of place altogether: current geographies have 'reference to nothing'. As a result, books will have to be rewritten, maps remade, and standards of inquiry and description reconceived. And they were.²⁹ Rewritten to accommodate the railway, these books had to reckon with all

---

²⁷ 'The Present State of the Railway Interest', 4.
²⁸ 'Railway Geography', *Punch*, 1847, 59.
²⁹ Churton's guidebook exemplifies how 'this lateral Babylon' required new modes of description and bibliographic design: for each railway line, the book offers capsule descriptions of notable scenes under the headings 'Left of Railway' on verso pages and 'Right of Railway' on recto pages. Mileage markers run down the inside margins of each page. *The Railroad Book of England* is part of an amazingly diverse set of textual technologies and bibliographic experiments deployed to make sense of the railway's expansiveness. Products of this print explosion included railway maps, Bradshaw's books of timetables, railway

it annihilated and imagine new ways to fill the gaps. Perhaps paradoxically, accidents offered some writers just such a space to reconstruct what the railway seemed to destroy.

ACCIDENTAL JUNCTIONS

> There is such a network of railways I do not think there is any one person in England... who knows what the different lines are. They run in such innumerable directions, and engines are passing along them at such angles at such various speeds, and with so much complication,... anybody... would suppose that they must all come to a general convergence and wreck, and that it will be the end of them all.
>
> Sir Sargeant Sargood, 1873[30]

In playing up the confusion of the railway network to his audience in Parliament, Sir Sargeant Sargood deploys some of the ingenuousness of a lawyer wishing to carry a point. Sargood uses hyperbole, but he only extends a readily available set of associations of the railway with complexity increasing to havoc. For many observers, the railway's expanding network seemed chaotic, a geographical expression of the speculative 'railway mania' which fuelled its incredible growth. In a sonnet protesting the railway's expansion into his beloved Lake District, 'On the Projected Kendal and Windermere Railway' (1844), William Wordsworth complains of the 'ruthless change' of the railway's 'false utilitarian lure / 'Mid his paternal fields at random thrown' (ll. 6, 7–8).[31] Freeman suggests that '[i]n the very early days, the array of lines appeared positively disjointed and haphazard. As more were opened, though, and as prospectors and surveyors pored over their maps, grander spatial strategies began to form'.[32] According to Freeman, the railway established a settled structure over time, but this progressive perspective was not shared by many Victorian observers. For *Punch*, the railway's grander spatial strategy looked like indiscriminate geographical domination. For Sargood, the 'innumerable directions' of tracks at 'such angles' created a tangled web which could only tend toward 'a general convergence and wreck'. Sargood

---

prints, cheap reprints at station bookstalls, newspapers, railway periodicals, and descriptive guidebooks, to name a few.

[30] Sir Sargeant Sargood quoted in Kellett, *Railways and Victorian Cities*, 294.
[31] William Wordsworth, 'On the Projected Kendal and Windermere Railway', *Morning Post*, 16 October 1844.
[32] Freeman, *Railways and the Victorian Imagination*, 1.

is also playing off anxieties about the danger of rocketing engines, as in this early complaint in the *Quarterly Review*: 'We should as soon expect the people to suffer themselves to be fired off upon one of Congreve's ricochet rockets, as trust themselves to the mercy of such a machine, going at such a rate'.[33] (The Liverpool–Manchester engine which struck Huskisson was named *Rocket*.) If early engines seemed like unguided missiles, the railway's extending tracks traced their crazy contrails. Near stations and cities, the apparent simplicity of a linear track could become enormously complicated with sidings, switching stations, and feeder tracks, many of which became vestigial over time. On a grander scale, these tracks stretched out into dendritic patterns which hardly looked strategic, but labyrinthine and inscrutable, becoming a lateral Babylon unto itself. The railway seemed to defy having been designed at all, randomly thrown and existing beyond the knowledge (as Sargood would have it) of 'any one person in England'.

Writing about nineteenth-century Chicago and the development of the American West, the historian William Cronon notes how the transformative power of the railway was often described in supernatural terms: 'Wherever the rails went, they brought sudden sweeping change to the landscape sand communities through which they passed . . . their power to transform landscapes partook of the supernatural, drawing upon a mysterious creative energy that was beyond human influence or knowledge'.[34] The American reaction to railways, as Leo Marx has shown, drastically differs from the British, especially in its accommodation of the railway as a feature of the landscape—and by extension its expansionist ideology.[35] That said, the 'mysterious creative energy that was beyond human influence or knowledge' points to a widely shared preoccupation with the forces designing and driving the railway's development, including its tracks as well as the metropolitan and regional communities through which they passed. Because England's geography was as constrained as America's was wide open, these mysterious forces were often characterized by British writers as 'compressionist' rather than expansionist. Such compression resulted in the railway's associations with the metropolis and with labyrinthine density as it concentrates within relatively narrow

[33] 'Commentary on the Projected Liverpool and Manchester Railway', *Quarterly Review* (March 1825): 361. William Congreve (not to be confused with the dramatist of the same name) devised the first system of rockets for use in war, initially used against the French navy in 1806. Propelled by gunpowder and lacking the tailfins of later rockets, these projectiles had commonly known guidance challenges. See Peter Macinnis, *Rockets: Sulfur, Sputnik and Scramjets* (Allen & Unwin, 2004).
[34] William Cronon, *Nature's Metropolis: Chicago and the Great West* (New York: W. W. Norton, 1991), 72.
[35] Leo Marx, *The Machine in the Garden: Technology and the Pastoral Ideal in America* (New York: Oxford University Press, 2000).

coastlines. Since the railway covered propertied and well-trodden ground in Britain, its 'mysterious creative energy' was just as frequently deplored as monstrously destructive. Like its centripetal and centrifugal effects on the metropolis, the Victorian railway was subject to the divergent forces of random expansion and highly compressed disorder, each of which seemed beyond human knowledge and potentially beyond control. To exemplify and interrogate these contradictions, many writers turned to scenes of junctions or of accidents.

The railway's 'powers of dispersal' are the central concern of the collected stories of *Mugby Junction*, authored by Dickens and other contributors for the extra Christmas number of *All the Year Round* in 1866.[36] The stories explore the logic of chance within the railway's disorderly development. Dickens's lead story follows a man in midlife crisis; as a recent editor of *Mugby Junction* explains, 'In flight from an old life of rigour and discipline, he boarded a train in London with the intention of alighting at a randomly chosen station'.[37] Into this disciplined life, the man, named Jackson, invites chance by climbing aboard a train. After arriving randomly at Mugby Junction, Jackson becomes known only as 'Barbox Brothers' because of the name on his luggage, or as 'the gentleman for Nowhere'. His identity is defined by his liminal status on the railway. Seeking some direction in his life, he looks for inspiration down the various lines of Mugby Junction, but he is baffled instead. For its elaboration of the junction's complexities, the passage describing his reaction deserves quoting at length:

> But there were so many Lines. Gazing down upon them from a bridge at the Junction, it was as if the concentrating companies formed a great industrial exhibition of the works of extraordinary ground spiders that spun iron. And then so many of the lines went such wonderful ways, so crossing and curving among one another, that the eye lost them. And then some of them appeared to start with the fixed intention of going five hundred miles, and all of a sudden gave it up at an insignificant barrier, or turned off into a workshop. And then others, like intoxicated men, went a little way very straight, and surprisingly slued round and came back again. And then others were so chock-full of trucks of coal, others were so blocked with trucks of casks,

---

[36] Charles Dickens, *Mugby Junction*, ed. Robert Macfarlane (London: Hesperus, 2005), viii. The title plays on 'Rugby Junction', which was at that time one of the more conspicuous railway junctions in England; see Norris Pope, 'Dickens's "The Signalman" and Information Problems in the Railway Age', *Technology and Culture* 42, no. 3 (July 2001): 436. According to Simmons, the stories 'arose out of a chance happening. That April [1866] he was travelling from London to Liverpool, and when the train stopped at Rugby his carriage was found to be on fire'; Simmons, *The Victorian Railway*, 199–200. *Mugby Junction* has accidental origins in many senses of the word.

[37] Dickens, *Mugby Junction*, viii.

others were so gorged with trucks of ballast, others were so set apart for wheeled objects like immense iron cotton-reels: while others were so bright and clear, and others were so delivered over to rust and ashes and idle wheelbarrows out of work, with their legs in the air (looking much like their masters on strike), that there was no beginning, middle, or end to the bewilderment.[38]

Dickens uses the Junction as a symbol for Jackson's emotional aimlessness. This life-at-a-crossroads trope might be a narrative cliché, except that the description of Mugby's spidery complexity is overwhelming. It echoes how Sargood characterizes the railway's confusion heading to general wreckage. In Dickens's opening story, that conceptual wreck gets localized as the scene of so many carts: chock-full, blocked, gorged, set apart, some new and some decaying, and strewn upon the tracks which Jackson cannot delineate. The passage traces the junction's confusion in conjunctions: 'and' leads to 'or'; another 'And then' leads to 'And then others' which leads elsewhere to 'while others' and other 'others'. The descriptive effort impedes its own goal; each attempt to straighten things out in prose adds another strand to the tangle. The clauses are subject to the switches, parallels, and dead ends of the junction itself. They aggregate and compile without sense, and Jackson decides that 'Mugby Junction must be the maddest place in England'.[39] Who is the genius of this place? Certainly no one at Mugby Junction. The only person Jackson meets is 'Lamps', a caricature of a dim-witted station attendant. Rather, the junction is the effect of 'concentrating companies'; it is a corporate exhibition lacking a coherent space; it is the legacy of 'extraordinary ground spiders that spun iron'. The railway does not derive from a definite agency, much as the 'gentleman for Nowhere' lacks his own identity. Instead, the railway web is an aggregate effect of concentrating forces which are, in Jackson's estimation, wonderful, sudden, surprising, and intoxicated.

Trollope explores questions about railway design and development at a similar junction in *The Prime Minister* (1876). Whereas Mugby Junction branches into seven lines, Trollope's 'Tenway Junction' arboresces even further.[40] Like Mugby, Tenway exists on the periphery of the metropolis it has profoundly expanded: 'some six or seven miles distant from London,

---

[38] Dickens, *Mugby Junction*, 11. [39] Dickens, *Mugby Junction*, 13.
[40] The notes to the Oxford edition suggest that Tenway is modelled after Willesden Junction which was also known as 'Bewildering Junction' or 'The Wilderness'. Anthony Trollope, *The Prime Minister* (Oxford; New York: Oxford University Press, 1983), 425. The anagrammatic names are literal tropes for the scrambling of the railway.

lines diverge east, west, and north, northeast, and north-west, round the metropolis in every direction, and with direct communication with every other line in and out of London'.[41] The junction exhausts the cardinal directions and the possibilities of railway travel. It forms the critical node of the blurry metropolitan network that Trollope described in *The Three Clerks*. In *The Prime Minister*, he describes the junction's confusing topography in familiar terms:

> these rails always run one into another with sloping points, and cross passages, and mysterious meandering sidings, till it seems to the thoughtful stranger to be impossible that the best trained engine should know its own line. Here and there and around there is ever a wilderness of wagons, some loaded, some empty, some smoking with close-packed oxen, and others furlongs in length black with coals, which look as though they had been stranded there by chance, and were never destined to get again into the right path of traffic.
>
> (2: 191)

At Tenway Junction, the compression of the railway network results in complete confusion. Tracks cross and meander mysteriously; the wagons upon them seem subject to the eternal misdirection of chance. The logic of the network is inscrutable even to an engine upon it which cannot 'know its own line'.[42] Where then does this mysterious knowledge exist? Dickens makes Jackson an outsider bound for nowhere, but Trollope is interested in the initiated, in seasoned travellers and commuters. He was one himself.

In his work for the post office, Trollope found himself extensively travelling across England on trains and, with time on his hands, he even fashioned a small tablet for writing: 'I could write as quickly in a railway-carriage as I could at my desk... In this way was composed the greater part of "Barchester Towers" and of the novel which succeeded it, and much also of others subsequent to them'.[43] That succeeding novel was *The Three Clerks*, which registered, seemingly first hand, the transformation of London into 'a great starfish'. In the 18 years between that novel and *The Prime Minister*, the railway had continued to expand; it was also entering in the 1870s, what Rolt calls 'a black decade in railway history'

---

[41] Trollope, *The Prime Minister*, 2: 191. Additional citations are inline to this edition.

[42] Like mother like son. In Frances Eleanor Trollope's novel *Veronica*, a passenger hears 'the whistle of some distant engine, screaming as though it had lost its way in the labyrinthine network of lines that converged just outside the great terminus, and were wildly crying for help and guidance'. See *Veronica* (London: Tinsley Brothers, 1870), 183, <http://books.google.com/books?id=ou4BAAAAQAAJ>.

[43] Trollope, *An Autobiography*, 93.

for its many accidents.⁴⁴ Thus, in the time between, the railway stretched farther with less of a sense of pattern than before. After decades of travel and writing on the rails, Trollope in *The Prime Minister* arrives at a more complicated understanding of the railway as a domain of self-organizing chaos.

The scale and complexity of Tenway Junction exceeds the knowledge of any individual, whether a seasoned traveller or not: 'It is a marvellous place, quite unintelligible to the uninitiated, and yet daily used by thousands who only know that when they get there, they are to do what some one tells them' (2: 191). Commuters and travellers go about their business, each like an atom in a larger mass, directed by 'some one' whom they do not expect to know. Whereas Mugby Junction was the maddest place in England, Tenway seems to have a *genius loci*: 'they all do get properly placed and unplaced, so that the spectator at last acknowledges that over all this apparent chaos there is presiding a great genius of order' (2: 192). Though nearly impossible to reason the mechanisms of this order, it reveals itself in the aggregate of apparent disorder. At Tenway, chaos becomes cosmos.⁴⁵ In the 1870s, the 'relativity imagination' was stirring in multiple Victorian contexts as Christopher Herbert suggests, but the railway came to encourage similar insights and lend explanatory power to Victorian writers interested in complex development. After years of travelling and writing on the rails, as well as surely remaining aware of its rising accidents, Trollope hints at a chaotic theory in which the mysterious meanderings of chance somehow aggregate into a stochastic order.

The dynamic works both ways. In the cosmos of Trollope's novel, this tenuous order can be shattered in a moment. Ferdinand Lopez, feeling the crushing weight of his ruined reputation and prospects, wanders perilously close to passing trains on the platforms. As railway pundits direct various individuals who know only to do what they are told, so Lopez is accosted by a pundit suspicious of his intentions.⁴⁶ But Tenway denies a totally disciplined order: 'Tenway Junction is so big a place, and so scattered, that it is impossible that all the pundits should by any combined activity

---

⁴⁴ *Red for Danger: A History of Railway Accidents and Railway Safety* (Newton Abbot, Devon: David & Charles, 1976), 61.
⁴⁵ Or perhaps 'chaosmos', the term Philip Kuberski borrows from *Finnegans Wake* to describe the 'play of determinacy and indeterminacy' in quantum science and modernist literature. Philip Kuberski, *Chaosmos: Literature, Science, and Theory* (Albany, NY: State University of New York Press, 1994), 2.
⁴⁶ Trollope's 'railway pundit' reveals the railway's global and colonial connections on the frontier of language. In India, 'pundit' ('pandit') referred to a learned or wise person. The term was also used for native surveyors the English hired for an ambitious geographical survey of India in the 1860s.

maintain to the letter that order of which our special pundit had spoken' (2: 193). The 'combined activity' produces both 'a great genius of order' and mass confusion which allows Lopez to slip across to another platform and, before anyone can prevent him, walk with calm deliberation down a ramp 'made for certain purposes of traffic' (2: 194). Traffic, in its inscrutable complexity, has still been designed to satisfy 'certain purposes'. Ironically, Lopez has 'certain purposes' of his own, taking advantage of the prevailing uncertainty of the Junction. He walks onto the tracks to be obliterated by an oncoming express. His fatal railway accident was certainly designed. Or was it? 'There was an inquest held of course,—well, we will say on the body,—and, singularly enough, great difference of opinion as to the manner, though of course none as to the immediate cause of the death. Had it been accidental, or premeditated?' (2: 195) The coroner's inquest lacks its primary evidence, the corpse. It can only conclude with a verdict of accidental death and a recommendation for better signalling in the station.[47] Neither forecloses upon the uncertainties embodied—well, we will say disembodied—by the railway and the unfortunate adventurer, Lopez.

'Accident, or suicide?' That question heads a small section in Ian Carter's analysis of the railway vignettes in *Dombey and Son*. At issue is the death of Mr Carker, the right-hand man of Mr Dombey who scandalously absconds with his money and wife. According to Dickens's outlines for the novel, Carker's death was planned all along. Carker himself realizes as much when, his scheme discovered, he flees from the pursuing Dombey: 'Death was on him. He was marked off'.[48] Like Lopez, he wanders into the path of an oncoming express engine and is obliterated:

> He heard a shout—another—saw the face change from its vindictive passion to a faint sickness and terror—felt the earth tremble—knew in a moment that the rush was come—uttered a shriek—looked round—saw the red eyes, bleared and dim, in the daylight, close upon him—was beaten down, caught up, and whirled away upon a jagged mill, that spun him round and round, and struck him limb from limb, and licked his stream of life up with its fiery heat, and cast his mutilated fragments in the air.
>
> (842)

---

[47] Nancy Henry puts Lopez in context of suicidal financiers whose ends offer moral justice. Lopez 'was the last of Trollope's speculator-suicides' and, like the inquest verdict, his death leaves justice suspended. See '"Rushing into Eternity": Suicide and Finance in Victorian Fiction', in *Victorian Investments: New Perspectives on Finance and Culture*, ed. Cannon Schmitt and Nancy Henry (Bloomington, IN: Indiana University Press, 2009), 174.

[48] Dickens, *Dombey and Son*, 842. Additional citations are inline to this edition.

Carter suggests this death is hardly ambiguous. The vile Mr Carker gets obliterated at the very moment he makes eye contact with his pursuer, the 'vindictive' Mr Dombey. Mr Carker, haunted by a 'nameless shock' which arrives *in propria persona* as a railway engine, realizes the answer to its persistent question of 'whither?' is the grave. But the disorientation of 'whither' the railway runs cannot be completely answered by the railway's association with death, as Carter concludes.[49] It is figured in Mr Carker who has been wandering near the tracks '[u]nable to rest, and irresistibly attracted' to the 'brink of it' (840). Mr Carker is as disoriented as Lopez. Did he wander into the train's path with certain purposes? Dickens tries to impose a moral framework on the scene, unconcerned with the question of accident or suicide. After all, neither Mr Carker nor the train causes the death: it seems providential. But the spectacle of the railway accident calls up more questions about causality and chance than Dickens cares to answer. For instance, 'whither' are Carker's remains headed? Dickens tries to cover up the problem of the body, as it were. The chapter ends with four men carrying away something heavy on a covered board. It does not say where they are going, delivering the body for another interpretive community to view and decide upon its demise. In this case, the coroner's jury could have only pronounced 'accidental death'.

Trollope, a novelist much more at home in a post-sacred world according to George Levine, includes an inquest not to solve the problem of why accidents happen but to complicate it.[50] Dickens strains to make the railway a vehicle for providential causality, but Trollope is interested in equally powerful though less distinct concepts of railway dis/order. If railway accidents raised the spectre of randomness within an orderly network, Lopez's suicide reveals its logical opposite: deliberation within a chaotic system.[51] Trollope joins these conditions at Tenway to make a both/and claim about the randomness and design operating in the railway's physical network and social dynamics. Lopez becomes a gruesome microcosm of the diffusion of atomized passengers throughout Tenway Junction: he 'in a moment had been knocked into bloody atoms' (2: 194).

---

[49] Certainly morbidity is the bass note of Dickens's critique of the railway in *Dombey and Son*, as in Chapter 20, 'Mr Dombey goes upon a Journey': 'The power that forced itself upon its iron way—its own—defiant of all paths and roads, piercing through the heart of every obstacle, and dragging living creatures of all classes, ages, and degrees behind it, was a type of the triumphant monster, Death' (311).
[50] George Levine, *Darwin and the Novelists: Patterns of Science in Victorian Fiction* (Cambridge, MA: Harvard University Press, 1988), 207.
[51] Lopez becomes 'a man of the crowd', in Poe's sense. The devious, deliberating mind within the railway crowd can be clearly related to urban detective fiction. See Carter, *Railways and Culture in Britain*, especially Chapter 8, 'Crime on the Line', and Chapter 9, 'Crime on the Train'.

Trollope anticipates the indecision of the inquest in his very syntax so that the reader, like the coroner's jury, is left to decide. He makes a curious switch of tenses from the simple past to a passive form of the past perfect: 'he walked down before the flying engine—and in a moment had been knocked'. The switch obscures any particular actor in the collision: Lopez walked, but the collision happened. It also renders grammatically invisible the moment of collision signified by the dash. The impact is an absent presence, indescribable except in anticipation or retrospect, and possessing a titanic force which blasts wholes into atoms without an intermediary state. Like the ingenious ways that Tenway's local chaos of railway tracks and individual passengers combine into sense, the railway accident diabolically renders things back, in a moment impossible to scrutinize, into nonsense. As passengers are 'properly placed and unplaced' into a greater whole, Lopez's body is vapourized into its smallest and unrecognizable parts.

With these state changes, Trollope lends a narrative body to attitudes about steam power. Boiler explosions preoccupied many nervous travellers in the early days of the railway. Steam also manifested a kind of atomic uncertainty in scientific discourse, especially in theories of gas after mid-century.[52] James Clerk Maxwell's kinetic theory of gases accepted the uncertainty of molecular motion into a new statistical model, basically making chance part of the equation. While such scientific abstraction rarely appears in railway discourse, it does show up in fascination with the railway's engineering challenges: how to orchestrate the complexity of crowds, cargo, and machinery into a working system. Even Williams, otherwise so boosterish about the railway, is awed:

> This immense number of passengers and enormous bulk of goods are drawn by engines of the most complicated mechanism, held together with millions of rivets, each engine containing an intricate network of tubes, numerous cranks, and other delicate pieces of workmanship, and the engines and

---

[52] To harness the expansive power of steam to propel a train engine is a material demonstration of the Newtonian physics of gas. Physicists since Robert Boyle had articulated with increasing sophistication the constant relationships between temperature, pressure, volume, and number of particles that define an 'ideal gas'. The mechanical interactions of individual particles or their particular pathways need not be considered; that they have non-reactive, elastic collisions is enough. In other words, molecules may careen around on random tracks, untraceable within the cloud, but their individual presence is subordinate to their aggregate effects as steam. However, by the mid-nineteenth century Maxwell and others were reconsidering how the mathematical rigors of the gas laws could actually be derived from the impossibly complex, random motion of molecules. Theodore M. Porter, *The Rise of Statistical Thinking, 1820–1900* (Princeton, NJ: Princeton University Press, 1986), 114. Maxwell came to formulate a statistical model, known as the kinetic theory of gases, which accepted the uncertainty of molecular motion through probability statements. The swerves of a particular particle had a new impact.

vehicles are connected by chains and couplings. In every separate item of all these innumerable parts lurk elements of danger, and the slightest fracture may produce disaster.[53]

Williams seems amazed that these individual components together assemble a steam-driven system which, for all its complexity and potential for accident, is so stable. He shares with Trollope a sense of mystery in the mass, a fascination with the 'complicated mechanism' or the improbable assembly of the network whose operation could be radically disrupted by 'the slightest fracture', the single elemental swerve. The dynamics of this dis/order may be unknowable even to the railway's engineers, much less to writers of the railway books of England. What Trollope and Dickens suggest is how other kinds of books stabilize such complexities in aestheticizing the accident, most conspicuously in scenes of accidents and junctions.

These were the scenes in which the Victorians explored the railway's dynamics of order and disorder. The railway's construction projects—particularly as it passed through cities—offered the same interpretive possibilities. Because these projects required significant demolition and bypass, they brought massive disruption into public view. Williams sketches what a resident living nearby might see: '[he] could look down on an infinite chaos of timber, shaft holes, ascending and descending chains and iron buckets which brought rubbish from below to be carted away'.[54] All these confused elements of construction are only productive of rubbish. Taken together, they create (or possibly reveal beneath the street) 'infinite chaos' within the railway's metropolitan dream of order.[55]

J. C. Bourne's lithograph of the railway's construction through London's Camden Town (see Figure 4) presents a cleaner, more orderly image than the description Dickens famously offers in *Dombey and Son*. Bourne's

---

[53] Williams, *Our Iron Roads*, 1968, 440. Such appreciation of mechanical complexity and ingenuity is a flavour of the industrial sublime; see Esther Moir, *The Discovery of Britain; the English Tourists, 1540 to 1840* (London: Routledge & Kegan Paul, 1964), 97 ff.

[54] Williams, *Our Iron Roads*, 1968, 166.

[55] Some critics have identified in this 'destruction and renewal of the pre-existing urban fabric' a principle of 'creative destruction' that defines the railway's urbanization of (the) capital. See Freeman, *Railways and the Victorian Imagination*, 122; David Harvey, *Consciousness and the Urban Experience: Studies in the History and Theory of Capitalist Urbanization* (Baltimore, MD: Johns Hopkins University Press, 1985), 28–9. Neil Smith argues that such uneven geographical development and stochastic growth is the signature of capital's 'production of space in its own image'; *Uneven Development: Nature, Capital, and the Production of Space* (New York: Blackwell, 1984), xi. If so, these zones of railway con/destruction were sites of contested interpretation about the very coherence of capital, particularly as a system that enfranchises (and in these places materializes) chance.

depiction seems placid compared to 'Staggs's Gardens', an urban landscape riven by an earthquake. Its full effects are best felt in a longer excerpt:

> The first shock of a great earthquake had, just at that period, rent the whole neighbourhood to its centre. Traces of its course were visible on every side. Houses were knocked down; streets broken through and stopped; deep pits and trenches dug in the ground; enormous heaps of earth and clay thrown up; buildings that were undermined and shaking, propped by great beams of wood. Here, a chaos of carts, overthrown and jumbled together, lay topsy-turvy at the bottom of a steep unnatural hill; there, confused treasures of iron soaked and rusted in something that had accidentally become a pond....
> There were a hundred thousand shapes and substances of incompleteness, wildly mingled out of their places, upside down, burrowing in the earth, aspiring in the air, mouldering in the water, and unintelligible as any dream. Hot springs and fiery eruptions, the usual attendants upon earthquakes, lent their contributions of confusion to the scene. Boiling water hissed and heaved within dilapidated walls, whence, also, the glare and roar of flames came issuing forth; and mounds of ashes blocked up rights of way, and wholly changed the law and custom of the neighbourhood.
> In short, the yet unfinished and unopened Railroad was in progress, and, from the very core of all this dire disorder, trailed smoothly away, upon its mighty course of civilization and improvement.
>
> (78–9)

The cutting which Bourne illustrates as a landscape sketch has become a 'steep unnatural hill' down which things have tumbled into wreckage. Dickens paints a tableau of the railway's 'progress' as 'dire disorder', the material demolition which accompanied every project of metropolitan improvement. If there is a great genius presiding, its name is disorder: objects are in 'chaos', 'wildly mingled', 'accidentally' recomposed, and radically undermined to the point they no longer signify, as 'unintelligible as any dream'. The distance between order and disorder is measured by the stylistic contrast of Dickens's adjacent paragraphs: from the near-exhaustion of apocalyptic language to the anticlimactic 'In short'. But the scene and sentiments are hardly reducible to summary. Laws and customs have been 'wholly changed' but into what we do not discover, save for the looming threat of death, the 'mounds of ashes'. Dickens overdetermines the railway-as-death to accommodate what is indeterminate, or what he, at least, cannot determine.

Later in the novel, after the construction is finished, Staggs's Gardens has 'vanished from the earth'; in its place stands a bustling railway town (244 ff.). As if getting to 'the heart of this great change', Dickens's elaborate description of the town concludes with the trains themselves: 'Night and day the conquering engines rumbled at their distant work,...

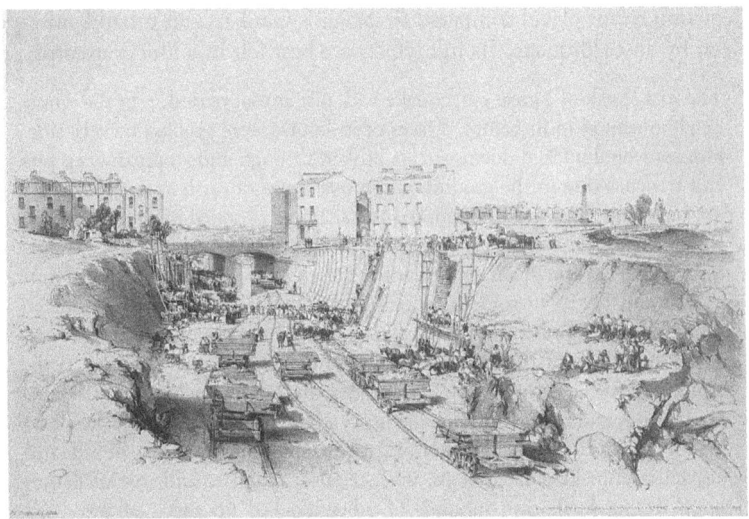

Fig. 4. J. C. Bourne, 'Building Retaining Wall near Park Street, Camden Town, Sept 17th 1838'

making the walls quake, as if they were dilating with the secret knowledge of great powers yet unsuspected in them, and strong purposes not yet achieved' (245–6). Having shaken and rent the earth, these engines still seem pregnant with power about which, in this later view, Dickens seems ambivalent. He may want to suspect 'great powers' and 'strong purposes' beyond the railway's death dealing, but this is 'secret knowledge'. Similarly, the description of the devastation to Staggs's Gardens cannot account for the principles of 'sudden sweeping change'.[56] We only learn the agent of that change: the railway, which is not even finished. The cause remains unknown. According to the narrator, the 'monster' which carries Mr Dombey through vertiginous scenes of devastation has only 'let the light of day in on these things: not made or caused them' (312). This invites a question, as Peter Sinnema points out: 'who, or what, is in

---

[56] In a sense, Tennyson was similarly confounded about the source of 'change'. He misunderstood the vehicle of his railway metaphor in 'Locksley Hall'—'Let the great world spin for ever down the ringing grooves of change.' Tennyson attended the opening of the Liverpool–Manchester railroad, but the crowd prevented a closer examination which would have revealed that train wheels did not, in fact, run in grooves. See Matthew Beaumont, 'The Railway and Literature: Realism and the Phantasmagoric', in *The Railway: Art in the Age of Steam*, ed. Ian G Kennedy and Julian Treuherz (New Haven, CT: Yale University Press, 2008), 35.

control, the technology or its inventors and mechanics?'[57] To arrest the heart of the railway's great change, to pry open the difficult dynamics of its creative destruction, Dickens makes the scene into a wreck.

While the dominant metaphor in the Staggs's Gardens scene is the catastrophic earthquake, the 'glare and roar of flames', dismembered objects, and the 'chaos of carts' resonate with contemporaneous descriptions of railroad accidents. In Staggs's Gardens, the railway has careened smack into London, reconfiguring its landscape 'accidentally'. Not just accidentally by chance, but accidentally in terms of material wreckage and injury. For Dickens and others, the aesthetics of accident offered a way of examining the railway's uneven developments, inscrutable complexity, seemingly haphazard growth, and radical challenges to geographic and sensory orientation. The Staggs's Gardens scene is conventionally accepted as critique, informing Dickens's greater ambivalence about progress or metropolitan improvement. And representations of accidents—whether in fiction, newspaper reports, or comic send-ups—have been similarly accepted as sceptical reactions to industrial modernity. However, these representations are also attempts to reformulate conventions of representation that the railway challenges. Writers like Trollope and Dickens do not merely describe complex or devastated landscape. Rather, they actively devastate their descriptions to pry open the stochastic or chaotic logic of the railway, perhaps, as so many critics want to suggest, as a figure for modernity itself.

COLLIDING INTERPRETATIONS

Accidents were the most striking manifestations of randomness on the railway. Harrington explains that the railway accident was 'characterised by an arbitrariness in the origins and effects of its violence' and that 'tales of narrow escapes and chance precipitation into disaster demonstrated the terrible randomness with which the railway accident claimed its victims'.[58] In this sense, accidents at once exemplified the randomness of the railway network and provided occasions to re-interpret it. Depictions of railway accidents in Victorian fiction have this double function. For example,

---

[57] Peter W. Sinnema, 'Representing the Railway: Train Accidents and Trauma in the *Illustrated London News*', *Victorian Periodicals Review* 31, no. 2 (Summer 1998): 162.
[58] Ralph Harrington, 'The Railway Accident: Trains, Trauma and Technological Crisis in Nineteenth-Century Britain', *Institute of Railway Studies, University of York*, 1999, <http://www.york.ac.uk/inst/irs/irshome/papers/rlyacc.htm>.

both Mugby Junction and Tenway Junction are marked by the degree of material disorder amounting to violence which also characterizes accident descriptions. Both Mugby Junction and Tenway Junction provide occasions for individuals to consider their relations to larger entities. Both emphasize the scene of the accident in part as commentary, in part as a tenuous solution to the challenges of representing the railway itself.

According to Matthew Beaumont, the railway proved to be 'an aesthetic problem' for literary representation, surprisingly resistant to the descriptive capacities of novelistic realism that the railway materially enabled. Beaumont is willing to link the generic dominance of the nineteenth-century novel to the expanding railway network, and is simultaneously curious as to its relative absence in novelistic representation.[59] Jack Simmons claims that 'there is no English novel of any importance in which the railway takes a central place'.[60] Instead, railway references are scattered over the corpus of nineteenth-century fiction. Citing a typical example, Beaumont suggests that railways get brief mentions as the passing impressions out of a passenger's window.[61] Even in *Dombey and Son*, as Carter points out, railways occupy only a sliver (8–9 pages) of its massive bulk.[62] The novel in general declines to interrogate the 'machine ensemble' for all the rich subject matter and thematic potential it seems to offer. Beaumont cites the variety of perceptual challenges that may have impeded description and more sustained meditation of the machine ensemble in prose. Because of this sensory scrambling, he claims that the primary response to the aesthetic problem of railways was, in written descriptions, the 'phantasmagoria, a fantastical or dream-like spectacle'.[63] Literary representation takes its cues, he argues, from the reports of railway passengers who deployed metaphors of the phantasmagoria, or magic lantern show, to compensate for the spatial and visual disorientation of the railway's scale and speed.

Beaumont finds an inaugural use of this metaphor in Stanley's account of the opening of the Liverpool–Manchester railroad:

---

[59] Beaumont, 'Railway and Literature', 36–7.
[60] Simmons, *The Victorian Railway*, 217. See also Carter, *Railways and Culture in Britain*, 3.
[61] Beaumont, 'Railway and Literature', 37.
[62] Carter, *Railways and Culture in Britain*, 75.
[63] Beaumont, 'Railway and Literature', 36. Schivelbusch argues that the railway reformed vision as panorama: 'The dissolution of reality and its resurrection as panorama thus became agents for the total emancipation from the traversed landscape' allowing the traveller to enter imaginary ones. See Schivelbusch, *The Railway Journey*, 64. With this in mind, Beaumont sees phantasmagoria on a trajectory towards aesthetic modernism and cinematic sensibilities.

I know not how to explain my meaning better, than by referring to the enlargement of objects in a phantasmagoria. At first the image is barely discernible, but as it advances from the focal point, it seems to increase beyond all limit. Thus an engine, as it draws near, appears to become rapidly magnified, and as if it would fill up the entire space between the banks, and absorb every thing within its vortex.[64]

The phantasmagoria lets Stanley telescope from local disorientation to the broader consequences of the railway's annihilation of time and space. As the railway fills 'the entire space', Stanley describes not just its visual magnification but its power to restructure the local through forces operating at a distance. As the engine 'seems to increase beyond all limit', so the railway blurs geographical and ontological boundaries to become the machine ensemble. Like a phantasmagoric dream sequence, Stanley's prose registers the 'optical deception' as a kind of apocalypse, a black hole consuming everything within its expanding horizon. Such a force is capable of obliterating the thinking subject or any narrative structure that stands in its way.

In his tight focus on phantasmagoria, Beaumont overlooks another response to the 'aesthetic problem' of the machine ensemble. If, for example, the Staggs's Gardens scene is phantasmagoric, it also explicitly alludes to the material wreckage of railway construction and accidents. If Carker's death by an onrushing train is a fantastical dream sequence, its waking reality invokes the threats of fatal accidents on the tracks. Beaumont even acknowledges that, in general, novelistic depictions of the railway tend 'to emblematise the destructive or apocalyptic energies of capitalist modernity quite as much as the progressive, supposedly "civilised" ones'.[65] In other words, prose fiction over-represents catastrophe as a feature of the railway network. If the railway remained resistant to realist frames of depiction, railway accidents and wreckage produced more than their fair share of what realism did frame. Beaumont accepts novels' conspicuous representations of railway dangers as *only* emblems of cultural critique. But we should see them as also solutions to the very aesthetic problems he identifies.

If the railway annihilated space and time, accident offered a paradoxical means of their recovery, though in catastrophic form.[66] Railway companies

---

[64] Stanley, 'Opening of the Liverpool and Manchester Railroad', 825.
[65] Beaumont, 'Railway and Literature', 35.
[66] For a related argument about the aesthetic consequences in depicting railway accidents in illustrated periodicals, see Paul Fyfe, 'Illustrating the Accident: Railways and the Catastrophic Picturesque in the *Illustrated London News*', *Victorian Periodicals Review* 46, no. 1 (2013): 61–91.

worked hard to do this reconstructive work on their own terms, using 'the rigour of timetables, the discipline of rulebooks, the grandiose architectural style of stations and the quasi-military uniforms of the great companies' as promises of perceptual stability, rigorous chronology, and the management of risk.[67] In the 1840s, companies migrated to a standardized 'railway time', kept in London (Greenwich) and broadcast telegraphically to stations for synchronization.[68] Promotional railway prints in the manner of Bourne's were likewise instrumental in depicting motionless scenes of travel, impressive company structures, and trains set among those pleasing topographical features which travellers could not easily perceive while underway.[69] However, the industry's very efforts to manage or aesthetically discipline the railway only accentuated its ruptures of order, its tenuous orchestration of complexity. Representations of railway accidents have largely been accepted on these terms as moments of critique. As Bloch suggests, 'the accident still reminds us of... a production that knows no civilized schedule'.[70] But Bloch's phrase suggests an alternative: accidents can also produce an uncivilized schedule. In other words, as much as they underscore chaotic disruption and damage, accidents also affix missing markers of periodicity, time, and place to the events they represent.

Depictions of accidents literally arrest the dizzying phantasmagoria of railway travel into moments for investigation and contemplation. They put people back outside the train and on foot, providing a switch of transport modes that recovers the scrutiny the train rendered impossible: of their place within the machine ensemble, of their location on a line that collapses distant points, of the intermediary moments of their passage. Anthony Giddens defines the phantasmagoria in this context: 'in conditions of modernity, place becomes increasingly *phantasmagoric*; that is to say, locales are thoroughly penetrated by and shaped in terms of social influences quite distant from them.'[71] For all their visual phantasmagoria, accidents also suggested ways in which place or the 'local' could be reconstructed given these conditions of distance. In this sense, representations of accidents are a darkly ironic response to a prevailing complaint about railway travel: not simply that it annihilates time and space, but

---

[67] Gareth Rees, *Early Railway Prints: British Railways from 1825–1850* (Ithaca, NY: Cornell University Press, 1980), 10.
[68] Simmons, *The Victorian Railway*, 345–57.
[69] Freeman, *Railways and the Victorian Imagination*, 230.
[70] Quoted in Schivelbusch, *The Railway Journey*, 132.
[71] Anthony Giddens, *The Consequences of Modernity* (Palo Alto, CA: Stanford University Press, 1990), 19. Emphasis original.

consequentially that it shifts the epistemology of travel away from the study of intermediate people, places, and their characteristics.

For many of the railway's critics, railway travel seemed either extremely dangerous or extremely boring. Nostalgic travellers yearned for the possibility of the picaresque, but found only a compartmentalized dullness relieved by reading or by circumscribed encounters with a few immediate persons whom they could not escape.[72] For some, the dullness of travel could not be relieved at all:

> The hours spent in a railway carriage are generally among the most tedious and uneventful hours in life. Hills, valleys, trees, cities, broad winding rivers, even at times glimpses of the great sea itself seem to fly past with such rapidity as to dazzle the eye and weary the brain. The loveliest scenery leaves no trace upon the memory; its picturesque beauty, shady nooks, and leafy bowers, so agreeable to the leisurely traveller, have no charm from the window of the railway carriage. We may fly from one end of the land to the other, with no feeling save that of profound weariness, and gratitude when the journey is over.[73]

This traveller is wearied by the railway's sensory assault and its collapse of geographical antipodes. They lament the loss of a picturesque country appreciable on more leisurely circuits. Of course, such a nostalgic landscape is itself differentially produced by Britain's urban-industrial changes.[74] Chandler and Gilmartin argue that 'the very act of laying

---

[72] This was the railway's great paradox, that it 'simultaneously annihilated space and compartmentalized it'; Freeman, *Railways and the Victorian Imagination*, 149. And so representations of the railway shifted toward scenes of social dynamics within train compartments; see Ellis and Hyman, *Railway Art*, 73; Freeman, *Railways and the Victorian Imagination*, 229–30. The sketches of character and place 'lost' to travel instead appear in railway stations or moving cars, apparent in paintings such as Robert Musgrave Joy's *Tickets Please!* (1851), Leopold Augustus Egg's *The Travelling Companions* (1862), and Frith's *The Railway Station*. Railway stations suited some authors just fine for sketching character at leisure; in a Dinah Craik novel from 1852 the protagonists 'drove on to that nucleus where so many diverse phases of human life converge, and may be at leisure studied or moralised over—a railway terminus'; Dinah Craik, *The Head of the Family* (London: Macmillan, 1890), 25, <http://books.google.com/books?id=uJBAAAAAIAAJ>. Stations and train compartments also offered the threats and titillation of unmanaged encounters, as seen in stories of crime and sexual danger.

[73] Iza Duffus [Mary-Anne] Hardy, *A Hero's Work* (London: Hurst and Blackett, 1868), 2: 67.

[74] In various ways, the railway augmented (or created) curiosity about the interstices it seemed to erase. Alan Everitt offers an interesting corollary: contrary to the railway's purely metropolitan influence, 'railways also did much to open up the historic riches of the countryside to a new generation of writers on rural society'. See Alan Everitt, 'The Railway and Rural Tradition, 1840–1940', in *The Impact of the Railway on Society in Britain: Essays in Honour of Jack Simmons*, ed. Jack Simmons, A. K. B. Evans, and John Gough (Aldershot, Hampshire; Burlington, VT: Ashgate, 2003), 181. Simmons finds a similar reaction regarding the railway's demolition of buildings and urban landscapes. Arguments about

claim to the rural sensibility, understood as a sensibility, is . . . a product of the metropolitan moment'.[75] So too the railway engendered a longing for slowness in places off the grid. In F. J. Hall's novel *The Next of Kin* (1854), one character complains of train travel that 'it whirled them away past hills and dales, villages and steeples, towns and woodlands, as if determined they should know as little about the country they travelled through as possible'.[76] The railway seemed to erase any knowledge of the intermediary landscapes through which it passed.[77] In a sense, the railway renders the characteristic features of the countryside into urban phenomena, experienced in such ephemeral abundance that the perceiving subject, as in Simmel's classic formulation, must screen out their unknowable noise.

Several writers, in reaction to the railway's impoverishment of place, retrofitted the stagecoach into an idealized vehicle for an epistemology of slower country travel.[78] In his novel *Norman Sinclair* (1861), William Aytoun laments the loss of character study that coach travel enabled:

> In a railway train you profit little by the scenery—you dash so rapidly past town and grange that you hardly have a glimpse of their outline—and you are utterly precluded from the grand old amusement of studying character on the road. The stage coach, on the contrary, carried you into the very heart of the country; gave you time to enjoy the scenery; brought under your notice many a curious specimen of life and manners; and enabled you, if the coachman or guard were disposed to be communicative, as was usually the

the destruction of the local 'stimulated a new consciousness of what was threatened, on the part of antiquaries, local councilors, and building developers'. *The Victorian Railway*, 155.

[75] James Chandler and Kevin Gilmartin, 'Introduction: Engaging the Eidometropolis', in *Romantic Metropolis: The Urban Scene of British Culture, 1780–1840*, ed. James Chandler and Kevin Gilmartin (Cambridge; New York: Cambridge University Press, 2005), 15.

[76] F. J. Hall, *The Next of Kin* (London: Thomas Cautley Newby, 1854), 1: 91, <http://books.google.com/books?id=F7YBAAAAQAAJ>.

[77] Nostalgia is a two-way street (or track), as writers within a century would pine for the loss or closing of railway stations which, for them, defined rural English places. Richards and MacKenzie suggest that the disappearance of country stations in the twentieth century heralds 'the slow, inexorable process of rural decay'; *The Railway Station*, 7.

[78] De Quincey offers the working model with 'The English Mail-Coach'. He sniffs at the 'blind insensate agencies' of modern train travel compared to the 'vital experience of the glad animal sensibilities' which deliver a thrilling sense of speed. See *The English Mail-Coach and Joan of Arc* (Boston, MA: Athenaeum Press, 1905), 16. The key difference for De Quincey is the unalienated vitalism of coach travel. Even so, he celebrates the mail-coach in ways that resemble phantasmagoric fascination about the railroad: its breakneck speed, the resulting phantasmagoric visual effects, and the distributed workings of a frenzied service which somehow harmonizes into a system: 'this post-office service spoke as by some mighty orchestra, where a thousand instruments, all disregarding each other, and so far in danger of discord, . . . terminate in a perfection of harmony like that of heart, brain, and lungs in a healthy animal organisation'; De Quincey, *The English Mail-Coach and Joan of Arc*, 2.

Chaos and Connections on the Victorian Railway   199

case, to form a tolerably accurate estimate of the peculiarities and history of the neighbourhood.[79]

As railway travel blurs the visual particulars of place, it also sacrifices knowledge of local particularity, the specimens and manners distinctive of that place and its peculiar history.[80] This is 'the very heart of the country'—not the placeless urban expanse the railway spans from topographical end to end. As the railway blurred the thresholds between country and city, it also became the occasion for writers like Aytoun to reproduce their differences. Seeking 'the very heart of the country', Aytoun looks for a national capital within a pastoral structure of feeling, as Raymond Williams says, and not within the metropolitan network that Churton's *Railway Book* inscribes. However, even Aytoun's traveller needs transportation and a guide. Aytoun and others imagined a ready alternative in the figure of the communicative coachman. Early in *Felix Holt* (1866), George Eliot brings on such a talkative, knowledgeable coachman as a narrative partner:

> The coachman was an excellent travelling companion and commentator on the landscape; he could tell the names of sites and persons, and explained the meaning of groups, as well as the shade of Virgil in a more memorable journey; he had as many stories about parishes, and the men and women in them, as the Wanderer in the 'Excursion', only his style was different.[81]

The coachman is an easy and stylish critic of the pastoral in a variety of forms, visual and narrative. He can discriminate sites and persons otherwise blurred on the rails. More than an oral historian, he is enthroned on his carriage as a kind of bard, heard in allusions to Virgil and Wordsworth's wanderer—who each, it should be noted, travel on foot.[82]

Felix Holt begins with slow journeys. The traveller discerns in this landscape 'an unchanging stillness as if Time itself were pausing'. Here, time is not annihilated but simply stopped, creating a rural stillness that

---

[79] William Edmondstoune Aytoun, *Norman Sinclair* (Edinburgh; London: William Blackwood and Sons, 1861), 250–1, <http://books.google.com/books?id=5NYOAAAAYAAJ>.
[80] It could be argued that 'the grand old amusement of studying character on the road' was not the legacy of country travel, but of the relatively new enterprise of studying urban populations on the street, as Chapter 2 suggests. In that sense, Aytoun's own curiosity about the country is a metropolitan export.
[81] George Eliot, *Felix Holt, the Radical*, ed. Fred C. Thomson (Oxford: Clarendon, 1980), 9.
[82] For discussions of walking as a technology of Romantic encounter, see Anne D. Wallace, *Walking, Literature, and English Culture: The Origins and Uses of Peripatetic in the Nineteenth Century* (Oxford: Clarendon, 1993); Gary Lee Harrison, *Wordsworth's Vagrant Muse: Poetry, Poverty, and Power* (Detroit, MI: Wayne State University Press, 1994).

the narrator contrasts to urban-industrial space: 'it was easy for the traveller to conceive that town and country had no pulse in common'.[83] The very heart of the country beats its own sinus rhythm. Or, in its stoppage of time, it has no pulse: no periodic ticking of the clock: no railway lines or telegraphs dictating a metropolitan cadence. For Neil Hertz, the word 'pulse' signals the 'perspectival contrasts' and paradoxes with which Eliot refigures the sublime.[84] The contrasts of *Felix Holt* sound out this systole and diastole as 'town and country', fast and slow travel, places in and out of time. Eliot changes the traveller's perspective from a railway 'tube journey'[85] to a carriage ride:

> the slow old-fashioned way of getting from one end of our country to the other is the better thing to have in the memory. The tube-journey can never lend much to picture and narrative; it is as barren as an exclamatory O! Whereas the happy outside passenger seated on the box from the dawn to the gloaming gathered enough stories of English life, enough of English labours in town and country, enough aspects of earth and sky, to make episodes for a modern Odyssey.[86]

Eliot makes railway travel into an antagonist of depiction and narrative: a zero, a vacuum, an empty 'O' like the tunnel mouth from which it emerges. By contrast, the country seen in slow motion produces narrative episodes in sufficiently varied aspect and quantity to produce a national epic. This epic is no strictly tracked linear narrative, but a gathering of episodes. The railway's barren journey does not allow for the collections of stories or the sketches of characters and places that together assemble a national life.[87]

---

[83] Eliot, *Felix Holt*, 8.

[84] Neil Hertz, *George Eliot's Pulse* (Palo Alto, CA: Stanford University Press, 2003), 13. Eliot's pulse alternates two 'vocabularies of motivation' which Hertz maps onto Kant's notions of the sublime: the 'dynamical' sublime which translates into the 'force' of fictions on Eliot's readers, and the 'mathematical' sublime concerned with how they might assimilate all the proliferating elements of her complex depictions; Hertz, *George Eliot's Pulse*, 2. In another instance, Hertz describes this alternation between design and chance, willed intention and random dissemination: 'one stresses the chancy workings of dissemination, the other refigures the event as voluntary'; Hertz, *George Eliot's Pulse*, 7.

[85] Eliot experienced such a 'tube journey' as a demonstration of a pneumatic or 'atmospheric' railway. For background on the story and a fuller technical description, see Henry Atmore, 'Railway Interests and the "Rope of Air"', *The British Journal for the History of Science* 37, no. 3 (September 2004): 245–79.

[86] Eliot, *Felix Holt*, 5.

[87] For some, the railway station also provided slow passage or stationary ground upon which to build notions of English place and character. Writing in 1908, Hilaire Belloc seems to respond almost explicitly to Eliot's critique: 'What is more English than the country railway station? I defy the eighteenth century to produce anything more English, more full of home and rest, and the nature of the country than my junction' in Sussex. The junction 'is a theme for English idylls', Belloc declares, and goes on to quickly sketch the

The jocular coachman in *Felix Holt* has his own perspective on the deleterious consequences of the railway network. His critique covers some familiar ground, including the anxieties of innkeepers and coachmen left behind by the runaway railway economy:

> the recent initiation of railways had embittered him: he now, as in a perpetual vision, saw the ruined country strewn with shattered limbs, and regarded Mr Huskisson's death as a proof of God's anger against Stephenson. 'Why, every inn on the road would be shut up!' and at that word the coachman looked before him with the blank gaze of one who had driven his coach to the outermost edge of the universe, and saw his leaders plunging into the abyss.[88]

This passage has its own pulse: the narrator describes the coachman's tone deflecting from familiar 'narrative' to 'high prophetic strain'. The railway radically distorts the coachman's chronotope from a moment of stillness to an indiscriminate 'now, as in a perpetual vision'. Paralleling this shift, his ability to discriminate persons and places deteriorates into an apocalyptic blank. His entire reaction is structured (and scattered) by references to accidents and damage. The railway network produces a 'ruined country strewn with shattered limbs'. The fatal injury of Huskisson proves the folly of railway engineer George Stephenson who built the infamous engine, *Rocket*. The coachman, transported in his apocalyptic reverie, imagines his own coach plummeting into the abyss of chaos, like the iconic train in the background of John Martin's painting *The Last Judgement* (1853). In the coachman's imagination, the technological accident becomes a sublime catastrophe, or what Hertz calls the 'drive to the end of the line'.[89] Nothing is left. Like the railway's erasure of picture and narrative to an absolutely barren 'exclamatory O!'—an empty cry of terror—the railway disaster represents total annihilation.

The power of Eliot's metaphor is itself overwhelming. But, if the railway seems to evacuate mimetic particularity and disable the knowledge of place, its very accidents could ironically restore them. They salvaged, without recourse to a nostalgic transportation history, a particularity of character and chronotope, though in grotesque form. In this sense, it is less surprising that *accidents* are one of the predominant forms of representing the railway in Victorian fiction. If Victorian writers overlook or even denigrate the railway in general, they seize upon its accidents to explore the very conditions of their art. As Levine argues, Victorian realists

---

characters there he loves. See Hilaire Beloc, *On Nothing and Kindred Subjects* (London: Methuen, 1908), 71–2.

[88] Eliot, *Felix Holt*, 9.   [89] Hertz, *George Eliot's Pulse*, 3.

came to compromise with the accidental and the arbitrary, reflecting the 'disruptive irrationality of experience', a paradigm of flux, and an emphasis on particularity and contingency as constitutive of meaning.[90] Furthermore, realism cashiered the providential understanding of chance in favour of meaningless accident, or the 'nonstructural detail' that Barthes would analyse as 'the reality effect'.[91] Literary realism may even represent the technologizing of accident in generic form. Significantly, Levine points not to George Eliot but to Trollope as the exemplar of the accidental realist. Eliot might reject the railway's apocalyptic crash, but Trollope embraced it as a conceptual and generic extreme. Particularly in the case of Lopez's accident and inquest, Trollope uses the accident to interrogate the complex interactions of persons, motives, and events that constitute the everyday.

Only a year before the publication of *Felix Holt*, Eliot had written very differently about the railways in a book review of William Lecky's *Rationalism in Europe*. To complement the book's argument about the rise of rational thinking, Eliot offers a related theory about historical consciousness which responds to 'an external Reason—the sum of conditions resulting from the laws of material growth, from changes produced by great historical collisions shattering the structures of ages and making new highways for events and ideas'.[92] Rationalism evolves within the aggregate material and ideological changes of history's progressive march. Notably, Eliot's metaphor for history includes great shattering collisions on new highways. Within only a few sentences, she elaborates how the 'external Reason' makes itself felt: not through the discovery of coincidence, but by the impact of impressions of connectedness:

> If right reason is a right representation of the co-existences and sequences of things, here are co-existences and sequences that do not wait to be discovered, but press themselves upon us like bars of iron. No séances... can annihilate railways, steam-ships, and electric telegraphs, which are demonstrating the inter-dependence of all human interests, and making self-interest a duct for sympathy.[93]

---

[90] George Lewis Levine, *The Realistic Imagination: English Fiction from Frankenstein to Lady Chatterley* (Chicago, IL: University of Chicago Press, 1981), 141.

[91] Levine, *The Realistic Imagination*, 151. Barthes begins by complaining that structural analysis has not been sufficiently concerned with the 'superfluous' or 'filling' detail; see 'The Reality Effect', in *The Rustle of Language*, trans. Richard Howard (New York: Hill and Wang, 1986), 141. In the first chapter, I argue the same about newspaper history and its inattention to accident news—including what Barthes (not coincidentally) defines as the *faits divers*.

[92] 'The Influence of Rationalism', *The Fortnightly Review*, 1846, 46.

[93] 'The Influence of Rationalism', *The Fortnightly Review*, 1846, 46.

Here, railways do not annihilate, but instead produce powerful impressions of 'inter-dependence' as ineluctable as 'bars of iron' or perhaps the rails themselves. The co-existences, sequences, and sympathetic relations of things are all subordinate to an 'external Reason' which, though not tantamount to divinity, answers similar arguments as natural theology with a materialist, rationalist worldview. Eliot's own 'right representation' of those things leads into the unique sense of particularities and contingencies of her realism, sharing here a surprising affinity with Victorian transportation networks and the connections they can dramatically reveal.

Laura Otis has claimed that Eliot internalizes these Victorian networks to model social interconnections and the dimensions of sympathy. Especially in *Middlemarch*, Eliot 'offers the communications web as an epistemological and moral model'.[94] It would be a mistake to make Eliot's web synonymous with the Victorian railway as she wants to develop a more embodied, organic model of mutual dependence and contingency. However, other novelists did turn to the railway to represent similar qualities of a complex network, as even Eliot hints. But rather than theorizing an 'external Reason', these novelists considered the emergent properties of the system itself. To represent them, they turned to the paradoxically generative scenes of accidents, allowing them to restore the particularity, chronotopes, and connections that Eliot elsewhere argued the railway had annihilated.

TERMINAL CONNECTIONS

In his history of railway disasters, Rolt recalls the first accident he ever heard anything about: the Dee Bridge disaster. Growing up near the area, Rolt experienced first-hand how 'the disaster impressed itself indelibly on local memory'. People were still giving 'graphic accounts' about it 75 years later.[95] The accident creates a traumatic memory of place, powerful enough to recur long into the future in 'graphic accounts'. If Aytoun's traveller seeks the heart of the country and stillness, the accident here provokes a heart attack whose effects are strangely similar: indelibly impressing local memory and the memory of the local. If railway time synchronized the country with the pulse of the town, accidents arrested that pulse to recover a peculiar uniqueness of place and an abiding

---

[94] Laura Otis, *Networking: Communicating with Bodies and Machines in the Nineteenth Century*, Studies in Literature and Science (Ann Arbor, MI: University of Michigan Press, 2001), 81.
[95] Rolt, *Red for Danger*, 95.

curiosity about its connections with the network at large. Rolt's history is hardly equivalent with what writers like Hardy, Aytoun, and Eliot declare the railway has undone: picturesque country scenes, stories producing intimate local knowledge, or richly textured episodes for a modern Odyssey. But there are other examples of its literary expression in which accident transforms from destructive event into a new context for reimaging complexity and development. In 1865, a year and a half before he published *Mugby Junction*, Dickens was involved in a serious train accident which became known (for its place) as the Staplehurst Disaster (see Figure 5). Perhaps because he was travelling with his mistress, perhaps because of the carnage he witnessed as he struggled to help the dying, Dickens would scarcely mention that event and its lasting impact. Its most notable references come in private letters and in the closing paragraph to the postscript of *Our Mutual Friend*, published later that same year.[96] Instead, the accident shows up elsewhere, casting shadows over mind and body. Studies of neuroses and trauma tend to dominate recent commentary about the cultural resonance of such railway accidents, such as in the

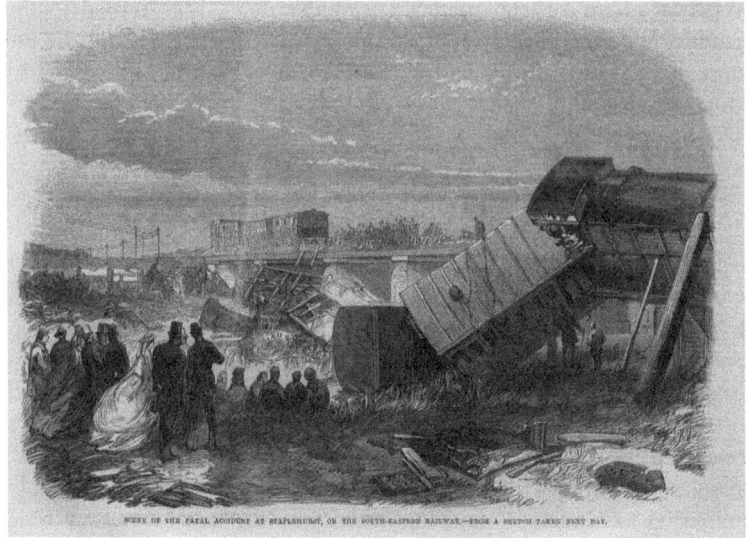

Fig. 5. 'Scene of the Fatal Accident at Staplehurst'
Illustrated London News, 17 June 1865, 572.

[96] See Jill L. Matus, 'Trauma, Memory, and Railway Disaster: The Dickensian Connection', *Victorian Studies* 43, no. 3 (2001): 413–36.

exemplary treatments by Nicholas Daly and Jill Matus. But curiously, the post-catastrophe stories of *Mugby Junction* are not as post-apocalyptic as *Dombey and Son*, a novel published well before the Staplehurst disaster. Rather, they create ambivalence about the railway's complex and often random effects.

Mugby Junction resembles Staggs's Gardens for how the railway's intricacy gets described as material catastrophe. Like the observers flocking to an accident's scene, Jackson surveys Mugby's chaos in awe, noting how 'so many lines' decompose into a catastrophic landscape of wreckage. Carts are haphazardly scattered in various states of decay; some rails stop at barriers, some run into buildings: and 'there was no beginning, middle, or end to the bewilderment'. The junction's complexity only resolves in metaphors of collisions, wreckage, and disfigurement. It is telling that Jackson's developing love interest is a young invalid named Phoebe, who feels herself very much a part of the junction: 'It seems to join me, in a way, to I don't know how many places and things that *I* shall never see' (18, original emphasis). Phoebe feels joined to an invisible network she knows only by chance: her father, Lamps the railway worker, tells her stories about passing people and 'collects chance newspapers and books' for her to read (23). Phoebe is a local fixture thrilled by chance connections to the transportation network, mediated by texts. But she cannot travel; she is affixed to the local by her unexplained paralysis. She is joined to the railway, nevertheless, in a darker affiliation with its chances: as a disabled body in its accidental disfigurement of place and personae.

The Staplehurst accident returns more explicitly in Dickens's gothic short story 'The Signalman'. As Jackson wanders the nearby landscape hoping to discover its peculiarities, he comes upon a deep cutting and sees a signalman stationed at the mouth of a tunnel below. He interviews the highly capable but haunted signalman, who describes how his signal house was the very site of an impromptu morgue for a 'beautiful young lady' killed in 'the memorable accident on this line' (60).[97] Railway trauma impresses its memory on the local, and this place becomes haunted by the eternal return of the accident victim in the signalman's mind, manifesting as a spectre standing next to the red warning light of the tunnel. Though unmentioned in the story, the signal house as morgue would also have become the ready site for viewing the deceased body, a stage for the coroner's inquest on the accident, then as always an attempt to communicate with the ghost of causality.

---

[97] For the historical background to this specific accident and problems of signalling, see Pope, 'Dickens's "The Signalman".'

'The Signalman' seems to reanimate a nightmare about the Staplehurst Disaster, an alternate reality in which Ellen Ternan, the 'beautiful young lady' with whom Dickens was travelling, did not survive. The haunting spectre may also be the intertextual ghost of Phoebe, a bright mythical beacon of prophecy who becomes a light in the tunnel to warn the signalman of impending danger. But the railway employee who should be most sensitive to these signs cannot grasp either the supernatural or material signals eluding him. He is baffled by the looming but unlocatable potential for catastrophe characteristic of accident: 'What is the danger? Where is the danger? There is danger overhanging, somewhere on the line. Some dreadful calamity will happen.... What can *I* do?' (63, original emphasis) Mistaking the warnings of an oncoming train for the pleadings of this ghost, the signalman is struck and killed on the tracks. That accident, like the haunted house of the signalman's box, marks the place of its occurrence, substantiating one of the missing narratives of the lines out of Mugby Junction.

In contrast to the unfortunate signalman, Jackson does follow Phoebe's signals in seeking richer connections through the railway network. When, after considering the madness of Mugby Junction, 'the gentleman for Nowhere' finally decides to go somewhere, he chooses one of the branch lines leading to 'the great ingenious town'—an easy mark for Manchester, the city that steam built. Here, he has a Dickensian urban epiphany:

> [He] went out for a walk in the busy streets. And now it began to be suspected by him that Mugby Junction was a Junction of many branches, invisible as well as visible, and had joined him to an endless number of byways. For, whereas he would, but a little while ago, have walked these streets blindly brooding, he now had eyes and thoughts for a new external world. How the many toiling people lived, and loved, and died; ... how good it was to know that such assembling in a multitude on their part ... engendered among them a self-respect ... 'I too am but a little part of a great whole'.
> (29)

Dickens's urban sensibilities help to shed a better light on what we have already seen: that Jackson, previously known for his luggage bound for nowhere, is already part of the undifferentiated multitude walking the streets 'blindly' or circulating on the railway network by chance. Only after Jackson subjects himself to the vagaries of Mugby Junction can he realize his connections to other people; only after Jackson rides the rails can he walk the streets sensitive to their lessons of populace and community. Strikingly, the city and the railway mutually decode their inscrutable complexities. Each context allows Dickens to imagine connections, epiphanies, and tragedies which emerge as little random parts of great if unstable multitudes. This late epiphany was only possible after Dickens experiences a railway accident that he had previously overdetermined as a symbol of death. Like Trollope, Dickens arrives at an understanding of the network that involves randomness as a constitutive feature rather than as an anomaly.

Thematically and materially in *Mugby Junction*, accidents are bound up with design. In a wonderful piece of bibliographic irony, the original issue of *Mugby Junction* was actually printed with an advertisement for accident insurance on its back cover (see Figure 6). *Mugby Junction* came wrapped in the characteristic blue paper that Chapman & Hall used for Dickens's part issues. The title appears on the front; on the back, a promise that 'Accidents Will Happen!' from the Railway Passengers Assurance Company—the first insurance company to offer passenger accident insurance, bundled into the cost of special tickets, starting in the late 1840s. Not long after, the company expanded its insurance policies to cover accidents in general, or what the back cover explains as 'accidents of every description'. The cover shows a canny bit of marketing for the insurance company and an opportunistic ad sale for the publisher. It also models what this chapter has sought to demonstrate: the links between junctions and accidents, the generalization of railway accidents into descriptive opportunities, and the acceptance of chance—by the risk management industry as well as Victorian novelists—as the flipside of integrated order, a potentially structuring rather than destructive principle.

In this light, the ruminations on the railway network in *Mugby Junction* recast Dickens's earlier sketches of the city, wherein accidents are the interpretive moments of chance. I began this project with an observation by Raymond Williams of 'a contradiction, a paradox' wherein the nineteenth-century metropolis reveals 'the coexistence of variation and apparent randomness with...a determining system'.[98] Accidents offered the Victorians explanatory power for that strange coexistence, making the metropolis an important catalyst for paradigmatic changes in probability thinking over the century. They are moments to scrutinize and reimagine relations in human environments, whether restructured by metropolis or machine ensemble, as contingently connected. They are moments to join

---

[98] Raymond Williams, *The Country and the City* (New York: Oxford University Press, 1973), 154.

ACCIDENTS WILL HAPPEN!

EVERYONE SHOULD THEREFORE PROVIDE AGAINST THEM!

£1000 IN CASE OF DEATH,

Or £6 per Week while laid-up by Injury

CAUSED BY

ACCIDENT OF ANY KIND,

(RIDING, DRIVING, HUNTING, SHOOTING, FISHING, &c.)

MAY BE SECURED

BY AN ANNUAL PAYMENT OF FROM £3. to £6 5s. 0d.

TO THE

RAILWAY PASSENGERS
ASSURANCE COMPANY.

OFFICES:

64, CORNHILL, & 10, REGENT STREET, LONDON.

The oldest established and largest Company in the World insuring against

ACCIDENTS OF EVERY DESCRIPTION.

For particulars apply to the Clerks at any of the Railway Stations, to the Local Agents, or at the Head Office,

64, CORNHILL, LONDON, E.C.

WILLIAM J. VIAN, Secretary.

RAILWAY PASSENGERS ASSURANCE COMPANY,
Empowered by Special Acts of Parliament, 1849 and 1864.

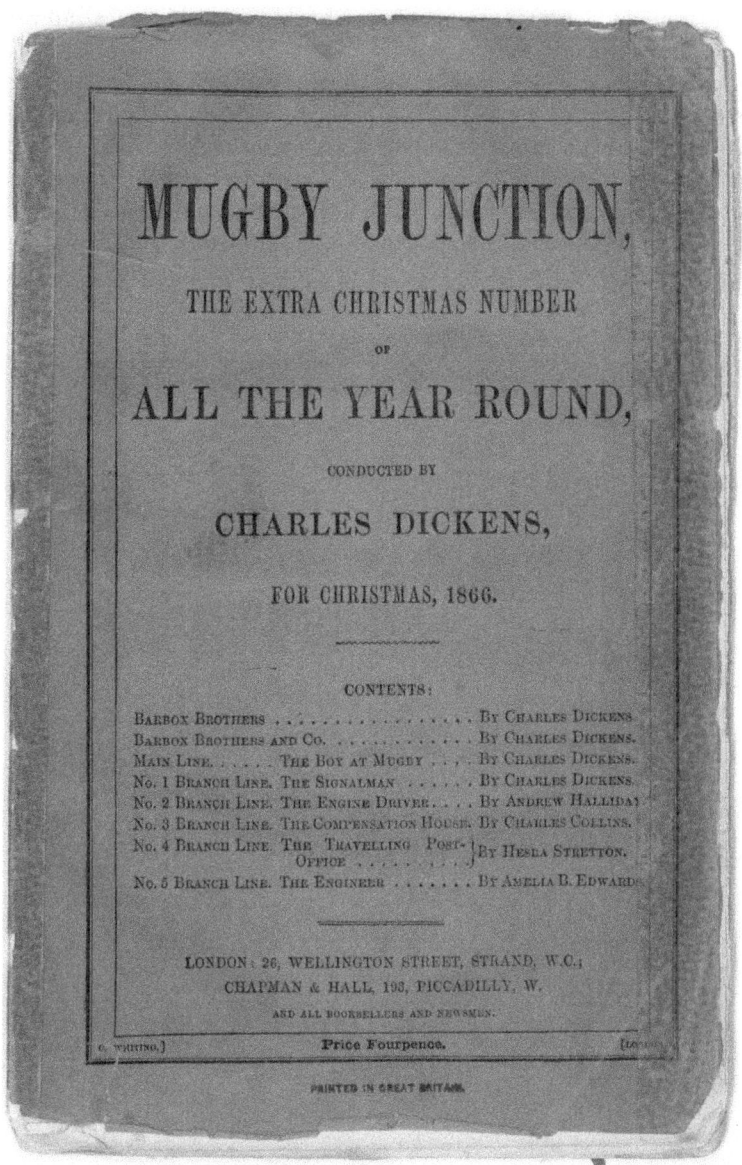

Fig. 6. Front and back cover of *Mugby Junction*, the Christmas issue of *All the Year Round* for 1866

textual production to a complex cultural field in which chance and risk were being reconceived. They are moments to assert that though this interdisciplinary field is anything but certain, accidents can go a long way in describing its development. Those changes are also a function of texts in all the diversity of their representations and in the material circumstances of their production and circulation. It is entirely possible to consider haphazardness and complexity with precision and conviction. So too is it possible to consider the accidental for its particular theoretical and textual designs.

Afterword: An Accidental Excursion

The arc of this book's argument about accident and design in the metropolis bends towards relativity thinking, the enfranchisement of chance, and the uneven development of modernity that various scholars date to the century's end. In exploring the development of such a modernity, Anthony Giddens actually suggests why accident may be a good place to look.[1] His culminating image is 'the juggernaut':

> a runaway engine of enormous power which, collectively as human beings, we can drive to some extent but which also threatens to rush out of our control and which could rend itself asunder. The juggernaut crushes those who resist it, and while it sometimes seems to have a steady path, there are times when it veers away erratically in directions we cannot foresee.[2]

Giddens has been rightly critiqued for overdetermining modernity as a totalizing condition. But the dynamic he identifies has some explanatory power in more specific historical terms.[3] Instead of representing a totalized risk society, the juggernaut runs the risk of accident, which, in Victorian contexts, better reveals its tenuous relationships with control and chaos, design and chance.

Consider the example of an 1845 cartoon (see Figure 7) in which *Punch* satirizes the idolatry of 'railway mania' and clarifies what the 'juggernaut' looks like in early Victorian England. A steam engine, running without any rails and piloted by a demon not at the controls, ploughs into a worshipping crowd whose most zealous members throw themselves in its

---

[1] Anthony Giddens, *The Consequences of Modernity* (Palo Alto, CA: Stanford University Press, 1990), 9.

[2] As Giddens explains, juggernaut derives 'from the Hindi *Jagannāth*, "lord of the world", and is a title of Krishna; an idol of this deity was taken each year through the streets on a huge car, which followers are said to have thrown themselves under, to be crushed beneath the wheels'. *The Consequences of Modernity*, 139.

[3] Modernity's runaway engine is strikingly similar to the enduring final image of Zola's *La Bête humaine*: while wrestling in a jealous fight, an engine driver and stoker fall off their speeding engine and are sundered into pieces; the driverless train full of passengers roars away on the tracks with unchecked speed to an accident that is waiting, somewhere, to happen.

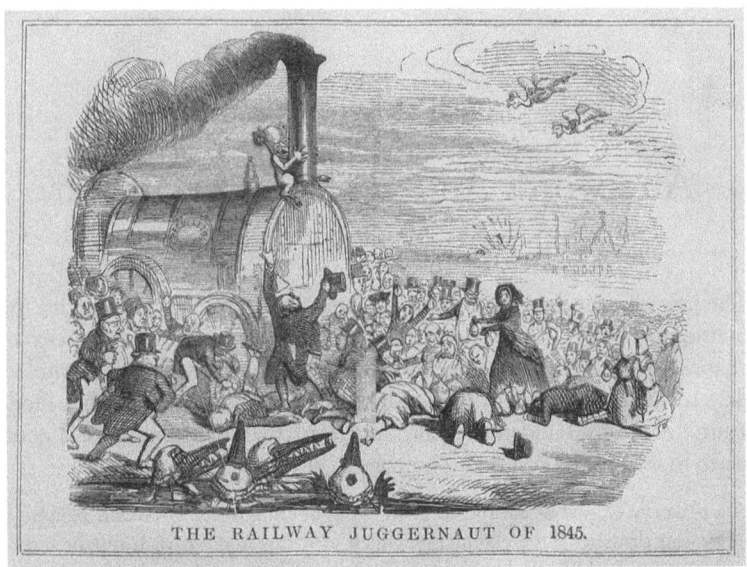

Fig. 7. 'The Railway Juggernaut of 1845'
[John Leech,] *Punch*, 26 July 1845, 47.

path. *Punch* makes the 1840s financial bubble of railway speculation tantamount to religious mania, showing investors seduced by what was sure to crash—and crush them as well. The cartoon gets additional satirical power from its visual association with train accidents, a source of so much anxious preoccupation, by evoking a scene of scattered victims and an onlooking crowd. The mass of people stretches back to the city skyline whose metropolitan boundaries the railway has profoundly stretched. The image animates questions of intent and victimization, fiscal responsibility and wild speculation, control and runaway trains, particularity and crowds, all on the terrain of changing metropolitan geographies. Like the array of Giddens's examples, like the cartoon in *Punch*, *By Accident or Design* spans the city and the railway, tracking the function of accidents in generating (and also resisting) the particular conditions of an emergent modernity in nineteenth-century English metropoles.

Within these metropolitan spaces, accident allows Victorian writers to engage design and chance for a variety of formal and cultural goals. In *Martin Chuzzlewit* (1843–4), Tom Pinch meets his sister Ruth and John Westlock together seemingly by chance in a London 'public thoroughfare':

'What an extraordinary meeting!' said Tom. 'I should never have dreamed of seeing you two together here.'
'Quite accidental,' John was heard to murmur.
'Exactly,' cried Tom; 'that's what I mean, you know. If it wasn't accidental, there would be nothing remarkable in it.'[4]

Tom is, of course, not all that surprised. John and Ruth are embarrassed because it looks as if their meeting in a public thoroughfare might have been planned. Suffice to say it was a happy coincidence. But Tom's jovial irony suggests something to take seriously: that accidents are indeed remarkable events, not just fascinating but subject to continual remarking or rewriting as the Victorians reconfigure their significance. This book has argued for the conspicuousness of accidents in representations of the metropolis which itself was under conceptual renovation. In considering what makes that metropolis remarkable, these writers are hardly enshrining its new cultural and imperial hegemony. Rather, using accidents to explore the capital city, they also introduce uncertainties about the metropolis as a 'dominant social form' and about the logic of its exchanges.[5]

Accident carries or is used to express causal instabilities in a variety of contexts. These are not limited to metropolitan concerns, but the Victorians frequently looked to accident for its explanatory power in the uncertain logic of urban development and exchange. While William Blake aphorized in 1809 that 'Great things are done when Men & Mountains meet; / This is not done by Jostling in the Street', the Victorians invested urban jostling, calamity, and coincidence with great significance in attempting to understand the mass phenomena characteristic of their increasingly metropolitan century.[6] They adapted such accidents to explore the cultural effects of indeterminacy on social taxonomies, urban topologies, transportation technologies, media production, and agency and liability. In so doing, they reinvented the ethical and epistemological significance of chance for an uncertain era.

This book has taken Henry James at his word, conceiving the metropolis as 'a tremendous chapter of accidents' whose particular plotlines and digressions sketch out how unstable notions of causality are deployed and reformed in Victorian culture. The mass phenomena, industrial transformation, and contingent networks of the nineteenth-century metropolis

---

[4] Charles Dickens, *The Life and Adventures of Martin Chuzzlewit* (London: Oxford University Press, 1966), 689.
[5] Raymond Williams, *The Country and the City* (New York: Oxford University Press, 1973), 154.
[6] William Blake, *The Complete Writings of William Blake; with Variant Readings*, ed. Geoffrey Keynes (London; New York: Oxford University Press, 1966), 550.

serve as muse for Victorian writers to imagine narratives and to publish texts that partake of the accidental, the spontaneous, and the chaotic. The preceding chapters have pursued this dynamic over and over: between ideas of accident and the written forms they generate, from the newspaper to the novel. What happens when something so seemingly insurgent and unpredictable as an accident gets systematized, whether in stylized prose, in ideas about public space, in networks of production, or as a congeries of textual features? The result, this book suggests, is an ambiguous middle ground between design and chance which is concretized in texts and metropolitan spaces. Conceived in this way, the Victorian metropolis stages the century's own transitions between providential and relativistic worldviews. Or, to describe this less teleologically, these interpretive paradigms collide in Victorian representations of urban phenomena with lasting effects for the genres of writing about the metropolis and the texts circulating through it.

By Accident or Design has presented selective examples of an extremely complex phenomenon in the service of this broad historical claim. It has risked the pursuit of chameleonic chance across disciplinary boundaries, through the grey areas of discourse formation, and into the bright, busy intersection of various streams of criticism. It has risked its own coherence to keep faith with the interpretive dynamics and contradictions of accidents themselves. At the close, it seems only appropriate to risk speculation beyond the book's own purview, to adopt the dispersive trajectory of accidents themselves. How does this model of accident pertain in contexts very different from the metropolitan, or in literary genres this book has not addressed? What happens to accident when we peer into the twentieth century, the supposed historical horizon for the epistemological integration of chance? Does accident continue to offer a useful analytical framework, or does it lose some of its dialectical edge? By way of closing this book and opening its toolbox for other considerations, I will hazard to depart from its primary focus on prose and offer the following experiment in reading a few turn-of-the-century poems: one about chance, another about accident.

In the Introduction, I argued that the metropolis presents an alternative pathway for the enfranchisement of chance and risk over the nineteenth century, running in parallel to developments in evolutionary biology which have attracted so much critical attention. Thomas Hardy has consistently been identified as a literary exemplar in this context, a 'post-Darwinian' writer who dramatizes in his works 'the full implications of the Darwinian rejection of natural theology and teleology'.[7] Sceptical

---

[7] Gillian Beer, *Darwin's Plots: Evolutionary Narrative in Darwin, George Eliot, and Nineteenth-Century Fiction*, 3rd edn (Cambridge: Cambridge University Press, 2009),

about design and pessimistic about the implications for human life, Hardy became committed instead to a 'provisional view of the universe' in which 'the generating power of the new is chance'.[8] In several ways, Hardy presents an interesting limit case for this book. His example is a challenge to when, historically speaking, the eclipse of providential with provisional views about causality registers in British literature; what sorts of genres best express or embody the 'probabilistic revolution' as it comes home to cultural production; how significant are metropolitan contexts in provoking these paradigmatic and generic developments; and, considering Hardy's own slippage across the boundaries of 'Victorian' and 'modernist' literary histories, how useful are those categories in telling this story. In the face of these challenges, does accident hold up as an explanatory framework? What might Hardy's poems confirm, deny, or further suggest about the transformations of accident as the century turns?

A major change in attitude seems immediately apparent in his poem 'Hap', first composed in 1866, as the speaker pines for a deity—any deity—to blame for his suffering. Like Wordsworth, he would rather be a pagan suckled in a creed outworn, but the universe of chance is too much with him. The closing sestet asks a question about causality: 'How arrives it joy lies slain, / And why unblooms the best hope ever sown?' (ll. 9–10) The final four lines answer with reference to the poem's title, downgrading the chance of 'Hap' into something crass, the 'dicing' gambles of 'purblind Doomsters':

> —Crass Casualty obstructs the sun and rain,
> And dicing Time for gladness casts a moan...
> These purblind Doomsters had as readily strown
> Blisses about my pilgrimage as pain.
> (ll. 11–14)

Even with the personification of 'Doomsters', gone are the suspicions of a designing providence which moments of 'hap' might have previously manifested. But Hardy's scepticism is not fatalism; we can find in his verse residual strains of spontaneous play within an otherwise deterministic framework. In other words, Hardy invites us to consider the hap of form, the potential providence of his poetic designs. If Time plays dice to gamble with the speaker's emotions, 'dicing Time' may also suggest how

---

200; George Levine, *Darwin and the Novelists: Patterns of Science in Victorian Fiction* (Cambridge, MA: Harvard University Press, 1988), 231.

[8] Florence Emily Hardy, *The Life and Work of Thomas Hardy*, ed. Michael Millgate (London; Basingstoke, Hampshire: Macmillan, 1984), 214; Levine, *Darwin and the Novelists*, 250.

Time dices or splits the chronological progression of verse into metrical feet: discrete, if sometimes unpredictable, units of time.[9] But this line, chopped into five iambs, is the most regular of the entire poem. With his characteristically inescapable irony, Hardy suggests simultaneously the pre-determined regularities and the hap of his poetic meter. The ironic persistence of regularity amid chance's scattering force registers a 'formal expression of his humanism', as Gillian Beer has suggested of Hardy's plots.[10] Within even a purblind universe of chance, design is persistently imposed.

Similar ironies appear in the rhyme of 'Hap'. The 'purblind Doomsters' are the agents of the speaker's arbitrary fate; theirs are the inexplicable 'labours—logicless' which God confesses to in Hardy's poem 'New Year's Eve'. Incidentally, the doomsters are also responsible for selecting the poem's final end rhymes, about which they 'had as readily strown' other sounds. They decide on the archaic 'strown' over 'strewn'; we might see this as Hardy's signature 'unexpected vocabulary' and the 'semimodern' opacity of his language.[11] But 'strown' is also expected as the rhyme word, invoked by logical labour of the sonnet form. In *The Chances of Rhyme*, Donald Wesling argues (via Gérard Genette) that poetic creation is energized by such a 'chance encounter with a blank space...in the table of forms'.[12] By writing 'Hap' into one of the most recognizable poetic forms, Hardy restrings the tension between design and chance into a generic conceit; he relieves some—but not all—of his thematic pessimism by the hap of rhyme. Beer identifies a similar dynamic as she listens closely to Hardy's prose: 'the reconciling pleasures of the ear sustain but do not disguise the semantic leaps'.[13] In Hardy's verse, the rhyme reconciles as well as accentuates the poem's emotional crisis, its search for the agency it cannot find. Instead, Hardy integrates 'chance and change' as structuring, repetitive features of experience and language.[14]

If 'Hap' is a poem about chance, what about accident? Hardy takes up the subject in 'The Convergence of the Twain', his commemorative lines

---

[9] Or what Tennyson calls 'The steps of Time—the shocks of Chance—' which measure out his cadences in *In Memoriam* (95, l. 142).

[10] *Darwin's Plots*, 223. For a related reading of enchantment and form in Hardy's novels, see George Levine, 'Hardy and Darwin: An Enchanting Hardy?', in *A Companion to Thomas Hardy*, ed. Keith Wilson, Blackwell Companions to Literature and Culture (Chichester, West Sussex: Wiley-Blackwell, 2009), 36–53.

[11] Jahan Ramazani, Richard Ellman, and Robert O'Clair, eds, *The Norton Anthology of Modern and Contemporary Poetry. Volume 1: Modern Poetry*, 3rd edn (New York: W. W. Norton, 2003), 43.

[12] Donald Wesling, *The Chances of Rhyme: Device and Modernity* (Berkeley, CA: University of California Press, 1980), 112.

[13] Beer, *Darwin's Plots*, 230.   [14] Beer, *Darwin's Plots*, 229.

on the sinking of the Titanic. For Hardy as for many others, the tragedy is so monumental, so symbolically overwhelming as to hardly seem accidental at all.[15] His poem reimagines the event in mythical terms. 'The Convergence of the Twain' sends on a collision course two elements from William Cowper's pastoral aphorism: what God and what man hath wrought. The 'smart ship' which vain humans 'designed' (destination New York City) collides head-on with the 'Shape of Ice' which, in the cosmos of the poem, was 'prepared' by 'The Immanent Will'. God made the sea, and man made the boat—a trans-Atlantic metropolitan vessel. Bert Hornback claims that their collision, as a form of coincidence, 'is not a matter of chance, nor is it a matter of arbitrarily determined fate'. This is no accident but expresses 'the essential moral relationship between cause and consequence'.[16] As this book has suggested, earlier writers had used accidents to split this 'essential' philosophical pairing in twain, to pry apart what Hardy calls the 'intimate welding' revealed by the accident itself (l. 26). If the accident is Hardy's muse, it no longer seems to inspire the *in*essential or arbitrary relationships which previous writers had found so provocative.

Or does it? Like 'Hap', 'The Convergence of the Twain' reanimates the chances of this accident with its play of form and deviation. Like the ship and iceberg, mortal ignorance and cosmic knowledge converge in the last several stanzas, each moving toward an 'intimate welding' whose significance we can only realize afterwards. 'No mortal eye could see' the looming iceberg or the import of the collision to follow, which is set up by the poem's penultimate stanza:

> Or sign that they were bent
> By paths coincident
> On being anon twin halves ‖ of one august event,
>
> (ll. 28–30)

Marking the last line's caesura helps to illustrate how Hardy formalizes the 'convergence' of his poem's theme. The first two lines of each stanza each have six syllables, three beats. The last line combines them into a single line of iambic hexameter. Line 30 calls attention with a spondee to the caesural suture of 'twin halves' into 'of one'. An alternative stanza could have been built with these same parts, splitting the last long line of each

---

[15] On their faked front-page for that day in history, the satirical newspaper *The Onion* announces: 'World's Largest Metaphor Hits Ice-berg; Titanic, Representation of Man's Hubris, Sinks in North Atlantic; 1,500 Dead in Symbolic Tragedy', *The Onion*, 16 April 2007, <http://www.theonion.com/articles/april-16-1912,10645/>.

[16] Bert G. Hornback, *The Metaphor of Chance: Vision and Technique in the Works of Thomas Hardy* (Athens, OH: Ohio University Press, 1971), 11, 10.

stanza to make four short trimetric lines with the rhyme scheme a–a–x–a. Seen also in line 26, '[t]he intimate welding of their later history', Hardy makes the moment of unrhyming, 'x', a hotspot for thematic convergence: the 'intimate welding' of difference into controlling structure, 'twin halves' combining into a metrical and rhyming whole.

Still, stanza 10 shows that, much though parallel paths converge, something can still veer surprisingly away. Echoing the meeting of iceberg and ship, what gets 'bent' into 'paths coincident' are two rhyming lines; they aurally converge in the last word of the stanza: 'event'. The 'one august event' refers to the collision itself, calling to mind a word and concept only present as a ghost rhyme: 'accident'. If accident was anywhere in this poem, it would be right here. Perhaps Hardy avoids the word to further insist that this was no accident at all, but an 'event' which discloses hidden meaning. If so, Hardy keeps faith with a hermeneutical tradition of accident which, according to Ross Hamilton, has predominated in modern thought. Or perhaps 'accident' escapes from the very spot upon which deterministic forces—of fate, of form—converge. The binary Hardy builds to frame the unknowable complexities of causation fails to secure this third term. Accident, on the one hand, can support Hardy's cosmic binary as a metaphor, an event which reveals the meaningful convergence of two apparently unrelated things. On the other hand, accident haunts the structure as its exception, the unmotivated and even arbitrary problem of inessential qualities, as Hamilton wants us to remember.[17] For instance, perhaps 'accident' just wouldn't have fit the line, but its metrical resistance to the pattern of stresses made by 'dicing Time' is another example of its contingency manifest in verse. We can imagine an alternative which might fit, and might better fit the historical circumstances, as this 'august event' occurred in chilly April. In line 30, could twin halves converge in 'one spring accident'? Of course not. That circumstantial detail splinters the mythical tone and timeline Hardy wants to use. The poem's final stanza describes the event as a 'consummation', a harvest of meaning in humanity's fall. It is caused by the 'Spinner of the Years'—the accidental muse, as it were—who says '"Now!" And each one hears, / And consummation comes, and jars two hemispheres'. The collision of 'twin halves' echoes in the jarring of hemispheres. The collision, like the command, is something heard. 'No mortal eye could see', but 'each one hears'. If we have been listening, we

---

[17] Annmarie Drury makes such an argument about Fitzgerald's *Rubáiyát* whose 'aesthetic of accident privileges chance and randomness over predictability and determinacy and prizes interruption and rapid metamorphosis over continuity'. See 'Accident, Orientalism, and Edward FitzGerald as Translator', *Victorian Poetry* 46, no. 1 (2008): 40.

have already heard such jarring or dissonance between formal commands, deviations, and contingencies.

We can find in these two poems evidence of the historical transformations of accident as well as its continuing usefulness as context and investigative lens. Foregrounded by urban life in the high Victorian era, sent across the countryside by the railway, accident has escaped its metropolitan environs to become a universal condition—the very condition Hardy invokes to hazard cosmic pronouncements. Taken together, the poems imply how the 'universe of chance' declared by C. S. Peirce at the turn of the century is simultaneously the enfranchisement and the taming of chance; chance is everywhere and hence nowhere.[18] Indeterminacy becomes newly subordinate to probabilistic and relativistic regimes; God does not play dice, Einstein famously declares.[19] Yet Hardy's poetry still does, even considering his philosophical assimilation of chance into its deterministic opposite. Seen (and heard) in the formal dynamics of his verse, the dialectics of accident continue to play in the margins of causality, a game in which earlier Victorian literature had raised the stakes on discourses which were folding chance into tamer epistemologies. Accident keeps providential and provisional views on the table; it makes their contest anything but certain. Although *By Accident or Design* has located this dynamic within a particular historical context, the English metropolis in the mid-nineteenth century, Hardy's poems are suggestive of a broader array of contexts, genres, and philosophical debates about which one might, with purpose, accidentally muse. So also do these poems suggest what one might expect to learn: how accidents remake the forms devised to account for them, imprinting these forms with questions about the chances of their making.

---

[18] Theodore M. Porter, *The Rise of Statistical Thinking, 1820–1900* (Princeton, NJ: Princeton University Press, 1986), 150.

[19] Mallarmé would disagree, declaring in his eponymous poem 'Un coup de dés jamais n'abolira le hasard': a throw of the dice will never abolish chance. His scattered, fragmented poem prominently features a shipwreck, perhaps a coincidental result of his own exploration of, as he declared in a letter, 'les plus purs glaciers de l'Esthétique'. See *Correspondance de Stéphane Mallarmé. Vol. 1: 1862–1871*, ed. Henri Mondor (Paris: Gallimard, 1959), 220. Mallarmé's poem is the dispersion to Hardy's convergence.

Bibliography

'19th Century British Library Newspapers'. *Gale Cengage Learning*, 2007. <http://infotrac.galegroup.com/itweb/viva_uva?db=BNCN>.
'A Railway Map of England'. *Punch*, 27 September 1845.
'Accident the Father of Improvement'. *Belfast News-Letter*, 19 February 1839.
Ackroyd, Peter. 'London Luminaries and Cockney Visionaries'. In *The Collection*, 341–51. London: Chatto & Windus, 2001.
Agathocleous, Tanya. *Urban Realism and the Cosmopolitan Imagination in the Nineteenth Century: Visible City, Invisible World*. Cambridge; New York: Cambridge University Press, 2011.
'Alarming Fire in Manchester—Suspected Case of Incendiarism'. *The Times*. 14 December 1836.
Alborn, Timothy. 'The Moral of the Failed Bank: Professional Plots in the Victorian Money Market'. *Victorian Studies* 38, no. 2 (1995): 199–226.
'Alleged Incendiarism'. *The Times*. 19 March 1846.
Allen, Peter M. *Cities and Regions as Self-Organizing Systems: Models of Complexity*. Amsterdam: Gordon and Breach, 1997.
Altick, Richard D. *The English Common Reader: A Social History of the Mass Reading Public, 1800–1900*. 2nd edn. Columbus, OH: Ohio State University Press, 1998.
Altick, Richard D. *The Presence of the Present: Topics of the Day in the Victorian Novel*. Columbus, OH: Ohio State University Press, 1991.
Anderson, Amanda. *Tainted Souls and Painted Faces: The Rhetoric of Fallenness in Victorian Culture*. Ithaca NY: Cornell University Press, 1993.
Anderson, Benedict R. *Imagined Communities: Reflections on the Origin and Spread of Nationalism*. London: Verso, 1983.
'Another Alarming Fire in Manchester. (From Our Own Correspondent.)'. *The Times*. 8 January 1842.
Arata, Stephen. *Fictions of Loss in the Victorian Fin de Siècle*. Cambridge: Cambridge University Press, 1996.
Aristotle. 'Poetics'. In *The Basic Works of Aristotle*, edited by Richard McKeon. New York: Random House, 1941.
Arscott, Caroline, and Griselda Pollock. 'The Partial View: The Visual Representation of the Early Nineteenth-Century Industrial City'. In *The Culture of Capital: Art, Power, and the Nineteenth-Century Middle Class*, edited by Janet Wolff and John Seed, 191–233. Manchester; New York: Manchester University Press, 1988.
Ashton, John. *Modern Street Ballads*. London: Chatto & Windus, 1888.
Atmore, Henry. 'Railway Interests and the "Rope of Air".' *The British Journal for the History of Science* 37, no. 3 (September 2004): 245–79. <http://www.jstor.org/stable/4028424>.

Bibliography

Aytoun, William Edmondstoune. *Norman Sinclair*. Edinburgh; London: William Blackwood and Sons, 1861. <http://books.google.com/books?id=5NYOAAAAYAAJ>.

Babbage, Charles. 'A Comparative View of the Various Institutions for the Assurance of Lives (1826)'. In *The History of Insurance*, edited by Henry Jenkins and Takau Yoneyama, 4: 241–383. London: Pickering & Chatto, 2000.

Babbage, Charles. *The Ninth Bridgewater Treatise: A Fragment*. 2nd edn. London: John Murray, 1838. <http://books.google.com/books?id=y_ERAAAAYAAJ>.

Baddeley, William. 'London Fires in 1847'. *Mechanics Magazine*, 29 July 1848. <http://books.google.com/books?id=ihkFAAAAQAAJ>.

Bagehot, Walter. 'Charles Dickens'. *The National Review* 7 (October 1858): 458–86. <http://books.google.com/books?id=NGBFAAAAYAAJ>.

Bagehot, Walter. *The English Constitution*. Edited by Miles Taylor. Oxford; New York: Oxford University Press, 2001.

Barlow, John Perry. 'A Declaration of the Independence of Cyberspace'. *Electronic Frontier Foundation*, 8 February 1996. <https://projects.eff.org/~barlow/Declaration-Final.html>.

Barthes, Roland. 'Structure of the Fait-Divers'. In *Critical Essays*, translated by Richard Howard, 185–96. Evanston, IL: Northwestern University Press, 1972.

Barthes, Roland. 'The Reality Effect'. In *The Rustle of Language*, translated by Richard Howard, 141–8. New York: Hill and Wang, 1986.

Baucom, Ian. *Specters of the Atlantic: Finance Capital, Slavery, and the Philosophy of History*. Durham, NC: Duke University Press, 2005.

Beaumont, Matthew. 'The Railway and Literature: Realism and the Phantasmagoric'. In *The Railway: Art in the Age of Steam*, edited by Ian G Kennedy and Julian Treuherz, 35–43. New Haven, CT: Yale University Press, 2008.

Beaumont, Matthew, and Michael J. Freeman, eds, *The Railway and Modernity: Time, Space, and the Machine Ensemble*. Oxford; New York: Oxford University Press, 2007.

Beer, Gillian. *Darwin's Plots: Evolutionary Narrative in Darwin, George Eliot, and Nineteenth-Century Fiction*. 3rd edn. Cambridge: Cambridge University Press, 2009.

Beer, Gillian. *Open Fields: Science in Cultural Encounter*. Oxford; New York: Oxford University Press, 1996.

Beetham, Margaret. 'Towards a Theory of the Periodical as a Publishing Genre'. In *Investigating Victorian Journalism*, edited by Laurel Brake and Aled Jones, 19–32. New York: St. Martin's Press, 1990.

Bell, David F. *Circumstances: Chance in the Literary Text*. Lincoln, NE: University of Nebraska Press, 1993.

Beloc, Hilaire. *On Nothing and Kindred Subjects*. London: Methuen, 1908.

Benjamin, Walter. *Charles Baudelaire: A Lyric Poet in the Era of High Capitalism*. Translated by Harry Zohn. New York: Verso, 1997.

Benkler, Yochai. *The Wealth of Networks: How Social Production Transforms Markets and Freedom*. New Haven, CT: Yale University Press, 2006.

Bennett, Deborah J. *Randomness*. Cambridge, MA: Harvard University Press, 1998.
Bernstein, Peter. *Against the Gods: The Remarkable Story of Risk*. New York: Wiley, 1996.
Blair, Ann. *Too Much to Know: Managing Scholarly Information Before the Modern Age*. New Haven, CT: Yale University Press, 2010.
Blake, William. *The Complete Writings of William Blake; with Variant Readings*. Edited by Geoffrey Keynes. London; New York: Oxford University Press, 1966.
Boehm, Katharina, and Josephine McDonagh. 'New Agenda. Urban Mobility: New Maps of Victorian London'. *Journal of Victorian Culture* 15, no. 2 (August 2010): 194–200.
Bolter, Jay David, and Richard Grusin. *Remediation: Understanding New Media*. Cambridge, MA: MIT Press, 1999.
Bowlby, Rachel. *Just Looking: Consumer Culture in Dreiser, Gissing, and Zola*. New York: Methuen, 1985.
'Braham's Delight'. J. Pitts, 1844 1819. Harding B 11(436). Bodleian Library Broadside Ballads. <http://bodley24.bodley.ox.ac.uk/cgi-bin/acwwweng/ballads/image.pl?ref=Harding+B+11(436)&id=01324.gif&seq=1&size=1>.
Brake, Laurel. 'The Longevity of "Ephemera": Library Editions of Victorian Periodicals and Newspapers'. Yale University, 2008.
Brantlinger, Patrick. *The Reading Lesson: The Threat of Mass Literacy in Nineteenth Century British Fiction*. Bloomington, IN: Indiana University Press, 1998.
Brewer, Ebenezer Cobham. 'Chapter of Accidents (A)'. *Dictionary of Phrase and Fable*. Philadelphia, PA: Henry Altemus Company, 1898. <http://www.bartleby.com/81/3380.html>.
'British Newspapers 1800–1900'. *British Library*, 2009. <http://newspapers11.bl.uk/blcs/>.
Bronstein, Jamie L. *Caught in the Machinery: Workplace Accidents and Injured Workers in Nineteenth-Century Britain*. Palo Alto, CA: Stanford University Press, 2008.
Brown, Lucy. *Victorian News and Newspapers*. Oxford; New York: Oxford University Press, 1985.
Brown, Samuel. 'On the Fires in London'. In *The Assurance Magazine*, 1: 31–62. London: Charles & Edwin Layton, 1851. <http://books.google.com/books?id=Fj0DAAAAYAAJ>.
Burney, Ian A. *Bodies of Evidence: Medicine and the Politics of the English Inquest, 1830–1926*. Baltimore, MD: Johns Hopkins University Press, 2000.
Butler, Joseph. *The Analogy of Religion Natural and Revealed to the Constitution and Course of Nature*. Dublin: George Ewing, 1736. <http://find.galegroup.com/ecco/infomark.do?&source=gale&prodId=ECCO&userGroupName=tall85761&tabID=T001&docId=CW121666346&type=multipage&contentSet=ECCOArticles&version=1.0&docLevel=FASCIMILE>.
Butt, John, and Kathleen Tillotson. 'Dickens as a Serial Novelist'. In *Dickens at Work*, 13–34. London: Methuen, 1957.

Butterworth, C. H. 'Overfeeding'. *Victoria Magazine*, November 1869.
Buzard, James. *Disorienting Fiction: The Autoethnographic Work of Nineteenth-Century British Novels.* Princeton, NJ: Princeton University Press, 2005.
Byerly, Alison. 'Effortless Art: The Sketch in Nineteenth-Century Painting and Literature'. *Criticism* 41, no. 3 (Summer 1999): 349–64.
Capuano, Peter. 'Maneuvering Between Early Nineteenth-Century Science, Religiosity, and Industrialization,' 2013.
Capuano, Peter. 'Novel Hands: Manual Activity and Victorian Fiction'. Ph.D. Dissertation, University of Virginia, 2009.
Capuano, Peter. 'On Sir Charles Bell's The Hand, 1833'. *BRANCH: Britain, Representation and Nineteenth-Century History.* Romanticism and Victorianism on the Net, 2012. <http://www.branchcollective.org/?ps_articles=peter-capuano-on-sir-charles-bells-the-hand-1833>.
Carey, James W. *Communication as Culture: Essays on Media and Society.* Boston, MA: Unwin Hyman, 1989.
Carlyle, Thomas. 'Letter to John Sterling,' 4 June 1835. The Carlyle Letters Online. <http://carlyleletters.dukejournals.org>.
Carlyle, Thomas. 'Signs of the Times'. In *The Spirit of the Age: Victorian Essays*, edited by Gertrude Himmelfarb. New Haven, CT: Yale University Press, 2007.
Carter, Ian. *Railways and Culture in Britain: The Epitome of Modernity.* Manchester; New York: Manchester University Press, 2001.
Castells, Manuel. *The Informational City: Information Technology, Economic Restructuring, and the Urban-Regional Process.* Oxford, UK; Cambridge, MA: Blackwell, 1989.
Cawthon, Elizabeth. 'New Life for the Deodand: Coroners' Inquests and Occupational Deaths in England, 1830–46'. *The American Journal of Legal History* 33, no. 2 (April 1989): 137–47.
de Certeau, Michel. *The Practice of Everyday Life.* Translated by Steven Rendall. Berkeley, CA: University of California Press, 1984.
Chandler, James, and Kevin Gilmartin. 'Introduction: Engaging the Eidometropolis'. In *Romantic Metropolis: The Urban Scene of British Culture, 1780–1840*, edited by James Chandler and Kevin Gilmartin, 1–41. Cambridge; New York: Cambridge University Press, 2005.
Chandler, James, and Kevin Gilmartin, eds. *Romantic Metropolis: The Urban Scene of British Culture, 1780–1840.* Cambridge; New York: Cambridge University Press, 2005.
Chapple, J. A. V, and Arthur Pollard, eds. *The Letters of Mrs. Gaskell.* Cambridge: Harvard University Press, 1967.
Chapple, J. A. V, and Anita C. Wilson, eds. *Private Voices: The Diaries of Elizabeth Gaskell and Sophia Holland.* Keele, Staffordshire: Keele University Press, 1977.
'Cheap Literature'. *British Quarterly Review*, April 1859.
Chittick, Kathryn. *Dickens and the 1830s.* Cambridge; New York: Cambridge University Press, 1990.

Chorley, Henry Fothergill. 'Review of Mary Barton'. *Athenæum* 1095 (21 October 1848): 1050–1.

Churton, Edward. *The Railroad Book of England: Historical, Topographical and Picturesque; Descriptive of the Cities, Towns, Country Seats, and Other Subjects of Local Interest, With a Brief Sketch of the Lines in Scotland and Wales*. London: Sidgwick and Jackson, 1973.

Clark, Geoffrey. *Betting on Lives: The Culture of Life Insurance in England*. Manchester: Manchester University Press, 1999.

Clarke, Bob. *From Grub Street to Fleet Street: An Illustrated History of English Newspapers to 1899*. Aldershot, Hampshire; Burlington: Ashgate, 2004.

Cobbett, William. 'Sussex Journal'. *Cobbett's Weekly Register*, 12 January 1822. <http://books.google.com/books?id=MS8FAAAAQAAJ>.

Cockerell, H. A. L, and Edwin Green. *The British Insurance Business 1547–1970*. London: Heinemann, 1976.

Collins, Charles. 'The Value of Accident'. *The Atlantic Monthly*, February 1870. <http://books.google.com/books?id=bEUwAQAAMAAJ&pg=PA172>.

Collins, Wilkie. 'The Unknown Public'. *Household Words*, 21 August 1858.

'Commentary on the Projected Liverpool and Manchester Railway'. *Quarterly Review*, March 1825, 361–2.

Cooter, Roger. 'The Moment of the Accident: Culture, Militarism and Modernity in Late-Victorian Britain'. In *Accidents in History: Injuries, Fatalities, and Social Relations*, edited by Roger Cooter and Bill Luckin, 107–57. Amsterdam; Atlanta, GA: Rodopi, 1997.

Cooter, Roger, and Bill Luckin, eds. *Accidents in History: Injuries, Fatalities, and Social Relations*. Amsterdam; Atlanta, GA: Rodopi, 1997.

Courtemanche, Eleanor. *The 'Invisible Hand' and British Fiction, 1818–1860: Adam Smith, Political Economy, and the Genre of Realism*. Houndmills, Basingstoke, Hampshire; New York: Palgrave Macmillan, 2011.

Cowper, William. *The Task*. London: John Sharpe, 1817.

Craik, Dinah. *The Head of the Family*. London: Macmillan, 1890. <http://books.google.com/books?id=uJBAAAAAIAAJ>.

Cronon, William. *Nature's Metropolis: Chicago and the Great West*. New York: W. W. Norton, 1991.

Dallas, E. S. 'Popular Literature—The Periodical Press. [Part 1]'. *Blackwood's*, January 1859.

Dallas, E. S. 'Popular Literature—The Periodical Press. [Part 2]'. *Blackwood's*, February 1859.

Dallas, E. S. 'Popular Literature—Tracts'. *Blackwood's*, May 1859.

Daly, Nicholas. 'Railway Novels: Sensation Fiction and the Modernization of the Senses'. *English Literary History* 66, no. 2 (1999): 461–87. <http://muse.jhu.edu/journals/elh/v066/66.2daly.html>.

Darwin, Charles. 'Darwin, C. R. to Lyell, Charles', 10 December 1859. Letter 2575. Darwin Correspondence Project. <http://www.darwinproject.ac.uk/letter/entry-2575>.

Darwin, Charles. *The Origin of Species*. Edited by Gillian Beer. Oxford: Oxford University Press, 1996.
Daston, Lorraine J. 'The Domestication of Risk: Mathematical Probability and Insurance 1650–1830'. In *The Probabilistic Revolution. Volume 1: Ideas in History*, edited by Lorenz Krüger, Lorraine J. Daston, and Michael Heidelberger, 237–. Cambridge, MA: MIT Press, 1987.
Daston, Lorraine, and Katherine Park. *Wonders and the Order of Nature, 1150–1750*. New York: Zone Books, 1998.
Davidson, Cathy N. 'Humanities 2.0: Promise, Perils, Predictions'. *PMLA* 123, no. 3 (May 2008): 707–17.
De Quincey, Thomas. *The English Mail-Coach and Joan of Arc*. Boston, MA: Athenaeum Press, 1905.
Denton, William. *Is Darwin Right? Or, The Origin of Man*. Wellesley, MA: Mrs. E. M. F. Denton, 1881. <http://books.google.com/books?id=_d04AAAAMAAJ>.
Dickens, Charles. *Bleak House*. Oxford: Oxford University Press, 1987.
Dickens, Charles. *Dombey and Son*. Edited by Andrew Sanders. London; New York: Penguin, 2002.
Dickens, Charles. *The Life and Adventures of Martin Chuzzlewit*. London: Oxford University Press, 1966.
Dickens, Charles. *Mugby Junction*. Edited by Robert Macfarlane. London: Hesperus, 2005.
Dickens, Charles. *The Posthumous Papers of the Pickwick Club*. Oxford; New York: Oxford University Press, 1987.
Dickens, Charles. *Sketches by Boz: Illustrative of Every-Day Life and Every-Day People*. London; New York: Oxford University Press, 1966.
Dickson, P. G. M. *The Sun Insurance Office, 1710–1960; The History of Two and a Half Centuries of British Insurance*. London: Oxford University Press, 1960.
Dimock, Wai Chee. 'Introduction: Genres as Fields of Knowledge'. *PMLA* 122, no. 5 (October 2007): 1377–88.
Dimock, Wai Chee. *Through Other Continents: American Literature Across Deep Time*. Princeton, NJ: Princeton University Press, 2006.
Dixon, J. Hepworth. 'Literature of the Lower Orders (Batch the First)'. *Daily News*. 26 October, 1847.
Dobraszczyk, Paul. 'Useful Reading? Designing Information for London's Victorian Cab Passengers'. *Journal of Design History* 21, no. 2 (Summer 2008): 121–41.
'Dreadful Fire at Manchester. Melancholy Loss of Several Lives'. *The Times*. 29 August 1838.
'Dreadful Fire in Manchester, With Loss of Life'. *The Times*. 28 August 1838.
Drury, Annmarie. 'Accident, Orientalism, and Edward FitzGerald as Translator'. *Victorian Poetry* 46, no. 1 (2008): 37–53.
Duty Keeper of Records. 'Original Fire Inquests,' 7 December 1976. Original Fire Inquests. CLA/041/F1/01/01/068 1845–1885. Corporation of London Records Office.

Dyos, H. J., and Michael Wolff. 'The Way We Live Now'. In *The Victorian City: Images and Realities*, edited by H. J Dyos and Michael Wolff, 2: 893–907. London: Routledge & Kegan Paul, 1973.
Egan, Pierce. 'Life in London'. In *Unknown London: Early Modernist Visions of the Metropolis, 1815–45*, edited by John Marriot, Masaie Matsumura, and Judith R. Walkowitz, V. London: Pickering & Chatto, 2000.
Eliot, George. *Felix Holt, the Radical*. Edited by Fred C. Thomson. Oxford: Clarendon, 1980.
Eliot, George. 'The Influence of Rationalism'. *The Fortnightly Review* 1 (1846): 43–55. <http://books.google.com/books?id=CO1GAAAAcAAJ&pg=PA43>.
Ellis, C. Hamilton, and Susan Hyman. *Railway Art*. Boston, MA: New York Graphic Society, 1977.
Elwin, Rev. Fountain. *Personal Danger, and Providential Deliverance. A Sermon Preached at the Octagon Chapel, Bath, on the Occasion of a Fatal Accident Which Happened to the Express Train, on the Great Western Railway, May 10, 1848*. London: J. Hatchard and Son, 1848.
Engels, Friedrich. *The Condition of the Working Class in England*. Translated by W. O. Henderson and W. H. Chaloner. New York: Macmillan, 1958.
Engels, Friedrich. *The Condition of the Working Class in England*. Edited by Victor Kiernan. Harmondsworth; New York: Penguin, 1987.
Everitt, Alan. 'The Railway and Rural Tradition, 1840–1940'. In *The Impact of the Railway on Society in Britain: Essays in Honour of Jack Simmons*, edited by Jack Simmons, A. K. B. Evans, and John Gough, 181–98. Aldershot, Hampshire; Burlington, VT: Ashgate, 2003.
Farber, Paul Lawrence. *Finding Order in Nature: The Naturalist Tradition from Linnaeus to E. O. Wilson*. Baltimore, MD: Johns Hopkins University Press, 2000.
Faulk, Barry J. *Music Hall & Modernity: The Late-Victorian Discovery of Popular Culture*. Athens, OH: Ohio University Press, 2004.
Feltes, N. N. 'Community and the Limits of Liability in Two Mid-Victorian Novels'. *Victorian Studies* 17, no. 4 (1974): 355–69.
Ferguson, Christopher. 'Inventing the Modern City: Urban Culture and Ideas in Britain, 1780–1880'. Ph.D. Dissertation, Indiana University, 2008.
Folsom, Ed. 'Database as Genre: The Epic Transformation of Archives'. *PMLA* 122, no. 5 (October 2007): 1572–9.
Forster, John. *The Life of Charles Dickens*. Philadelphia, PA: J. B Lippincott & Co., 1872. <http://books.google.com/books?id=r00YAAAAYAAJ>.
Foucault, Michel. 'Nietzsche, Genealogy, History'. In *Language, Counter-Memory, Practice*, edited by Bouchard, Donald F., translated by Donald F. Bouchard and Sherry Simon, 139–64. Ithaca, NY: Cornell University Press, 1977.
Foucault, Michel. *The Order of Things: An Archaeology of the Human Sciences*. New York: Pantheon Books, 1970.
Fowles, John. *Shipwreck*. London: Cape, 1974.
Franklin, J. Jeffrey. *Serious Play: The Cultural Form of the Nineteenth-Century Realist Novel*. Philadelphia, PA: University of Pennsylvania Press, 1999.

Freedgood, Elaine. *Victorian Writing About Risk: Imagining a Safe England in a Dangerous World.* Cambridge; New York: Cambridge University Press, 2000.

Freedman, Jonathan, N. Katherine Hayles, Jerome McGann, Meredith L. McGill, Peter Stallybrass, and Ed Folsom. 'Responses to Ed Folsom's "Database as Genre: The Epic Transformation of Archives"'. *PMLA* 122, no. 5 (October 2007): 1580–612.

Freeman, Michael J. *Railways and the Victorian Imagination.* New Haven, CT: Yale University Press, 1999.

Frith, Christopher D. *Making Up the Mind: How the Brain Creates Our Mental World.* Malden, MA: Blackwell, 2007.

Fryckstedt, Monica Correa. *Elizabeth Gaskell's Mary Barton and Ruth: A Challenge to Christian England.* Acta Universitatis Upsaliensis 43. Uppsala: Stockholm: [Uppsala universitet] ; Distributor, Almqvist & Wiksell International, 1982.

Fyfe, Paul. 'Illustrating the Accident: Railways and the Catastrophic Picturesque in the *Illustrated London News*'. *Victorian Periodicals Review* 46, no. 1 (2013): 61–91.

Fyfe, Paul. 'On the Opening of the Liverpool and Manchester Railway, 1830'. *BRANCH: Britain, Representation and Nineteenth-Century History.* Romanticism and Victorianism on the Net, 2012. <http://www.branchcollective.org/?ps_articles=paul-fyfe-on-the-opening-of-the-liverpool-and-manchester-railway-1830>.

Gagnier, Regenia. *Subjectivities: A History of Self-Representation in Britain, 1832–1920.* New York: Oxford University Press, 1991.

Gallagher, Catherine. *The Industrial Reformation of English Fiction: Social Discourse and Narrative Form, 1832–1867.* Chicago, IL: University of Chicago Press, 1985.

Garcha, Amanpal. *From Sketch to Novel: The Development of Victorian Fiction.* Cambridge; New York: Cambridge University Press, 2009.

Garfield, Simon. *The Last Journey of William Huskisson.* London: Faber, 2002.

Garnica, Alicia. 'The Curious Life of the Corpse in Nineteenth-Century English Literature and Culture'. Ph.D. Dissertation, University of Southern California, 2009.

Gaskell, Elizabeth. *Cranford.* Edited by Elizabeth Porges Watson. New York: Oxford University Press, 2011.

Gaskell, Elizabeth Cleghorn. *Mary Barton: A Tale of Manchester Life.* Edited by Jennifer Foster. Peterborough, Ont.; Orchard Park, NY: Broadview, 2000.

Gaskell, Elizabeth Cleghorn. *North and South.* Edited by Patricia Ingham. London: Penguin, 1995.

Giddens, Anthony. *The Consequences of Modernity.* Palo Alto, CA: Stanford University Press, 1990.

Giddens, Anthony. *Runaway World: How Globalisation Is Reshaping Our Lives.* New York: Routledge, 2000.

Gilbert, Pamela K. *Mapping the Victorian Social Body.* Albany, NY: State University of New York Press, 2004.

Gilroy, Paul. *The Black Atlantic: Modernity and Double Consciousness*. Cambridge, MA: Harvard University Press, 1993.
Green, Judith. 'Accidents: The Remnants of a Modern Classificatory System'. In *Accidents in History: Injuries, Fatalities, and Social Relations*, edited by Roger Cooter and Bill Luckin, 35–58. Amsterdam; Atlanta, GA: Rodopi, 1997.
Green, Judith. *Risk and Misfortune: A Social Construction of Accidents*. London; Bristol, PA: University College of London Press, 1997.
Grillo, Virgil. *Charles Dickens' Sketches by Boz: End in the Beginning*. Boulder, CO: Colorado Associated University Press, 1975.
Grossman, Jonathan H. *Charles Dickens's Networks: Public Transport and the Novel*. Oxford; New York: Oxford University Press, 2012.
Hacking, Ian. *The Emergence of Probability: A Philosophical Study of Early Ideas About Probability, Induction and Statistical Inference*. 2nd edn. Cambridge; New York: Cambridge University Press, 2006.
Hacking, Ian. *The Taming of Chance*. Cambridge; New York: Cambridge University Press, 1990.
Hadley, Elaine. *Melodramatic Tactics: Theatricalized Dissent in the English Marketplace, 1800–1885*. Palo Alto, CA: Stanford University Press, 1995.
Hall, F. J. *The Next of Kin*. London: Thomas Cautley Newby, 1854. <http://books.google.com/books?id=F7YBAAAAQAAJ>.
Hamilton, Ross. *Accident: A Philosophical and Literary History*. Chicago, IL: University of Chicago Press, 2007.
Hancher, Michael. 'From Street Ballad to Penny Magazine: "March of Intellect in the Butchering Line"'. In *Nineteenth-Century Media and the Construction of Identities*, edited by Laurel Brake, Bill Bell, and David Finkelstein, 93–103. Basingstoke, Hampshire: Palgrave, 2000.
Handley, Graham. *An Elizabeth Gaskell Chronology*. Basingstoke, Hampshire; New York: Palgrave Macmillan, 2004.
Hardy, Florence Emily. *The Life and Work of Thomas Hardy*. Edited by Michael Millgate. London; Basingstoke, Hampshire: Macmillan, 1984.
Hardy, Iza Duffus [Mary-Anne]. *A Hero's Work*. London: Hurst and Blackett, 1868.
Harrington, Ralph. 'The Railway Accident: Trains, Trauma and Technological Crisis in Nineteenth-Century Britain'. *Institute of Railway Studies, University of York*, 1999. <http://www.york.ac.uk/inst/irs/irshome/papers/rlyacc.htm>.
Harris, Michael. *London Newspapers in the Age of Walpole: A Study of the Origins of the Modern English Press*. Rutherford, NJ: Fairleigh Dickinson; Associated University Presses, 1987.
Harrison, Gary Lee. *Wordsworth's Vagrant Muse: Poetry, Poverty, and Power*. Detroit: Wayne State University Press, 1994.
Hartman, Charles O. *Virtual Muse: Experiments in Computer Poetry*. Hanover, NH: University Press of New England, 1996.
Harvey, David. *The Condition of Postmodernity: An Enquiry into the Origins of Cultural Change*. Oxford; Cambridge, MA: Blackwell, 1989.

Harvey, David. *Consciousness and the Urban Experience: Studies in the History and Theory of Capitalist Urbanization*. Baltimore, MD: Johns Hopkins University Press, 1985.
Head, Sir Francis Bond. 'Railroads in Ireland'. *Quarterly Review* 63 (January 1839): 1–60.
Hemestedt, Geoffrey. 'Inventing Social Identity: *Sketches by Boz*'. In *Victorian Identities: Social and Cultural Formations in Nineteenth-Century Literature*, edited by Ruth Robbins and Julian Wolfreys, 215–29. Basingstoke, Hampshire: Macmillan, 1996.
Henry, Nancy. '"Rushing into Eternity": Suicide and Finance in Victorian Fiction'. In *Victorian Investments: New Perspectives on Finance and Culture*, edited by Cannon Schmitt and Nancy Henry, 161–81. Bloomington, IN: Indiana University Press, 2009.
Hepburn, James. *A Book of Scattered Leaves: Poetry of Poverty in Broadside Ballads of Nineteenth-Century England* 2 vols. Lewisburg, PA: Bucknell University Press, 2000.
Herbert, Christopher. *Victorian Relativity: Radical Thought and Scientific Discovery*. Chicago, IL: University of Chicago Press, 2001.
Hertz, Neil. *George Eliot's Pulse*. Palo Alto, CA: Stanford University Press, 2003.
Hindley, Charles, ed. *Curiosities of Street Literature*. New York: Augustus M. Kelley, 1970.
Hobbs, Andrew. 'The Deleterious Dominance of *The Times* in Nineteenth-Century Scholarship'. *Journal of Victorian Culture* 18, no. 4 (2013): 472–97.
Hobbs, Andrew. 'When the Provincial Press Was the National Press (*c*.1826–*c*.1900)'. *International Journal of Regional and Local Studies* 5, no. 1 (Spring 2009): 16–43.
Hollington, Michael. 'Dickens the Flâneur'. *Dickensian* 77, no. 2 (Summer 1981): 71–87.
Holloway, John, and Joan Black, eds. *Later English Broadside Ballads*, II. London: Routledge & Kegan Paul, 1979.
Hornback, Bert G. *The Metaphor of Chance: Vision and Technique in the Works of Thomas Hardy*. Athens, OH: Ohio University Press, 1971.
Huett, Lorna. 'Among the Unknown Public: *Household Words, All the Year Round* and the Mass-Market Weekly Periodical in the Mid-Nineteenth Century'. *Victorian Periodicals Review* 38, no. 1 (2005): 61–82. <http://muse.jhu.edu/journals/victorian_periodicals_review/v038/38.1huett.html>.
Hume, David. *An Enquiry Concerning Human Understanding*. Edited by Stephen Buckle. Cambridge: Cambridge University Press, 2007.
Humpherys, Anne. 'Popular Narrative and Political Discourse in Reynolds's Weekly Newspaper'. In *Investigating Victorian Journalism*, edited by Laurel Brake and Aled Jones, 33–47. New York: St. Martin's Press, 1990.
'Illustrated Periodical Literature'. *Bookseller*, November 30, 1861.
'Inquests on Fires'. *The Times*. 22 April 1850.
'Insurance Against Accidents of All Kinds'. *Chambers's Edinburgh Journal*, 19 April 1854.

Jacobs, Jane. *The Death and Life of Great American Cities*. New York: Random House, 1961.
Jaffe, Audrey. *Vanishing Points: Dickens, Narrative, and the Subject of Omniscience*. Berkeley, CA: University of California Press, 1991.
Jakobson, Roman. 'Closing Statement: Linguistics and Poetics'. In *Style in Language*, edited by Thomas A. Sebeok. Cambridge, MA: MIT Press, 1960.
James, Henry. 'London'. *Century Magazine*, December 1888. <http://cdl.library.cornell.edu/cgi-bin/moa/pageviewer?coll=moa&root=/moa/cent/cent0037/&tif=00229.TIF&view=50&frames=1>.
James, Henry. 'Preface'. In *The Tragic Muse*, VII. *The Novels and Tales of Henry James*. London: Macmillan, 1908.
Jenkins, David Trevor, and Takau Yoneyama, eds. *The History of Insurance*, I. 8 vols. London: Pickering & Chatto, 2000.
Jenkins, David Trevor, and Takau Yoneyama, eds. 'Instructions for the Agents of the Sun Fire Office'. In *The History of Insurance*, 1: 247–93. London: Pickering & Chatto, 2000.
Jervis, John. *Sir John Jervis on the Office and Duties of Coroners: With Forms and Precedents*. Edited by C. W. Lovsy. 3rd edn. London: Sweet, Maxwell, and Stevens & Sons, 1866.
Jewett, Hilary. 'The Scene of the Accident in the Nineteenth Century'. Ph.D. Dissertation, Yale University, 1996.
Johns, Bennett G. 'The Poetry of Seven Dials'. *Quarterly Review* 122 (April 1867): 382–406.
Johnson, Steven. *Emergence: The Connected Lives of Ants, Brains, Cities, and Software*. New York: Scribner, 2001.
Johnson, Steven. *The Ghost Map: The Story of London's Most Terrifying Epidemic—and How It Changed Science, Cities, and the Modern World*. 1st edn. New York: Riverhead, 2006.
Johnstone, Christian. 'On Periodical Literature'. *Tait's Edinburgh Magazine*, 1 July 1833.
Jones, Aled. *Powers of the Press: Newspapers, Power and the Public in Nineteenth-Century England*. Aldershot, Hampshire: Ashgate, 1996.
Kavanagh, Thomas M. *Enlightenment and the Shadows of Chance: The Novel and the Culture of Gambling in Eighteenth-Century France*. Baltimore, MD: The Johns Hopkins University Press, 1993.
Kellett, John R. *Railways and Victorian Cities*. London: Routledge & Kegan Paul, 1979.
Kern, Stephen. *A Cultural History of Causality: Science, Murder Novels, and Systems of Thought*. Princeton, NJ: Princeton University Press, 2004.
Kern, Stephen. *The Culture of Time and Space 1880–1918*. Cambridge, MA: Harvard University Press, 1983.
Keyes, Ralph. 'Who Said That?' *Bark Magazine*, August 2006. <http://www.ralphkeyes.com/quote/press-quote-primer>.
Killick, Tim. *British Short Fiction in the Early Nineteenth Century: The Rise of the Tale*. Aldershot, Hampshire; Burlington, NJ: Ashgate, 2008.

King, Andrew. 'A Paradigm of Reading the Victorian Penny Weekly: Education of the Gaze and *The London Journal*'. In *Nineteenth-Century Media and the Construction of Identities*, edited by Laurel Brake, Bill Bell, and David Finkelstein, 77–92. Basingstoke, Hampshire: Palgrave, 2000.

King, Andrew, and John Plunkett, eds. *Victorian Print Media: A Reader*. Oxford; New York: Oxford University Press, 2005.

Koven, Seth. *Slumming: Sexual and Social Politics in Victorian London*. Princeton, NJ: Princeton University Press, 2004.

Kuberski, Philip. *Chaosmos: Literature, Science, and Theory*. Albany, NY: State University of New York Press, 1994.

Kyburg, Henry Ely, and Mariam Thalos. *Probability Is the Very Guide of Life: The Philosophical Uses of Chance*. Chicago, IL: Open Court, 2003.

Landow, George P. *Images of Crisis: Literary Iconology, 1750 to the Present*. Boston, MA: Routledge & Kegan Paul, 1982.

Lane, Roger. *Violent Death in the City: Suicide, Accident, and Murder in Nineteenth-Century Philadelphia*. Cambridge, MA: Harvard University Press, 1979.

Lauster, Martina. *Sketches of the Nineteenth Century: European Journalism and Its Physiologies, 1830–50*. Basingstoke, Hampshire; New York: Palgrave Macmillan, 2007.

Lay, M. G. *The Ways of the Road: A History of the World's Roads and of the Vehicles That Used Them*. New Brunswick, NJ: Rutgers University Press, 1992.

Lee, Maurice S. *Uncertain Chances: Science, Skepticism, and Belief in Nineteenth-Century American Literature*. New York: Oxford University Press, 2012.

Lefebvre, Henri. *The Production of Space*. Oxford; Cambridge, MA: Blackwell, 1991.

Legge, James. *The Sacred Books of China: The Texts of Confucianism*. New York: Scribners, 1899.

Levine, Caroline. 'Strategic Formalism: Toward a New Method in Cultural Studies'. *Victorian Studies* 48, no. 4 (Summer 2006): 625–57. <http://muse.jhu.edu/journals/victorian_studies/v048/48.4levine.html>.

Levine, George. *Darwin and the Novelists: Patterns of Science in Victorian Fiction*. Cambridge, MA: Harvard University Press, 1988.

Levine, George. 'Hardy and Darwin: An Enchanting Hardy?' In *A Companion to Thomas Hardy*, edited by Keith Wilson, 36–53. Chichester, West Sussex: Wiley-Blackwell, 2009.

Levine, George Lewis. *The Realistic Imagination: English Fiction from Frankenstein to Lady Chatterley*. Chicago, IL: University of Chicago Press, 1981.

Levinson, Marjorie. *The Romantic Fragment Poem: A Critique of a Form*. Chapel Hill, NC: University of North Carolina Press, 1986.

Liddle, Dallas. *The Dynamics of Genre: Journalism and the Practice of Literature in Mid-Victorian Britain*. Charlottesville, VA: University of Virginia Press, 2009.

Liu, Alan. 'Transcendental Data: Toward a Cultural History and Aesthetics of the New Encoded Discourse'. *Critical Inquiry* 31, no. 1 (Autumn 2004): 49–84.

Bibliography

Lukács, György. *The Theory of the Novel; A Historico-Philosophical Essay on the Forms of Great Epic Literature*. Translated by Anna Bostock. Cambridge, MA: MIT Press, 1971.
Macinnis, Peter. *Rockets: Sulfur, Sputnik and Scramjets*. Crows Nest, NSW: Allen & Unwin, 2004.
McDowall, William. *History of the Burgh of Dumfries*. Edinburgh: Adam and Charles Black, 1867. <http://books.google.com/books?id=D7QHAAAAQAAJ>.
MacKay, Charles. 'On Popular and National Poetry'. *Bentley's Miscellany*, March 1838.
McGann, Jerome J. 'The Rationale of Hypertext'. In *Radiant Textuality: Literature After the World Wide Web*, 53–74. New York: Palgrave, 2001.
MacPherson, Sandra. *Harm's Way: Tragic Responsibility and the Novel Form*. Baltimore, MD: Johns Hopkins University Press, 2010.
Maidment, Brian. '"Penny" Wise, "Penny" Foolish?: Popular Periodicals and the "March of Intellect" in the 1820s and 1830s'. In *Nineteenth-Century Media and the Construction of Identities*, edited by Laurel Brake, Bill Bell, and David Finkelstein, 104–21. Basingstoke, Hampshire: Palgrave, 2000.
Mallarmé, Stéphane. *Correspondance de Stéphane Mallarmé. Vol. 1: 1862–1871*. Edited by Henri Mondor. Paris: Gallimard, 1959.
Manovich, Lev. *The Language of New Media*. Cambridge, MA: The MIT Press, 2002.
Marcus, Sharon. *Apartment Stories: City and Home in Nineteenth-Century Paris and London*. Berkeley, CA: University of California Press, 1999.
Marcus, Steven. 'Reading the Illegible'. In *The Victorian City: Images and Realities*, edited by H. J. Dyos and Michael Wolff, 1: 257–76. London: Routledge & Kegan Paul, 1973.
Martyn, William Frederic. *A Dictionary of Natural History*. London: Longman et al., 1806.
Marx, Leo. *The Machine in the Garden: Technology and the Pastoral Ideal in America*. New York: Oxford University Press, 2000.
Matus, Jill L. *The Cambridge Companion to Elizabeth Gaskell*. Cambridge: Cambridge University Press, 2007.
Matus, Jill L. 'Trauma, Memory, and Railway Disaster: The Dickensian Connection'. *Victorian Studies* 43, no. 3 (2001): 413–36. <http://muse.jhu.edu/journals/victorian_studies/v043/43.3matus.html>.
Maxwell, Richard. 'Dickens, the Two Chronicles, and the Publication of *Sketches by Boz*'. *Dickens Studies Annual* 9 (1981): 21–32.
May, Trevor. *Gondolas and Growlers: The History of the London Horse Cab*. Phoenix Mill, Gloucestershire: Alan Sutton, 1995.
Mayhew, Henry. *London Labour and the London Poor*. London: G. Woodfall, 1851.
Mays, Kelly J. 'The Disease of Reading and Victorian Periodicals'. In *Literature in the Marketplace: Nineteenth-Century British Publishing and Reading Practices*, edited by John O. Jordan and Robert L. Patten, 165–94. Cambridge; New York: Cambridge University Press, 1995.

Merrill, Lynn L. *The Romance of Victorian Natural History*. New York: Oxford University Press, 1989.
'Metropolitan Municipalities'. *Illustrated London News*, 5 May 1866.
'Metropolitan Press'. *Dictionary of Nineteenth-Century Journalism*. ProQuest LLC, 2011 2005. <http://gateway.proquest.com/openurl?url_ver=Z39.88-2004& res_dat=xri:c19index-us&rft_dat=xri:c19index:DNCJ:955>.
Mill, John Stuart. *On Liberty and Other Essays*. Edited by John Gray. Oxford; New York: Oxford University Press, 1991.
Miller, J. Hillis. *The Disappearance of God: Five Nineteenth-Century Writers*. Cambridge, MA: Belknap Press, 1963.
Miller, J. Hillis. 'The Fiction of Realism: *Sketches by Boz, Oliver Twist*, and Cruikshank's Illustrations'. In *Charles Dickens and George Cruikshank: Papers Read at a Clark Library Seminar on May 9, 1970*, 1–69. Los Angeles, CA: William Andrews Clark Memorial Library, University of California, 1971.
Miller, J. Hillis. *Victorian Subjects*. Durham: Duke University Press, 1991.
Millstein, Roberta Lynn. 'The Chances of Evolution: An Analysis of the Roles of Chance in Microevolution and Macroevolution'. Ph.D. Dissertation, University of Minnesota, 1997.
Moir, Esther. *The Discovery of Britain; the English Tourists, 1540 to 1840*. London: Routledge & Kegan Paul, 1964.
Monk, Leland. *Standard Deviations: Chance and the Modern British Novel*. Palo Alto, CA: Stanford University Press, 1993.
Moore, Henry Charles. *Omnibuses and Cabs: Their Origin and History*. London: Chapman & Hall, 1902. <http://books.google.com/books?id=i33tAAAAMAAJ>.
More, Hannah. *Turn the Carpet; Or, the Two Weavers: A New Song in a Dialogue between Dick and John*. London: J. Marshall, 1796. <http://find.galegroup.com/ecco/infomark.do?&source=gale&prodId=ECCO&userGroupName=tall85761&tabID=T001&docId=CW3316021656&type=multipage&contentSet=ECCOArticles&version=1.0>.
Mudie, Robert. *Babylon the Great: A Dissection and Demonstration of Men and Things in the British Capital*. 2 vols. London: Charles Knight, 1825.
Mussell, James. *The Nineteenth-Century Press in the Digital Age*. New York: Palgrave Macmillan, 2012.
Mussell, James. 'The Passing of Print: Digitising Ephemera and the Ephemerality of the Digital'. *Media History* 18, no. 1 (February 2012): 77–92.
Mussell, James, and Suzanne Paylor. 'Mapping the "Mighty Maze": Nineteenth-Century Serials Edition'. *19: Interdisciplinary Studies in the Long Nineteenth Century* 1 (2005). <http://19.bbk.ac.uk/index.php/19/article/view/437>.
Nead, Lynda. *Victorian Babylon: People, Streets, and Images in Nineteenth-Century London*. New Haven, CT: Yale University Press, 2000.
Neal, Wendy. *With Disastrous Consequences: London Disasters 1830–1917*. Enfield Lock, Middlesex: Hisarlik, 1992.
Newman, John Henry. *An Essay in Aid of a Grammar of Assent*. Oxford; New York: Clarendon Press, 1985.

Newsom, Robert. *A Likely Story: Probability and Play in Fiction*. New Brunswick, NJ: Rutgers University Press, 1988.

Nord, Deborah Epstein. *Walking the Victorian Streets: Women, Representation, and the City*. Ithaca, NY: Cornell University Press, 1995.

'Of All the Various and Useful Institutions'. *Illustrated London News*, 30 August 1845.

Ogborn, Miles. *Spaces of Modernity: London's Geographies, 1680–1780*. New York: Guilford Press, 1998.

Oliphant, Margaret. 'The Byways of Literature: Reading for the Million'. *Blackwood's* 84 (August 1858): 200–16.

Oliphant, Margaret. 'New Books'. *Blackwood's Edinburgh Magazine* 108 (August 1870): 166–88.

'Omnibus Conductors'. *The Times*. 29 January 1841.

'Omnibus Conductors and Cab-Drivers'. *The Times*. 2 September 1836.

'Omnibus Law'. *The Times*, 30 January 1836.

Otis, Laura. *Networking: Communicating with Bodies and Machines in the Nineteenth Century*. Ann Arbor, MI: University of Michigan Press, 2001.

Owens, Alastair, Nigel Jeffries, Karen Wehner, and Rupert Featherby. 'Fragments of the Modern City: Material Culture and the Rhythms of Everyday Life in Victorian London'. *Journal of Victorian Culture* 15, no. 2 (August 2010): 212–25.

Paley, William. *Natural Theology: Or, Evidences of the Existence and Attributes of the Deity, Collected from the Appearances of Nature*. Houston, TX: St. Thomas Press, 1972.

Pardoe, (Julia). *Reginald Lyle*. New York: Burgess & Day, 1854. <http://books.google.com/books?id=CwQnAAAAMAAJ>.

Parejo Vadillo, Ana. *Women Poets and Urban Aestheticism: Passengers of Modernity*. Basingstoke, Hampshire; New York: Palgrave Macmillan, 2005.

Parker, Simon. *Urban Theory and the Urban Experience: Encountering the City*. Abingdon, Oxfordshire; New York: Routledge, 2004.

Parsons, Deborah L. *Streetwalking the Metropolis: Women, the City, and Modernity*. Oxford; New York: Oxford University Press, 2000.

Patey, Douglas Lane. *Probability and Literary Form: Philosophic Theory and Literary Practice in the Augustan Age*. Cambridge; New York: Cambridge University Press, 1984.

Patmore, Coventry. 'Popular Serial Literature'. *North British Review* 7 (May 1847): 110–36.

Payne, William. 'Inquests on Fires'. *The Times*. 28 June 1851.

Payne, William. 'Letter to the Right Hon. John Musgrove, Lord Mayor of London,' April 1851. Original Fire Inquests. CLA/041/F1/01/01/068 1845–1885. Corporation of London Records Office.

Pearson, Robin. *Insuring the Industrial Revolution: Fire Insurance in Great Britain, 1700–1850*. London: Ashgate, 2004.

Pearson, Robin. 'Moral Hazard and the Assessment of Insurance Risk in Eighteenth- and Early-Nineteenth-Century Britain'. *Business History Review* 76, no. 1 (2002): 1–35.
'Penny-a-Liners'. *Chambers's Edinburgh Journal* NS 57 (1 February 1845): 65–8.
Pike, David L. *Metropolis on the Styx: The Underworlds of Modern Urban Culture, 1800–2001*. Ithaca, NY: Cornell University Press, 2007.
Plotz, John. *The Crowd: British Literature and Public Politics*. Berkeley, CA: University of California Press, 2000.
Poe, Edgar. *Essays and Reviews*. New York: Library of America, 1984.
Poovey, Mary. 'Figures of Arithmetic, Figures of Speech: The Discourse of Statistics in the 1830s'. *Critical Inquiry* 19, no. 2 (1993): 256–76. <http://www.jstor.org/stable/1343876>.
Poovey, Mary, ed. *The Financial System in Nineteenth-Century Britain*. New York: Oxford University Press, 2003.
Poovey, Mary. 'Forgotten Writers, Neglected Histories: Charles Reade and the Nineteenth-Century Transformation of the British Literary Field'. *English Literary History* 71, no. 2 (Summer 2004): 433–53. <http://www.jstor.org/stable/30030057>.
Poovey, Mary. *A History of the Modern Fact: Problems of Knowledge in the Sciences of Wealth and Society*. Chicago, IL: University of Chicago Press, 1998.
Poovey, Mary. *Making a Social Body: British Cultural Formation, 1830–1864*. Chicago, IL: University of Chicago Press, 1995.
Pope, Norris. 'Dickens's "The Signalman" and Information Problems in the Railway Age'. *Technology and Culture* 42, no. 3 (July 2001): 436–61. <http://www.jstor.org/stable/25147745>.
'Popular Literature of the Day'. *British and Foreign Review; Or, European Quarterly Journal* 10 (January 1840): 223–46.
Porter, Theodore M. *The Rise of Statistical Thinking, 1820–1900*. Princeton, NJ: Princeton University Press, 1986.
Porter, Theodore M. *Trust in Numbers: The Pursuit of Objectivity in Science and Public Life*. Princeton, NJ: Princeton University Press, 1995.
Pratt, Edwin A. *A History of Inland Transport and Communication in England*. London: K. Paul, Trench, Trübner & Co., 1912.
Pratt, Mary Louise. 'Arts of the Contact Zone'. *Profession*, 1991, 33–40.
'Preface'. *Penny Magazine*, December 1832.
Progress of British Newspapers. London: Swan Electric Engraving Company, 1901.
Puskar, Jason. *Accident Society: Fiction, Collectivity, and the Production of Chance*. Palo Alto, CA: Stanford University Press, 2012.
'Railway Geography'. *Punch*, 1847.
Ramazani, Jahan, Richard Ellman, and Robert O'Clair, eds. *The Norton Anthology of Modern and Contemporary Poetry. Volume 1: Modern Poetry*. 3rd edn. New York: W. W. Norton, 2003.
'Reading as a Means of Culture'. *Sharpe's London Magazine*, December 1867.
Rees, Gareth. *Early Railway Prints: British Railways from 1825–1850*. Ithaca, NY: Cornell University Press, 1980.

'Rev. of Sketches by "Boz," Illustrative of Every-Day Life and Every-Day People'. *The Monthly Review*, March 1836. <http://books.google.com/books?id=koweAQAAMAAJ>.
Richards, Jeffrey, and John M. MacKenzie. *The Railway Station: A Social History*. Oxford: Oxford University Press, 1986.
Richardson, Brian. *Unlikely Stories: Causality and the Nature of Modern Narrative*. Newark, DE: University of Delaware Press, 1997.
'Riding and Reading'. *Punch*, 1851. <http://books.google.com/books?id=wJNEAAAAcAAJ>.
Ritvo, Harriet. *The Platypus and the Mermaid, and Other Figments of the Classifying Imagination*. Cambridge, MA: Harvard University Press, 1997.
Robbins, Bruce. 'Telescopic Philanthropy: Professionalism and Responsibility in Bleak House'. In *Nation and Narration*, edited by Homi Bhabha, 213–30. London; New York: Routledge, 1990.
Robinson, Alan. *Imagining London, 1770–1900*. Basingstoke, Hampshire; New York: Palgrave Macmillan, 2004.
Rolt, L. T. C. *Red for Danger: A History of Railway Accidents and Railway Safety*. Newton Abbot, Devon: David & Charles, 1976.
Rose, Jonathan. *The Intellectual Life of the British Working Classes*. New Haven, CT: Yale University Press, 2001.
Rubery, Matthew. *The Novelty of Newspapers: Victorian Fiction After the Invention of the News*. Oxford; New York: Oxford University Press, 2009.
Ruskin, John. 'The Study of Architecture in Our Schools'. In *On the Old Road. Volume 1—Art*. Orpington, Kent: George Allen, 1885.
Sanders, Mike. 'Manufacturing Accident: Industrialism and the Worker's Body in Early Victorian Fiction'. *Victorian Literature and Culture* 28, no. 2 (2000): 313–29. <http://www.jstor.org/stable/25058521>.
Schivelbusch, Wolfgang. *The Railway Journey: The Industrialization of Time and Space in the 19th Century*. Berkeley, CA: University of California Press, 1986.
Schlicke, Paul. '"Risen Like a Rocket": The Impact of *Sketches by Boz*'. *Dickens Quarterly* 22, no. 1 (March 2005): 3–18.
Schwarzbach, Frederic. '*Sketches by Boz*: Fiction for the Metropolis'. *Dickensian* 72 (13–20): 1976.
Sennett, Richard. *The Uses of Disorder: Personal Identity & City Life*. New York: Knopf, 1970.
Shattock, Joanne, and Michael Wolff, eds. *The Victorian Periodical Press: Samplings and Soundings*. Leicester: Leicester University Press, 1982.
'Shocking Cab Accident'. *The Times*. 14 October 1836.
Sicher, Efraim. *Rereading the City, Rereading Dickens: Representation, the Novel, and Urban Realism*. New York: AMS Press, 2003.
Simmons, Jack. *The Railway in Town and Country, 1830–1914*. Newton Abbot, Devon; North Pomfret, VT: David & Charles, 1986.
Simmons, Jack. *The Victorian Railway*. New York: Thames and Hudson, 1991.

Sinnema, Peter W. 'Representing the Railway: Train Accidents and Trauma in the *Illustrated London News*'. *Victorian Periodicals Review* 31, no. 2 (Summer 1998): 142–68. <http://www.jstor.org/stable/20083063>.

'Sketchability, *n.*'. *Oxford English Dictionary*. Oxford University Press, 2012. <http://www.oed.com.proxy.lib.fsu.edu/view/Entry/180768?redirectedFrom=sketchability#eid>.

Slater, Michael. *Charles Dickens*. New Haven, CT: Yale University Press, 2009.

Smiles, Samuel. *The Life of George Stephenson, Railway Engineer*. London: John Murray, 1857. <http://books.google.com/books?id=yjkBAAAAQAAJ>.

Smith, Charles Manby. 'The Press of the Seven Dials'. In *The Little World of London; Or, Pictures in Little of London Life*, 251–66. London: A. Hall, Virtue & Co., 1857.

Smith, Neil. *Uneven Development: Nature, Capital, and the Production of Space*. New York: Blackwell, 1984.

Soja, Edward W. *Postmodern Geographies: The Reassertion of Space in Critical Social Theory*. London; New York: Verso, 1989.

Sommerville, C. John. *The News Revolution in England: Cultural Dynamics of Daily Information*. New York: Oxford University Press, 1996.

Stanley, Rev. Edward. 'Opening of the Liverpool and Manchester Railroad'. *Blackwood's Edinburgh Magazine* 28 (November 1830): 823–30.

Stokes, John. '"Encabsulation": Horse-Drawn Journeys in Late-Victorian Literature'. *Journal of Victorian Culture* 15, no. 2 (August 2010): 239–53.

Studer, Patrick. 'Textual Structures in Eighteenth-Century Newspapers: A Corpus-Based Study of Headlines'. *Journal of Historical Pragmatics* 4, no. 1 (2003): 19–44.

Tambling, Jeremy. *Going Astray: Dickens and London*. Harlow, Essex: Pearson Longman, 2009.

Taylor, Frank. *The Newspaper Press as a Power in Both the Expression and Formation of Public Opinion*. Oxford: B. H. Blackwell, 1898.

Taylor, William Cooke. 'The Moral Economy of Large Towns'. *Bentley's Miscellany*, 1840.

Tebbutt, Melanie. *Making Ends Meet: Pawnbroking and Working-Class Credit*. New York: St. Martin's Press, 1983.

Thackeray, William M. 'Half a Crown's Worth of Cheap Knowledge'. *Fraser's Magazine*, March 1838.

'The Catastrophe in Regent's-Park. The Inquest and Verdict of the Jury'. *The Times*. 29 January 1867.

'The Chapter of Accidents'. *Oxford English Dictionary*. Oxford University Press, 1989. <http://www.oed.com/view/Entry/30613?rskey=s3HOXw&result=2&isAdvanced=false#eid216078486>.

'The Late Fire in Aldermanbury'. *The Times*. 22 August 1845.

'The Money Market'. *The Times*. 14 December 1825.

'The Present State of the Railway Interest'. *The Times*. 12 January 1850.

'The Railway Traveller's Farewell to His Family'. *Punch*, 1851.

'The Step Taken by Mr. Payne'. *The Times*. 27 August 1845.

Thomas, Keith. *Religion and the Decline of Magic*. New York: Scribners, 1971.
Trebilcock, Clive. *Phoenix Assurance and the Development of British Insurance*. 2 vols. Cambridge: Cambridge University Press, 1985.
Trollope, Anthony. *An Autobiography*. New York: Harper, 1883. <http://books.google.com/books?id=u4YIAAAAQAAJ>.
Trollope, Anthony. *The Prime Minister*. Oxford; New York: Oxford University Press, 1983.
Trollope, Anthony. *The Three Clerks*. New York: Harper, 1860. <http://books.google.com/books?id=GBoGAAAAQAAJ>.
Trollope, Frances Eleanor. *Veronica*. London: Tinsley Brothers, 1870. <http://books.google.com/books?id=ou4BAAAAQAAJ>.
Trotter, David. *Cooking with Mud: The Idea of Mess in Nineteenth-Century Art and Fiction*. Oxford; New York: Oxford University Press, 2000.
Tschumi, Bernard. *Architecture and Disjunction*. Cambridge, MA: MIT Press, 1994.
Ure, Andrew. *The Philosophy of Manufactures: Or, An Exposition of the Scientific, Moral, and Commercial Economy of the Factory System of Great Britain*. London: Charles Knight, 1835.
Valpola, Harri. 'Bayesian Ensemble Learning for Nonlinear Factor Analysis'. Ph.D. Dissertation, Finnish Academies of Technology, 2000.
Vargish, Thomas. *The Providential Aesthetic in Victorian Fiction*. Charlottesville, VA: University of Virginia Press, 1985.
Vicinus, Martha. 'Dark London'. *Indiana University Bookman* 12 (1977): 63–92.
Virilio, Paul. *Unknown Quantity*. London; New York: Thames & Hudson; Fondation Cartier pour l'art contemporian, 2003.
Walkowitz, Judith R. *City of Dreadful Delight: Narratives of Sexual Danger in Late-Victorian London*. Chicago, IL: University of Chicago Press, 1992.
Wall, Cynthia. *The Prose of Things: Transformation of Description in the Eighteenth Century*. Chicago, IL: University of Chicago Press, 2006.
Wallace, Anne D. *Walking, Literature, and English Culture: The Origins and Uses of Peripatetic in the Nineteenth Century*. Oxford: Clarendon, 1993.
Warren, Philip. *The History of the London Cab Trade: From 1600 to the Present Day*. London: Taxi Trade Promotions Ltd, 1995.
Weightman, Gavin, and Steven Humphries. *The Making of Modern London, 1815–1914*. London: Sidgwick & Jackson, 1983.
Weinberger, David. *Everything Is Miscellaneous: The Power of the New Digital Disorder*. New York: Times Books, 2007.
Welsh, Alexander. *The City of Dickens*. London: Clarendon, 1971.
Wertheimer, Eric. *Underwriting: The Poetics of Insurance in America, 1722–1872*. Palo Alto, CA: Stanford University Press, 2006.
Wesling, Donald. *The Chances of Rhyme: Device and Modernity*. Berkeley, CA: University of California Press, 1980.
Whitman, Walt. 'To a Locomotive in Winter'. In *Leaves of Grass*, 358–9. Boston, MA: James Osgood and Co., 1881. <http://www.whitmanarchive.org/published/LG/1881/poems/269>.

Whitney, William Dwight, and Benjamin Eli Smith. 'Chapter, N'. *The Century Dictionary and Cyclopedia*. New York: The Century Co., 1911. <http://books.google.com/books?id=ownpAAAAMAAJ>.
Wiener, Joel H. 'Sources for the Study of Newspapers'. In *Investigating Victorian Journalism*, edited by Laurel Brake and Aled Jones, 155–65. New York: St. Martin's Press, 1990.
Wilkinson, Ian. 'Performance and Control: The Carnivalesque City and Its People in Charles Dickens's *Sketches by Boz*'. *Dickens Studies Annual* 35 (2005): 1–19.
Williams, Frederick Smeeton. *Our Iron Roads: Their History, Construction and Administration*. 2nd edn. London: Cass, 1968.
Williams, Frederick Smeeton. *Our Iron Roads: Their History, Construction and Social Influences*. London: Ingram, Cooke, and Co., 1852. <http://books.google.com/books?id=cycOAAAAQAAJ>.
Williams, Raymond. *The Country and the City*. New York: Oxford University Press, 1973.
Wilson, Elizabeth. *The Sphinx in the City: Urban Life, the Control of Disorder, and Women*. Berkeley, CA: University of California Press, 1992.
Winter, James. *London's Teeming Streets, 1830–1914*. London: Routledge, 1993.
Witmore, Michael. *Culture of Accidents: Unexpected Knowledges in Early Modern England*. Palo Alto, CA: Stanford University Press, 2001.
Wolfreys, Julian. *Writing London: The Trace of the Urban Text from Blake to Dickens*. Basingstoke, Hampshire: Macmillan, 1998.
Wordsworth, William. 'On the Projected Kendal and Windermere Railway'. *Morning Post*, 16 October 1844.
Wordsworth, William. *The Prelude, Or, Growth of a Poet's Mind: An Autobiographical Poem*. London: Edward Moxon, 1850.
'World's Largest Metaphor Hits Ice-Berg; Titanic, Representation of Man's Hubris, Sinks in North Atlantic; 1,500 Dead in Symbolic Tragedy'. *The Onion*, 16 April 2007. <http://www.theonion.com/articles/april-16-1912,10645/>.
Wright, Thomas. 'Concerning the Unknown Public'. *Nineteenth Century* 13 (February 1883): 279–96.
'Yesterday Morning the Various Fire Insurance Companies'. *The Times*. 28 January 1841.
Ziegler, Garrett. 'The City of London, Real and Unreal'. *Victorian Studies* 49, no. 3 (Spring 2007): 431–55.

Index

accident
  in broadsides and ballads 149–60
  cabs and busses 28, 31, 61, 67, 82–5, 91, 96–7
  concepts of 5, 16, 20–4, 26–7, 34–5, 37–40, 82–3, 109, 124–5, 128–31, 207–10
  financial 11–12, 120, 122, 211–12
  general examples of 3–4, 16, 31–2, 42, 47–50, 64–5, 112
  industrial 7, 29, 100–31, *see also* fire and injury 42, 49, 61, 65, 67, 85, 91, 120, 129–30, 154, 186–9, 201
  in newspapers 27–8, 31–3, 38–51, 96–7
  railway 26, 29, 38, 170–3, 186–8, 193–6, 201–10, 212
  Regent's Park ice accident 137, 153–8
  the technological accident 29, 37, 39, 172
  see also chapter of accidents
Ackroyd, Peter 19n63
actuary 11, 23, 38, 109–10, 127n98
Agathocleous, Tanya 15n48
Alborn, Timothy 11n35, 105n18, 113
aleatory 6, 26, 63–4
Altick, Richard 161
Anderson, Amanda 87
'annihilation of space and time' 172, 174–5, 196, 199–203
Arata, Stephen 101n3
archive 33–7, 163–9
Aristotle 22–3, 109, 127
Arscott, Caroline 13
Ashton, John 152
assurance, *see* insurance: life
Aytoun, William 198–9, 203–4

Babbage, Charles 8, 105n16
Babylon 2, 15, 69–70, 78, 104, 135, 139, 177, 179–80
Baddeley, William 110–11, 116, 118
Bagehot, Walter 96, 146n61
ballads and broadsides 29–30, 132–4, 138–40, 142, 149–60
  'cocks' 153
  Catnach Press 155–8
Barker, William, *see* 'omnibus cad'
Barthes, Roland 61, 63–4, 97, 202

Baucom, Ian 10–11, 23, 102, 106, 116n64
Baudrillard, Jean 129n107
Bayes, Thomas 127n98
Beaumont, Matthew 194–5
Beer, Gillian 5, 6n18, 23n77, 216
Beetham, Margaret 34, 135n13
Bell, David 21n69
Bell, Sir Charles 7–8, 10
Belloc, Hilaire 200n87
Benjamin, Walter 15, 17, 175
biology, *see* natural history
Blair, Ann 164n124
Blake, William 213
Bluebeard 89
Bolter, Jay, and Richard Grusin 149
Bourne, J.C. 190–2, 196
Bowlby, Rachel 144
Boz, *see* Charles Dickens
Brake, Laurel 34n9
Brantlinger, Patrick 135n10, 145n54
Bridgewater Treatises 7–8, 10
Bronstein, Jamie 170n2
Brown, Lucy 41n27, 43, 45, 46
Brown, Samuel 103–4, 110–11, 116, 118
Burney, Ian 46n43, 51–3, 58
Butler, Bishop (Joseph) 6, 8
Buzard, James 15n48
Byerly, Alison 97–8

cabs:
  accidents of 31, 61, 67, 82–5, 96–7
  history of 67–8, 79–81, 83–4
  licensing examination, *see* 'knowledge of London'
Capuano, Peter 7n21, 146n58
Carlyle, Thomas 139n24, 156n99
Carter, Ian 175n13, 187–8
Castells, Manuel 19, 169
causation 5–12, 15, 20–1, 33, 44–8, 53–8, 61–6, 89–90, 96–8, 118–19, 125, 127, 188, 215, 218
  problem of induction 90, 104
  see also natural theology; Providence
Cawthorn, Elisabeth 53n76
Chambers's Edinburgh Journal 31, 42, 46
chance 3, 101, 215
  historical interpretations of 5, 22–3, 121

chance (*cont.*)
  and insurance 107, 119–24, 207,
    see also actuary
  in mathematics 8–9, 121, 127n98
  in natural history 4–6, 136, 143
  in physics 9, 21, 189
  and the railway 171, 181–90, 205
  as reading practice 144, 156–7,
    164n124, 205, *see also* random
    selection
  in religion 6–8, 40–1, 122–3, 125–7,
    see also Providence
Chandler, James, and Kevin
  Gilmartin 17n55, 197–8
chaos 173, 186–90
  chaos theory 19n63
Chapple, J.A.V, and Anita Wilson 116n64
chapter of accidents 1, 4, 213
  ballad 158–60
  in newspapers 40–4, 60, 64
cheap literature 132–69
Chittick, Kathryn 72n17, 73
Churton, Edward 179–80
Clark, Geoffrey 119n72
Clarke, Bob 39n23, 48n50, 50, 54
classification 69n11, 70, 72–4, 87–9, 91,
  93, 98
  natural history 135n13, 137–8, 140–3,
    166, *see also* taxonomy
  sociology 141–2
  textual markup 166
Cobbett, William 2, 4, 177
Cockerell, H.A.L., and Edwin
  Green 118n69, 123n84
Collins, Wilkie 29, 134–5, 140n28,
  142–6, 158, 161, 164
'Convergence of the Twain' 216–19
Cooter, Roger 22–4, 35
coroner's inquest 31–2, 46–4, 50–61, 65,
  97, 101, 118–19, 132, 154,
  187–8, 205
  in newspapers 28, 46, 53–61
Courtemanche, Eleanor 122–3, 131
Cowper, William 1–2
Craik, Dinah 197n72
Cranford 11
Cronon, William 182
crowds 12, 132, 154, 189, 212
Cruikshank, George 98n88

Dallas, E.S. 29, 133, 137, 139, 142,
  157, 165
Daly, Nicholas 175, 205
Darwin, Charles 4–6, 215–16
Daston, Lorraine 119

database 162–9
  of newspapers 35, 39
de Certeau, Michel 18, 75–6, 78
De Quincey, Thomas 198n78
Denton, Williams 4
description, history of 101–2, 106–16,
  128, 130
design 4–12, 15–16, 93, 95–6, 98–9
  architecture 2, 19
  argument from design 6–8, 214
dialectic 14–16, 22, 30, 92, 94, 98, 104,
  214, 219
Dickens, Charles 30
  Bleak House 13, 51n58, 117n66,
    146n58
  coroners' inquests 51n58
  Dombey and Son 177n19, 187–8,
    191–4
  and insurance 116n64, 117n66
  Martin Chuzzlewit 212–13
  Mugby Junction 182–4, 205–9
  and the railway 173, 182–4, 204–9
  Sketches by Boz 70, 71–99
digital humanities 35–6, 138, 163–4,
  166–8
Dimock, Wai Chee 162, 167
Disraeli, Benjamin 119
Dixon, J. Hepworth 140
Dobraszczyk, Paul 68, 80n43, 81n44
Dombey and Son 177n19, 187–8, 191–4
Drury, Annmarie 218n17
Dyos, H.J. 48

Egan, Pierce 68, 69n10, 94n72
Eliot, George 29, 173, 199–204
  Felix Holt 199–202
emergence 19
empire 56, 174, 176–9, 213
Engels, Friedrich 2, 103
ephemera 29, 34n9, 45, 133–4, 141, 146,
  148, 151
Evelyn, John 153
Everitt, Alan 197n72
evolution 3–6, 91, 214
The Examiner 44, 49, 64

faits divers 28, 32–3, 61, 63–5, 97
Farr, William 111n43
Felix Holt 199–202
Feltes, N.N. 124n90
finance 11, 101, 120, 122, 212
fire 28–9, 56, 97, 101–2
  see also insurance: fire
flâneur 17, 28, 73–74, 143–4
Folsom, Ed 162

Foucault, Michel 22, 68, 69n11, 140n30
Franklin, Jeffrey 21n69
Freedgood, Elaine 11, 18, 70n12, 102n6
Freeman, Michael 174, 181, 197n72

Gagnier, Regenia 74n22, 82, 85, 159
Gallagher, Catherine 102n6, 116, 119, 126–7, 130
Garcha, Amanpal 78, 82n49, 84n53, 95
Gaskell, Elizabeth:
 Cranford 11
 and insurance 100–8, 116–31
 Mary Barton 29, 100–7, 116–32
 North and South 52n59, 105, 129n106
 and religion 126–7
 Ruth 116n64
Gaskell, William 126
Gauss, Carl Friedrich 8–9, 137n18
genre 4, 26, 214
 ballads and broadsides 29, 138–42, 150–60
 literary sketch 28, 71, 91, 94–9
 newspaper 28, 33–4, 60
 novel 29, 102–3, 116, 127–31
Giddens, Anthony 10, 211
Gilbert, Pamela 17n55
Gilroy, Paul 16–17
'Great Wen', the 2, 177
Green, Judith 22–4, 37n15
Grillo, Virgil 72n16, 73n18, 97–8
Grossman, Jonathan 76

Hacking, Ian 9, 121n75
hackney coach 79, 81, 83, 86
Hadley, Elaine 111n41, 113–14
Hamilton, Ross 20, 22–3, 218
Hancher, Michael 147n64
'Hap' 215–6
Hardy, Thomas 214–9
 'Convergence of the Twain' 216–9
 'Hap' 215–6
Harrington, Ralph 193
Head, Sir Francis Bond 174
Hemestedt, Geoffrey 74n22, 87
Henry, Nancy 187n47
Hepburn, James 152n88
Herbert, Christopher 21, 186
hermeneutics 20, 23, 26, 63, 148, 218
Hertz, Neil 200–1
Hewitson, Anthony 47–8
Hobbs, Andrew 48–9
Hollington, Michael 74n22
Hornbeck, Bert 217
Huett, Lorna 143–4
Hughes, Michael 151

Hume, David 90, 104
Humpherys, Anne 61n84
Huskisson, William 171, 182, 201

Illustrated London News 14, 55–6, 154, 204
industrial novel 101–2, 116, 127–31
insurance:
 development of 10–11, 29, 103–6, 109–16
 fire 57, 103–7, 110–16, 120
 fraud 103, 106, 117
 life 38, 105, 114
 railway 207–9
 and religion 10, 38
 see also actuary; liability; risk management

Jacobs, Jane 19
Jaffe, Audrey 89
Jakobson, Roman 108n31
James, Henry 1–2, 4, 103, 129–130, 213
Jervis, Sir John 52n61, 53n66
Jewett, Hilary 33, 45
Johns, Bennett 29, 138, 150–1, 155–7
Johnson, Steven 13, 19n63
Jones, Aled 34, 45, 53, 112
journalism, *see* newspapers
juggernaut 211–2

Kavanagh, Thomas 9, 21n69, 121n77, 128
Kay, James 126
Kern, Stephen 21n71, 175n13
Killick, Tim 95–6
King, Andrew 134n7, 144, 166, 168
Koven, Seth 17n55
'knowledge of London' 28, 67–8, 70–1, 73, 76–7, 80, 94, 98–9
Kyburg, Henry, and Mariam Thalos 121n75

Laplace, Pierre-Simon 8–9, 137n18
Lauster, Martina 75n27, 95n80
Lee, Maurice 21n70, 24n84
Levine, Caroline 26
Levine, George 4n8, 5–6, 21, 130n111, 188, 202, 216n10
Levinson, Marjorie 96
liability 11, 57–8, 105, 123n84, 124–5
liberalism 21n72, 93, 124
Liddle, Dallas 33, 66n98, 167
Life in London 68, 69n10, 94n72
London 1–2, 12–15, 46–51, 139–40, 153–8

London (cont.)
  'city of London' 12, 56, 58
  railway construction 172, 176–80, 184–7
  transportation, see transport: system
  see also 'knowledge of London'

machine ensemble, see railway: machine ensemble
Mackay, Charles 142, 150
MacPherson, Sandra 20n69, 93, 124
Maidment, Brian 134n7
Mallarmé, Stéphane 219n19
Manchester 2, 103–4, 126, 171, 206–7
Manovich, Lev 136n15, 163–5
manufacturing 7–8, 105–6, 112, 123
  accidents, see accidents: industrial
  reform 123n84
maps 80, 180
Marcus, Sharon 17n55
Marcus, Stephen 3
Marx, Leo 182
Mary Barton 29, 100–7, 116–32
mass media 137, 150
mathematics 8–9
  see also statistics
Matus, Jill 116n64, 129n108, 204–5
Maxwell, James Clerk 9, 91, 189
Mayhew, Henry 141–2, 152
Mays, Kelly 148
McGann, Jerome 162, 167–8
M'Diarmid, John 61–2
Mechanics' Magazine 110
melodrama 112–15
Merrill, Lynn 140–1
metropolis 6, 12–15, 48–51, 68–71, 139–40
  metropolitan improvement 15, 97, 190–1
  see also empire; London; railway: urbanization
Mill, John Stewart 28
Miller, J. Hillis 1n2, 89
modernity:
  theories of 3, 10–11, 18–19, 37, 173, 193, 196, 211
  urban modernity 15–20, 74–5, 77–8, 94, 175, 212
Monk, Leland 21n72
Moore, Henry Charles 80, 84, 85n55, 86
More, Hannah 9–10
Morning Chronicle 44, 72
Mudie, Robert 69, 86
Mugby Junction 182–4, 205–9
Mussell, James 36n14, 43n32, 66n97, 148, 162, 166

natural history 3, 6, 135n13, 136
natural theology 6–8, 214
Nead, Lynda 13, 15, 18, 70n14, 92, 104
Neal, Wendy 154n93
new formalism 26
new media 29, 138, 149–50, 164–9
Newman, John Henry 8, 147n65
newspapers 27–8, 151
  accident news 42, 44–51, 61–2, see also accidents: in newspapers
  coroners' inquests in 28, 46, 53–61
  headlines 39–40
  literary sketch 96–7, see also genre: literary sketch
  metropolitan 48–51
  miscellaneous news 47–8, 61–6, see also *faits divers*
  police news 44–5, 51, 64
  provincial press 47–8
  theories of genre 32, 34, 43–5, 53, 65
  see also *The Examiner*; *Illustrated London News*; *Morning Chronicle*; *The Times*
Nord, Deborah Epstein 17n54, 74n22
North and South 52n59, 105, 129n106

Ogborn, Miles 17n55, 18–19
Oliphant, Margaret 29, 133–7, 139, 146–9, 159
omnibus:
  accidents of 28, 82, 91
  development of 76–7
  'omnibus cad' 82, 85–6
Otis, Laura 203

Paley, William 6–8
Parker, Simon 1n1, 25, 75n27
Parsons, Deborah 17n54, 74n22
pastoral 2, 176, 199
Patey, Douglas 21n69, 121n75, 128n101
Patmore, Coventry 143
Payne, William 56–60, 101, 118
Pearson, Robin 103n8, 110
pedestrians 28, 74–6, 132, 156, 199
  see also *flâneur*
'penny a liners' 46, 85, 153n89, 157
penny journals 144–6
phantasmagoria 194–6
physics 9, 21, 189
the picturesque 84, 195n66, 197
Pierce, C.S. 30, 219
Pike, David 15n48, 17n55
Plotz, John 14n46
Poe, Edgar 95, 144n49
Pollock, Griselda 13

Index

Poovey, Mary 9, 11, 69n10, 89n64, 101, 110n35, 111, 133
Pope, Norris 183n36
popular literature 133–62
Porter, Theodore 9, 30n91, 104, 109, 121
The Prime Minister 184–90
probability:
  mathematics 20, 121
  relation to novel 121, 127–31
  in risk assessment 109–11, 118–24
  theories of 4, 8–9, 121, 125–7
Providence 7, 9–10, 20, 38, 122–31, 188
  and political economy 122–3
Punch 81, 170, 178–80, 211–12
Puskar, Jason 21n72, 107, 123

quantitative analysis 35–7, 54, 134n8
Quetelet, Adolphe 8–9

railway:
  accidents, *see* accident: railway
  illustrations and paintings 190–2, 196, 197n72, 201
  junctions 177–90, 205–7
  Liverpool and Manchester opening 171, 182
  machine ensemble 29, 173, 194–5
  'railway mania' 77, 181, 211–12
  railway time 195–6, 199–200, 203, *see also* 'annihilation of space and time'
  and urbanization 29, 174–83
  see also 'phantasmagoria'
randomness 9–10, 24, 94, 131
  and railway construction 173, 181–3
  random diffusion 148–9, 161–2
  random selection 29, 133–47, 164
  see also serendipity
'reading for the million' 29, 133–7
realism 89, 102–3, 128–30, 201–3
relativity 21, 186, 211
religion, *see* natural theology; Providence; Unitarianism
remediation 29, 137, 149–69
Reynolds, G.W.M. 69
risk 10–11, 119
  railway accidents 170–1, 207–9
  risk assessment 102–3, 106–11, 116–21, 125–7
  risk management 101–7, 109–16, 117–24, 207–9
Robbins, Bruce 129n104
Robinson, Alan 74n22
Rolt, L.T.C. 171, 203–4
Rose, Jonathan 161

Rubery, Matthew 32, 43n31, 49n54, 66n98
Ruskin, John 2

Sanders, Mike 123n84, 124–5
Schivelbusch, Wolfgang 29, 37, 105n20, 123n84, 172–3, 175, 194n63
Sennett, Richard 19
sensationalism 111–15, 135, 175
serendipity 162–3
Seven Dials 136, 140, 155
Shattock, Joanne 48n51, 162
Sicher, Ephraim 78
'The Signalman' 205–6
Simmel, Georg 17, 175, 198
Simmons, Jack 176–7, 183n36, 194
Sinnema, Peter 192–3
sketch, *see* genre: literary sketch
Sketches by Boz 28
  'Hackney-coach Stands' 79–82
  'The Last Cab-driver, and the First Omnibus Cad' 83–93
  'Love and Oysters' 71–2
  'Omnibuses' 73, 76–9, 97
  publication history 71–2
  relation to journalism 96–8
  'Seven Dials' 140
Slater, Michael 73, 85n54, 87n60
Smith, Charles Manby 134n10, 136, 150
social geography 17–18, 175–6
Society for the Diffusion of Useful Knowledge 147
sociology 93, 70
Sommerville, C. John 39n22, 62–3, 65
Staggs's Gardens 191–3, 195
  see also Dombey and Son
Stanley, Rev. Edward 171, 195
Staplehurst Disaster 204–6
statistics 9, 28, 37, 109–11, 114–15
  development of 3, 9
  statistical society 126
Stokes, John 76
the sublime 195, 200–1
suburbs 177–8
Sun Fire Office 106–7, 117

taxonomy 69n11, 72, 83, 91–3, 138, 140–3
Taylor, William Cooke 13, 114
Tebbutt, Melanie 120n73
Tennyson, Alfred 192n56, 216n9
Ternan, Ellen 206
Thackeray, William Makepeace 139n25
The Three Clerks 177, 185
Thomas, Keith 126